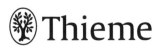

Procedural Dermatology

Volume I: Reconstruction

Postresidency and Fellowship Compendium

David H. Ciocon, MD
Director of Procedural Dermatology and Dermatologic Surgery
Associate Professor of Medicine
Director of Clinical Operations
Division of Dermatology
Montefiore Medical Center
Albert Einstein College of Medicine
Bronx, New York, USA

Yoon-Soo Cindy Bac, MD
Mohs Micrographic Surgeon and Dermatologic Oncologist
Cosmetic and Laser Surgeon
Laser & Skin Surgery Center New York;
Clinical Assistant Professor of Dermatology
New York University Grossman School of Medicine
The Ronald O. Perelman Department of Dermatology
New York, New York, USA

466 Illustrations

Thieme
Stuttgart • New York • Delhi • Rio de Janeiro

Library of Congress Cataloging-in-Publication Data is available from the publisher.

Georg Thieme Verlag KG
Rüdigerstrasse 14, 70469 Stuttgart, Germany
+49 [0]711 8931 421, customerservice@thieme.de

Cover design: © Thieme
Cover image source: © Thieme
Typesetting by TNQ Technologies, India

Printed in Germany by Beltz Grafische Betriebe   5 4 3 2 1

DOI: 10.1055/b000000252

ISBN: 978-3-13-242405-0

Also available as an e-book:
eISBN (PDF): 978-3-13-242406-7
eISBN (epub): 978-3-13-258256-9

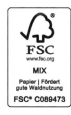

FSC
www.fsc.org
MIX
Papier | Fördert
gute Waldnutzung
FSC® C089473

Contents

1   Facial, Scalp, Neck, Hands, Lower Extremities, and Genital Anatomy.   1

Shauna Higgins, Marissa B. Lobl, and Ashley Wysong

2   Reconstruction of the Forehead Unit.   25

Ardeshir Edward Nadimi, Sonal A. Parikh, and Vishal Anil Patel

3   Reconstruction of the Nasal Unit   41

Ian Maher, Jamie L. Hanson, and Gabriel Amon

Contents

Contents

Preface

The history of dermatologic surgery has witnessed profound but sustained transformation over the past four decades. Prior to the 1980s, many complex surgical reconstructions after Mohs surgery were outsourced to plastic surgeons or head and neck surgeons because dermatologists lacked the training or comfort level to perform such difficult cases. As education has evolved at the postgraduate level in both residency and fellowship programs and through conferences offered by the American College of Mohs Surgery and the American Society of Dermatologic Surgery, dermatologists have increasingly assumed the reins of surgical reconstruction after Mohs micrographic surgery, whether it involves the head and neck, or the delicate areas of the hand, feet, and genitalia.

The aim of this compendium is to provide a comprehensive summary of the latest techniques in surgical reconstruction after Mohs surgery based on the location of the defect. Drawing on the expertise of internationally recognized experts in the field of reconstructive surgery, we adopt a concise but algorithmic approach tailored to the benefit of the fledgling surgeon fresh from training and the seasoned surgeon looking to hone and expand existing techniques. While we recommend algorithms as a way of forming logical and coherent surgical plans for challenging defects in difficult-to-treat areas, we caution against a "cookbook" approach. Like any other in the art of medicine, individual cases must be treated on an individual basis. Treatment plans should always be tailored to the individual patients with close consideration of their unique anatomy, their comorbidities, their age, their social situation, their short- and long-term goals, and their insights and expectations.

In the words of Isaac Newton, our humble efforts are made possible only by standing on the shoulders of giants. Many of the techniques described in this text were developed, modified, and perfected by pioneers such as Richard G. Bennett and John A. Zitelli, who graciously agreed to contribute to this endeavor, among others. We are grateful to all our contributors who gave their time and their wisdom selflessly. Ours is a collective effort whose ultimate reward comes from the sharing and distribution of knowledge. Finally, I would be remiss if I did not extend my deepest gratitude to my co-editor Dr. Yoon-Soo "Cindy" Bae who had the vision and courage to conceive this idea, which is a labor of friendship and deep mutual respect. Thank you for inviting me on this incredible journey.

David H. Ciocon, MD

Contributors

Saud Aleissa, MD, FAAD
Assistant Professor
Department of Dermatology
King Abdulaziz University Hospital
Jeddah, Saudi Arabia

Ziad M. Alshaalan, MD
Department of Internal Medicine
College of Medicine
Jouf University
Sakaka, Saudi Arabia

Gabriel Amon, MD
Resident
Department of Dermatology
University of Minnesota Medical School
Minneapolis, Minnesota, USA

Thomas S. Bander, MD
Director of Procedural Dermatology
Department of Dermatology
Maine Medical Partners
Portland, Maine, USA

Thomas K. Barlow, DO, DHEd
Mohs Surgeon
Deseret Dermatology
Saratoga Springs, Utah, USA

Anne Barmettler, MD
Director of Oculoplastics;
Associate Professor of Ophthalmology;
Associate Professor of Surgery
Department of Ophthalmology
Montefiore Medical Center, Albert Einstein
  College of Medicine
Bronx, New York, USA

Richard G. Bennett, MD
Professor of Clinical Dermatology
Department of Dermatology
UCLA and USC Schools of Medicine
University of Southern California
Los Angeles, California, USA

David G. Brodland, MD
Assistant Professor
Department of Dermatology
Zitelli & Brodland Skin Cancer Center
University of Pittsburgh
Pittsburgh, Pennsylvania, USA

Merrick A. Brodsky, MD
Mohs Micrographic Surgery and Dermatologic
  Oncology Fellow
Department of Dermatology
The Ohio State Medical Center
Columbus, Ohio, USA

David H. Ciocon, MD
Director of Procedural Dermatology and
  Dermatologic Surgery;
Associate Professor of Medicine;
Director of Clinical Operations
Division of Dermatology
Montefiore Medical Center
Albert Einstein College of Medicine
Bronx, New York, USA

Arjun Dayal, MD
Attending Dermatologist
Section of Dermatology
Rush Copley Medical Center
Aurora, Illinois, USA

Chloe Gianatasio, MS
Director
Department of Scientific Affairs
Efficient CME
Fort Lauderdale, Florida, USA

C. William Hanke, MD
Clinical Professor
Department of Otolaryngology
Indiana University School of Medicine
Indianapolis, Indiana, USA

Jamie L. Hanson, MD
Dermatologist (nonacademic)
Department of Dermatology
Associated Skincare Specialists
Blaine, Minnesota, USA

Shauna Higgins, MD
Resident Physician
Department of Dermatology
University of Southern California
Los Angeles, California, USA

Jenny C. Hu, MD, MPH
Associate Clinical Professor
Department of Dermatology
Keck School of Medicine
University of Southern California
Los Angeles, California, USA

Marissa B. Lobl, PhD
Medical Student
Department of Dermatology
University of Nebraska Medical Center
Omaha, Nebraska, USA

Ian Maher, MD
Professor;
Director of Dermatologic Surgery;
Program Director, Mohs Surgery and
 Dermatologic Oncology Fellowship
Department of Dermatology
University of Minnesota;
Medical Director for Dermatology
M Health Fairview
Minneapolis, Minnesota, USA

Shaun D. Mendenhall, MD
Assistant Professor of Surgery (Plastics) and
 Orthopaedic Surgery
Divisions of Plastic and Reconstructive Surgery and
 Orthopaedic Surgery
Children's Hospital of Philadelphia
Perelman School of Medicine
University of Pennsylvania
Philadelphia, Pennsylvania, USA

Kira Minkis, MD, PhD
Associate Professor of Dermatology
Department of Dermatology
Weill Cornell Medicine
New York, New York, USA

Vineet Mishra, MD
Associate Professor of Dermatology
Department of Dermatology
University of California San Diego
San Diego, California, USA

Ardeshir Edward Nadimi, MD, FAAD
Mohs Micrographic Surgeon/Cutaneous Oncologist
Private Practice
Centreville, Virginia, USA

Kristina Navrazhina, PhD
MD-PhD Student, MS3
Department of Dermatology
Weill Cornell Medicine
New York, New York, USA

Sonal A. Parikh, MD
Staff Dermatologist and Mohs Surgeon
DermSurgery Associates – The Woodlands
The Woodlands, Texas, USA

Parth Patel, MD
Dermatologist
Division of Dermatology
Montefiore Medical Center
Bronx, New York, USA

Vishal Anil Patel, MD, FAAD, FACMS
Director of Cutaneous Oncology
GW Cancer Center;
Director of Dermatologic Surgery
GW Department of Dermatology;
Associate Professor of Dermatology and
 Medicine/Oncology
George Washington University School of
 Medicine & Health Sciences
Washington DC, USA

Rebecca Lissette Quinonez, MD, MS
Research Fellow
Department of Research Division
Miami Dermatology and Laser Institute
Miami, Florida, USA

Evelyn R. Reed, MD
Plastic Surgery Resident
Division of Plastic Surgery
University of Utah
Salt Lake City, Utah, USA

Anthony Rossi, MD, FAAD, FACMS
Assistant Attending
Department of Medicine, Dermatology Service
Memorial Sloan Kettering Cancer Center
New York, New York, USA

Ethan T. Routt, MD
Staff Dermatologist and Mohs Surgeon
Golden Dermatology
Honolulu, Hawaii, USA

Madison E. Tattini, BS
Student
University of Utah
Salt Lake City, Utah, USA

Adam J. Tinklepaugh, MD
Assistant Professor of Medicine
Department of Dermatology
School of Medicine
University of Utah
Salt Lake City, Utah, USA

Anne Truitt, MD
Staff Dermatologist and Mohs Micrographic Surgeon
Skin Surgery Medical Group
San Diego, California, USA

Gian Vinelli, MD
Mohs Surgeon
Department of Dermatology
Rochester Regional Health
Rochester, New York, USA

Jill Waibel, MD
Subsection Chief
Department of Dermatology
Baptist Hospital;
Clinical Voluntary Assistant Professor
Dr. Phillip Frost Department of Dermatology and
    Cutaneous Surgery
University of Miami Miller School of Medicine
Miami, Florida, USA

Jenna Wald, MD
Fellow
Department of Dermatology
St. Vincent's Hospital
Indianapolis, Indiana, USA

Rachel Westbay, MD
Clinical Instructor
Mount Sinai School of Medicine
New York, New York, USA

Ramone F. Williams, MD, MPhil
Mohs Surgeon
Department of Dermatology
Harvard Medical School/Massachusetts
    General Hospital
Boston, Massachusetts, USA

Thomas J. Wright, MD
Plastic Surgery Resident
Division of Plastic Surgery
University of Utah
Salt Lake City, Utah, USA

Ashley Wysong, MD, MS
Professor and Founding Chair
Department of Dermatology
University of Nebraska
Omaha, Nebraska, USA

John A. Zitelli, MD
Adjunct Associate Professor
Departments of Dermatology, Otolaryngology, and
    Plastic Surgery
University of Pittsburgh Medical Center
Pittsburgh, Pennsylvania, USA

1 Facial, Scalp, Neck, Hands, Lower Extremities, and Genital Anatomy

Shauna Higgins, Marissa B. Lobl, and Ashley Wysong

Summary

This chapter discusses the anatomic areas of the face, scalp, neck, hands, lower extremities, and genitalia that are relevant to minimally invasive and surgical procedures performed for medical, oncologic, and cosmetic indications.

Keywords: dermatologic surgery, cosmetic procedures, anatomy, danger zones

1.1 Introduction

Dermatologic surgery has expanded significantly with advances in minimally invasive and surgical procedures for medical, oncologic, and cosmetic indications. Procedurally relevant knowledge of anatomy is crucial to planning procedures, achieving optimal outcomes, and minimizing adverse events.

1.2 Head and Neck

1.2.1 Cosmetic Units and Facial Fat Pads

The face is broken down into a number of cosmetic subunits that share common characteristics such as skin color, texture, thickness, and presence or absence of hair.[1] The cheek, temple, chin, and eyelids exist as their own well-defined units, with the nose and ear being subdivided into several smaller units (▶ Fig. 1.1).[1] At the borders of these units exist junction lines that include the melolabial fold that separates the cheek from the upper cutaneous lip, the mentolabial crease that divides the chin from the lower cutaneous lip, the nasolabial fold, the nasofacial sulcus, the hairline, and the jawline.[2] These cosmetic units and their junction lines have a number of surgical implications. For example, junction lines generally serve as ideal locations to place incisions and closures.[2] Surgical closures should also generally be confined to a single cosmetic subunit.[1] When not possible, skin should be recruited from adjacent subunits and scar lines should be placed within junction lines or parallel to relaxed skin tension lines.[1] When a defect involves several cosmetic subunits, consider repairing each subunit independently.[1] Additionally, when the majority of a cosmetic subunit has been removed, for example, in tumor extirpation, consider removing the remaining portion and replacing the entire unit.[1]

Cosmetic subunits and their corresponding junctions also reflect variations in tissue composition and three-dimensional structure and contour.[2] It is essential to thoroughly evaluate each patient for individual concavities, convexities, and transition zones. For example, variations in presence and density of fat pads such as the buccal and orbital pads can influence contour and may have implications for the depth and prominence of

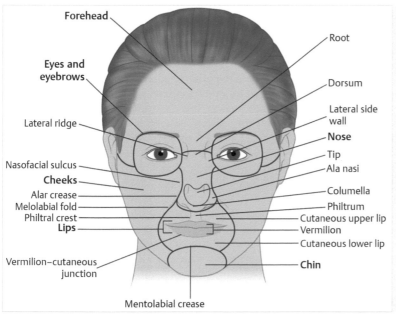

Fig. 1.1 Cosmetic subunits of the face.[2] (Reprinted with permission from Robinson JK, Arndt KA, LeBoit PE, Wintroub BU. Atlas of Cutaneous Surgery. Copyright Elsevier, 1995.)

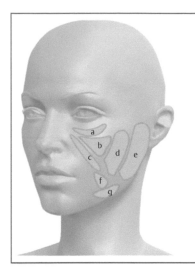

Superficial fat compartments:
  a) Infraorbital fat
  b) Medial cheek fat
  c) Nasolabial fat
  d) Middle cheek fat
  e) Lateral temporal-cheek fat
  f) Superior jowl fat
  g) Inferior jowl fat

Fig. 1.2 Superficial fat compartments of the face. (Image courtesy of Dr. Salvatore Piero Fundaro, Dr. Kwun Cheung Hau, and IMCAS Academy.)

junction lines. Results of a 2018 study of 30 cadaver specimens revealed 7 bilateral distinct superficial (subcutaneous) facial fat compartments (when excluding the 3 subcutaneous compartments of the forehead): superficial nasolabial, superficial medial cheek, superficial middle cheek, superficial lateral cheek, jowl, and superficial superior temporal and superficial inferior temporal.[3] Increased age was shown to have a significant influence on the inferior displacement of the superficial nasolabial and jowl compartments ($p < 0.001$).[3] Several of these compartments are illustrated (▶ Fig. 1.2). Wysong et al used magnetic resonance imaging scans of men and women to demonstrate measurable decreases in volume in the infraorbital area and the medial and lateral cheek areas, and concluded that facial soft tissue undergoes significant deterioration during the aging process and is different between men and women.[3,4,5] Thus, this inevitably manifests in changes in volume and tissue laxity that can be addressed with injectable soft-tissue fillers. Of note, a 2018 cadaveric study utilized upright computed tomographic scanning to simulate the effects of gravity and reported that the superficial (subcutaneous) fat compartments behave differently upon injection of filling material.[3] Whereas the inferior aspect of the nasolabial, middle cheek, and jowl compartments descended on filling, this effect was not observed for the medial or lateral cheek compartment or either of the superficial temporal compartments.[3] Thus, in a clinical setting, care must be taken when injecting volumizing material into the subcutaneous plane.[3] Targeting specific superficial fat compartments, such as the superficial nasolabial fat compartment, can result in an effect opposite to that desired: instead of reducing the nasolabial crease depth by the implantation of soft-tissue filler, a worsening of its appearance and a deepening of the crease can be noted.[3] On the contrary, injections of soft-tissue filler into the superficial temporal compartments or the superficial medial cheek compartment (also called the

malar fat pad) have been associated not with descent but with an increase in the local volume and an increase in the soft-tissue projection capable of inducing a lifting effect in the middle and/or lower face.[3]

The suborbicularis oculi fat (SOOF) has also been reported to be of particular clinical and procedural relevance, as nerves and vasculature such as the infraorbital and zygomaticofacial nerves course through the SOOF.[6] The infraorbital nerve travels through the medial SOOF or deep medial cheek fat, whereas the zygomaticofacial nerve and artery travel through the lateral SOOF.[6] Knowledge of this anatomy can help the surgeon accurately place nerve blocks and avoid bruising from bleeding complications.[6] Further, because nerves travel within the medial and lateral SOOF, it is important to avoid performing multiple or crisscross passes with the needle in this plane, a technique that increases risk of nerve injury.[6]

1.2.2 Superficial Landmarks

The frontal, maxillary, zygomatic, and mandibular bones give rise to the prominent bony surface landmarks on the face that include the orbital rim, the zygomatic arch, the mastoid process, and the mentum (▶ Fig. 1.3).[2] On the orbital rim, several important foramina can be located. This includes the supraorbital and infraorbital foramina, with the former being located and palpable on the underside of the superior orbital rim 2.5 cm or approximately one thumb-breadth from midline.[2] The supraorbital neurovascular bundle emerges from this foramen and includes the supraorbital artery, vein, and nerve.[2] The infraorbital foramen can generally be located 1 cm below the infraorbital rim and is where the infraorbital artery, nerve, and vein emerge from the skull.[2] The zygomatic arch serves as the prominent bone of the lateral cheek.[2] Its posterior aspect helps define the superior pole of the parotid gland, the superficial temporal artery, and the temporal branches of the facial nerve.[2] Of note, the

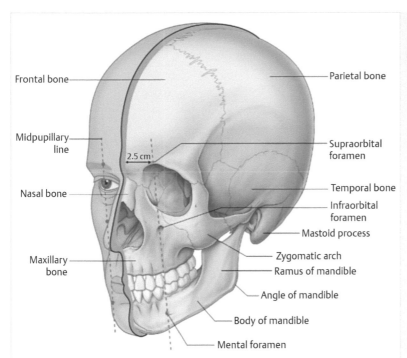

Fig. 1.3 Bony landmarks of the face. (Reprinted with permission from Robinson JK. Surgery of the Skin. Copyright Elsevier, 2015.)

Frontal bone

Parietal bone

Midpupillary line

2.5 cm

Supraorbital foramen

Nasal bone

Temporal bone

Infraorbital foramen

Mastoid process

Maxillary bone

Zygomatic arch

Ramus of mandible

Angle of mandible

Body of mandible

Mental foramen

temporal branch of the facial nerve is most superficial and vulnerable in the area around and just above the zygomatic arch. The mastoid process is the bony prominence palpated posterior and inferior to the postauricular sulcus.[2] It serves as the landmark for the emergence of the facial nerve trunk from the stylomastoid foramen.[2] After exiting the stylomastoid foramen, the trunk of the facial nerve travels through the nook of the neck for 1 to 1.5 cm, typically located midway between the cartilaginous tragal pointer of the external auditory canal and the posterior belly of the digastric muscle before entering the parotid gland. The mental protuberance of the mandible forms the prominence of the chin.[2] The mental foramina, which are found on either side of the mandible along a vertical plumb line with the supraorbital and infraorbital foramina, are the route by which the mental nerve and artery exit the skull.[2]

1.2.3 Muscles

There are two types of muscles in the face: the muscles of facial expression, also known as the mimetic muscles, and the muscles of mastication (▶ Fig. 1.4). The muscles of facial expression are unique in that they are the only muscles to insert directly into the skin and interdigitate with other muscles. They can be described by the cosmetic subunits on which they act.

The muscles acting around the eyelids include the frontalis, corrugators, and orbicularis occuli.[2] The frontalis muscle of the upper face/forehead acts as one unit to wrinkle the forehead and raise the eyebrows.[2] It secondarily works to raise the eyelids via its interdigitation with

the orbicularis oculi muscle.[2] Injury to the frontalis muscle results in ipsilateral flattening of the forehead and often brow depression.[2] The corrugator supercilii muscle is located underneath the bilateral eyebrows and is a common target of botulinum toxin injections.[2] It has a large transverse head and an oblique head, the latter of which inserts into and depresses the skin of the medial brow to form the scowl lines of the glabella.[2] The depressor supercilii has also been described as having a similar function.[2] The orbicularis oculi encircles the orbital region and is described as having outer orbital and inner palpebral components.[2] The palpebral component can be further divided into preseptal and pretarsal components.[2] It interdigitates with the frontalis, corrugator supercilii, and procerus muscles. The inner orbital component acts to tightly close the eye and depress the eyebrow, whereas the outer palpebral portion acts to more gently close the eye and blink.[2] It is innervated by temporal and zygomatic branches of the facial nerve.[2]

Muscles acting around the nose are minimal. The intrinsic muscle of the nose is the nasalis muscle, which functions to tense the skin over the dorsum and depress the septum to aid in deep inspiration. Superiorly, the procerus muscle extends down from the frontalis and aids in "scrunching" the nose. The levator labii superioris alaeque nasi also sends a few fibers to the lateral ala nasi and aids in dilating the nostril upon inspiration.

Muscles acting around the mouth include the orbicularis oris and the four lip elevators. The orbicularis oris muscle interdigitates with a number of other muscles of facial expression and functions to draw the lips together and also to pucker the lips. The four lip elevators are the

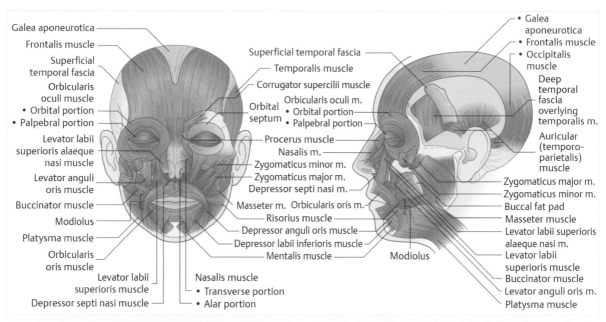

Fig. 1.4 Muscles of facial expression. (Reprinted with permission from Salasche SJ. Anatomy. In: Rohrer TE, Cook JL, Nguyen T, eds. Flaps and Grafts in Dermatologic Surgery. Copyright Elsevier, 2008.)

levator labii superioris alaeque nasi, levator labii superioris, zygomaticus major, and zygomaticus minor. They all function to aid with smiling and other oral movements. The upper lip and the corner of the mouth are elevated by the risorius and the levator anguli oris muscles. Muscles involved in movement of the lower lip include the mentalis muscle, the depressor anguli oris, and the depressor labii inferioris muscle. The mentalis muscle helps wrinkle the skin of the chin, the depressor anguli oris depresses the corner of the mouth, and the depressor labii inferioris muscle depresses the lower lip.

1.2.4 Innervation

The primary nerves of the head and neck are the trigeminal (cranial nerve V), facial (cranial nerve VII), and spinal accessory nerve (cranial nerve XI). The trigeminal nerve provides motor innervation to the muscles of mastication, the facial nerve supplies the muscles of facial expression, and the spinal accessory nerve supplies the sternocleidomastoid (SCM) and trapezius muscles. Both the trigeminal and facial nerves are comprised of both sensory and motor nerve components, whereas the spinal accessory nerve is predominantly comprised of motor fibers. Motor nerves of the head and neck become increasingly superficial as they near their target muscle, making the lateral borders of these muscles sites of potential nerve injury.[6] Sensory nerves generally course in neurovascular bundles with their respective arteries and veins and, relative to motor nerves, are more superficial and therefore more prone to injury and involvement by invasive skin cancers.[7]

The trigeminal nerve is a combined sensory and motor nerve, supplying sensory innervation to the face and anterior scalp and motor innervation to the muscles of mastication.[7] It also sends secretory fibers to the lacrimal, parotid, and mucosal glands.[7] Its three main sensory branches are the ophthalmic (V1), maxillary (V2), and mandibular (V3) branches (▶ Fig. 1.5).[7]

The ophthalmic nerve exits the skull at the supraorbital foramen and divides into three main branches: the nasociliary, the lacrimal, and the frontal nerves.[7] The nasociliary branch further divides into the infratrochlear nerve, which serves the medial canthus and the root of the nose, and the external nasal branch of the anterior ethmoidal nerve, which serves the dorsum, tip, and columella of the nose.[7] Both the infratrochlear and external nasal branches are amenable for nerve block and regional anesthesia, which can be useful in dermatologic surgery. The lacrimal nerve supplies the lateral upper eyelid.[7] The frontal nerve divides into the supratrochlear and supraorbital nerves.[7] The supratrochlear nerve exits the supratrochlear notch about 1 cm lateral to midline to serve the upper eyelid and forehead/scalp.[7] The supraorbital nerve exits the supraorbital foramen about 2.5 cm lateral to midline to also supply the upper eyelid and the forehead/scalp (▶ Fig. 1.5).[7]

The ophthalmic nerve emerges from the supraorbital foramen, a point 2.5 mm above the superior orbital margin, 23.9 mm from the facial midline, 25.89 mm from the nasion, and 30.08 mm from the frontozygomatic suture. The infraorbital foramen, from which the maxillary nerve emerges, is located 7.19 mm inferior to the infraorbital margin, approximately 45 mm from the nasion and

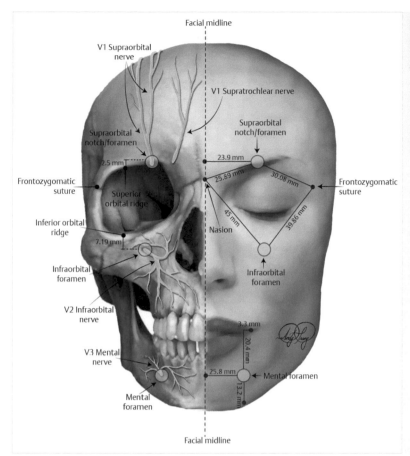

Fig. 1.5 The trigeminal nerve. (Image courtesy of Andy Trang, MD, Department of Psychiatry, University of Arizona, Tucson, Arizona, USA.)

39.86 mm from the frontozygomatic suture. The mental nerve arises from the mental foramen, which is 20.4 mm inferior and 3.3 mm medial to the cheilions, as well as 25.8 mm lateral to the midline and 13.2 mm above the inferior mandibular margin.

The maxillary nerve exits the cranial cavity via the foramen rotundum and divides into three main branches: the infraorbital, zygomaticofacial, and zygomaticotemporal nerves.[7] The infraorbital is the largest branch and exits the infraorbital foramen about 1 cm below the infraorbital rim in the mid-pupillary line.[7,8] It innervates the upper lip, medial cheek, lateral nose, and lower eyelid.[7] Injury can be minimized by avoiding injections at the junction of the nasojugal crease and lid–cheek crease.[6] The zygomaticofacial innervates the malar eminence, while the zygomaticotemporal innervates the temple region.[7]

The mandibular nerve is the largest of the three main trigeminal branches and is the only one to carry motor fibers, which innervate the muscles of mastication.[7] Its three main branches are the auriculotemporal, buccal, and mental nerves.[7] The auriculotemporal runs deep to the mandible and reaches the surface of the skin superior to the parotid gland, where it joins the superficial temporal artery and vein to supply sensory innervation to the

lateral ear, temple, and parietal/temporal scalp.[7] The buccal nerve provides sensory innervation to the cutaneous surface of the cheek in addition to the cheek mucosa and buccal gingiva and sulcus.[9] It typically courses between the two heads of the pterygoid muscle, below the inferior portion of the temporalis muscle to ultimately join with the buccal branches of the facial nerve and pierce the posterior portion of the buccinator to branch extensively on the buccal surface of the cheek.[9] On average, the buccal nerve was found in one cadaveric study to lie 3 cm lateral to the angle of the mouth.[9] The mental nerve is at the highest risk of injury of all the mandibular nerve branches.[1] It exits the mental foramen in the mid-pupillary line along with the mental artery and vein and innervates the chin and the inferior mucosal and cutaneous lip.[7,10,11,12] Whereas the mental branch and the infraorbital branch of the maxillary division are available for nerve block anesthesia, the buccal branch is not.[7] The buccal branch is also not subjected to the same degree of iatrogenic injury, as the nerve is often protected by the buccal fat pad or the superficial musculoaponeurotic system (SMAS).[13,14]

The facial nerve is a mixed sensory and motor nerve that may also be injured during a number of head and neck procedures such as tumor extirpation, liposuction, and parotid gland manipulation, thus requiring a strong

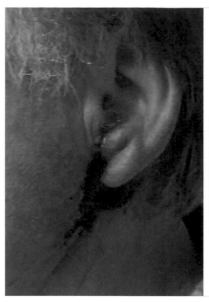 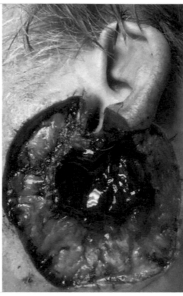

Fig. 1.6 Main trunk of the facial nerve.

knowledge of its course to mitigate negative surgical sequelae.[15] The facial nerve exits the cranial cavity via the stylomastoid foramen inferior to the tragus of the ear.[16] Its main branch is thus at risk of damage with removal with large and deep tumors near the inferior auricular attachment (▶ Fig. 1.6). After exiting the cranial cavity, the facial nerve travels through the fat between the SCM and digastric muscles to the parotid within which it splits into a superior temporofacial and an inferior cervicofacial trunk.[16] The trunk eventuates in the five major branches of the facial nerve that innervate the muscles of facial expression: the temporal, zygomatic, buccal, marginal mandibular, and cervical nerves.[1] All five branches course deep to the parotid and are prone to injury during dermatologic surgery.[16,17,18,19,20] Frequently used anatomic landmarks to identify the facial nerve and its branches include the tragal pointer, the tympanomastoid suture, the posterior belly of the digastric, the styloid process, and the retromandibular vein.[15] The consistency of soft-tissue landmarks, however, is influenced by age, prior surgeries, intrinsic scarring, and the extent of the existing pathology.[15] Bony landmarks have also been recently reported to be variable between the two sexes.[15] Thus, one group has introduced a new anatomic triangle called Borle's triangle for safer and more reliable operative identification of the trunk of the facial nerve, particularly during procedures involving manipulation of the parotid gland.[15] The triangle is outlined by joining the inferior tip of the mastoid process, the superior border of the posterior belly of the digastric muscle, and the posterior border of the ramus of mandible with imaginary lines.[15] The branches of the facial nerve most prone to clinically relevant iatrogenic injury are the temporal and marginal mandibular branches, as these represent terminal rami in approximately 85% of the population.[1] The remaining branches of the facial nerve have numerous branches that

minimize risk of permanent damage.[1] The zygomatic nerve and its numerous branches innervate the orbicularis oculi muscle, the corrugator supercilii muscle, and the procerus muscle.[21] The buccal nerve primarily innervates the levator labii superioris, the levator labii superioris alaeque nasi, buccinators, zygomaticus major and minor, levator anguli oris, and orbicularis oris muscles.[22] The cervical branch innervates the platysmal muscle and is rarely a clinical consideration.[7]

The inferior auricular attachment is in close proximity to the main trunk of the facial nerve. It courses anterior to the SCM, poster to the parotid fascia, and approximately 2 cm from the surface.

The course of the temporal branch of the facial nerve to the frontalis muscle can be approximated by a line connecting a point 0.5 cm below the tragus of the ear (near the inferior auricular attachment) to a point 2 cm above the lateral eyebrow.[23] Schwember et al showed that the branch emerges from the parotid gland at a point that is approximately 29 mm from the intertragal notch, 59 mm from the palpebral lateral commissure, and 98 mm from the labial commissure.[24] In a cadaveric study, Gosain et al found that it divides into an average of three several rami inferior to the zygomatic arch before reconnecting above the arch.[25,26] The posterior ramus was found to cross over the zygomatic arch at a range of 8 to 39 mm anterior to the external acoustic meatus.[27] The anterior most ramus has been estimated to be found at a distance of 35.4 ± 4.6 mm from the root of the helix.[28] According to Owsley et al, once the temporal branch of the facial nerve crosses the zygomatic arch, it begins to course more superficially.[29] Within a few centimeters superior to the zygomatic arch, the galeal layer is replaced by fibrofatty tissue making the nerve more vulnerable to damage, particularly in procedures such as a temporoparietal fascia flap or a brow or facelift.[1,30,31] In procedures in which the fascial plane has been exposed, however, if the plane easily moves side to side to the gloved finger, it is generally the superficial temporal fascia and the temporal nerve is likely intact.[1] If the tissue is an immovable, tightly bound glistening membrane, the temporal fascia over the temporal muscle has likely been reached and the nerve has been cut.[7] Damage to the temporal nerve results in paresis of the frontalis muscle with an ipsilateral inability to wrinkle the forehead or open the eye widely.[7]

The marginal mandibular branch of the facial nerve is responsible for supplying motor innervation to the depressor labii inferioris, depressor anguli oris, and mentalis muscles.[32] It is particularly prone to injury given its superficial position and only partial coverage by the platysma at the jaw line and at the anterior border of the masseter muscle and given the frequency with which skin cancers and deep acne scars occur in these locations.[7] Its course, however, has been reported to be highly variable.[31,33,34,35,36,37,38] Several studies have found that its branches within the parotid gland course superficially to the retromandibular vein. Therefore, surgeons should be cautious when operating in the vicinity of the retromandibular vein, particularly in the superficial plane.[39] In an anatomic study examining 40 cadavers, Basar et al found that the marginal mandibular branch exits from the parotid gland between 4.9 and 15.2 mm from the posterior border of the mandible and 0.2 and 15.1 mm from the inferior border of the mandible. Upon exiting the parotid gland, the nerve splits, giving off between one and four rami.[31,33,34,35] After exiting the parotid gland, the marginal mandibular branch courses roughly parallel to the mandible in an anteromedial direction before crossing the facial artery and migrating superiorly and anteromedially toward the target muscles of the lower lip and chin.[31,35] Most marginal mandibular rami are above the inferior border of the mandible once they have reached the facial artery, although it has been reported that it can cross the facial artery anywhere from 10.6 mm below to 30 mm above the inferior border of the mandible.[31,34] It is important to note that soft-tissue atrophy due to aging may result in inferior displacement of the nerve, a key consideration in elderly patients. A useful technique for avoiding marginal mandibular damage is placing incisions at least 3 cm or 2 fingerbreadths below the inferior border of the mandible, thus ensuring adequate clearance of the nerve. This technique is not infallible, as the nerve may remain within millimeters of the incision.

The spinal accessory nerve (CN XI) is responsible for providing motor innervation to the SCM and trapezius muscles. Iatrogenic injury to the accessory nerve is a well-documented complication of cutaneous oncological neck surgery and particularly neck dissections and lymph node biopsies.[22] Accessory nerve injury is also a potential complication of cosmetic procedures such as rhytidectomy.[40,41,42] The accessory nerve exits the SCM and enters the posterior triangle of the neck as it courses toward the trapezius. The posterior triangle of the neck is located between the SCM, trapezius, and clavicle. The spinal accessory nerve generally exits the SCM superior to Erb's point at a range of 1 to 20 mm above it.[43,44,45] This point is roughly 70 to 90 mm above the clavicle. After emerging from the SCM, the accessory nerve follows a posterolateral course within the posterior triangle toward the trapezius. At this point, the accessory nerve travels underneath the deep cervical fascia while remaining superficial to the levator scapulae muscle.[43] Several superficial landmarks can be utilized in approximating the course of the accessory nerve. A useful method is to draw a triangle comprised of three points: Erb's point, the inferior border of the upper one-third of the SCM, and the superior point of the lower one-third of the anterior trapezius (▶ Fig. 1.7). Of note, the great auricular nerve originates from the cervical plexus, which also emerges from Erb's point. It passes inferiorly to cross the SCM muscle about 6 cm inferior to the auditory canal, and courses just deep to the SMAS along the pathway of the external jugular vein.[19] If dissection is done beneath the thick lateral adipose layer at the same depth past the boundary beyond which it lies deep to the SCM fascia, the dissection will proceed beneath the greater auricular nerve.[6]

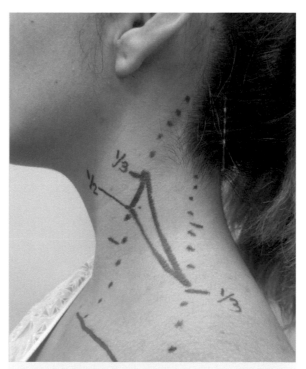

Fig. 1.7 Superficial landmarks that may be used to approximate the course of the accessory nerve. A useful method is to draw a triangle comprised of Erb's point, the inferior border of the upper one-third of the sternocleidomastoid (SCM), and the superior point of the lower one-third of the anterior trapezius.

1.2.5 Vasculature

The majority of the blood supply to the skull and its contents is derived from the common carotid artery, with the remainder coming from the vertebral artery[46]

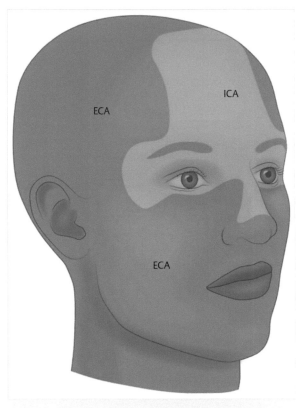

Fig. 1.8 Regions of the face supplied by the internal and external carotid arteries. (Reprinted with permission from von Arx T, Tamura K, Yukiya O, Lozanoff S. The Face: A Vascular Perspective. A literature review. Swiss Dent J. 2018; 128(5):382–392.)

(▶ Fig. 1.8, ▶ Fig. 1.9). At the level of the fourth cervical vertebral body/hyoid bone, the common carotid artery divides into the external and internal carotid arteries.[47] All vasculatures reaching the facial skin originate from either the external or internal branches of the common carotid artery.[7,48] The internal carotid artery system is predominantly dedicated to supplying the brain, although a few branches supply the head and neck region.[7] The external carotid system predominantly supplies the lower face, temple, and posterior scalp.[7] Its main branches are the inferior and superior labial arteries, facial artery, transverse facial, and infraorbital artery.[7,48]

The facial artery exits the submandibular gland at the anterior border of the masseter muscle at the jawline and curves around the inferior border of the mandible, where its pulse can be felt.[47] It then ascends toward the medial eye, giving off the inferior labial artery within the orbicularis oris muscle en route.[7] This artery in combination with the horizontal and vertical labiomental arteries comprise the majority of the perfusion to the lower lip.[47] The horizontal labiomental artery also arises from the facial artery and is located below the inferior labial artery.[47] The vertical labiomental artery is a branch of the submental artery.[47] All three arteries form a vascular network in the subcutaneous and submucosal tissues of the lower lip with tiny vessels branching to the skin, mucosa, and muscles.[47] In the upper lip, the superior labial artery is given off at the level of the commissure and follows a course similar to its lower lip counterpart.[7,47] Areas with minimal soft-tissue coverage over the blood supply, such as the lips, are at risk of skin necrosis even when minor injections are performed as injected volume may tamponade the vasculature and result in tissue ischemia.[6] This creates the need for extreme care when augmenting small anatomic units that have thin soft-tissue units.[6]

After giving off the superior labial artery, the facial artery becomes known as the angular artery, at which point it courses toward the alar base, along the lateral aspect of

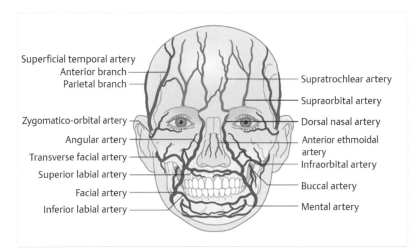

Fig. 1.9 Vascular supply to the face. (Reprinted with permission from Salasche SJ. Anatomy. In: Rohrer TE, Cook JL, Nguyen T, eds. Flaps and Grafts in Dermatologic Surgery. Copyright Elsevier, 2008.)

the nose, and ultimately anastomoses with the dorsal nasal artery, a branch of the ophthalmic artery of the internal carotid that emerges from the medial orbit and runs down the nasal dorsum to anastomose with the lateral nasal branch of the facial artery on each side.[7,47] This supplies the skin of the medial eye angle, the lacrimal sac, and the bridge of the nose.[47] The dorsal nasal artery (also known as the infratrochlear artery) also connects with the angular artery of the facial artery, and thus represents an anastomosis between the internal and external carotid artery systems.[47] It runs downward along the side of the nose to supply the bridge of the nose and connect with the angular artery of the external carotid system.[7] The anastomotic complex of the angular and dorsal nasal artery at the level of the medial canthus is an important vascular pedicle for the dorsal nasal or Rieger flap.[18] Additionally, small vessels from the inferior alar branch supply the alar base and nostril floor, whereas small twigs from the superior alar branch perfuse the nasal dorsum and superior rim of the nostril.[47] The external nasal artery, a terminal branch of the anterior ethmoidal artery, surfaces at the junction of the nasal bone and lateral nasal cartilage. This artery supplies the inferolateral areas of the nose and may also anastomose with the lateral nasal artery.[47]

Understanding the topography of the blood vessels distributed around the nasolabial fold region is essential for ensuring the safety of dermal filler injections into the area and avoiding vascular complications that include skin necrosis, embolism, or even blindness.[49] In patients with a congenital or acquired nondominant facial artery in the nasolabial region, there is a risk of damaging the thickened infraorbital artery during deep injections into the skin and subcutaneous tissue.[49] Superficial injections are thus recommended for removing rhytids of the nasolabial fold.[49] Injection of dermal filler materials into the deep dermis is only recommended after preoperatively checking for contact of the needle or cannula with the bone[49] (▶ Fig. 1.10).

Additional branches of the external carotid include the postauricular artery, the occipital artery, the superficial temporal artery, and the internal maxillary artery.[7] The postauricular artery curves around the styloid process to innervate the posterior ear and portions of the adjacent scalp above and behind the ear.[7] The occipital artery courses posteriorly and superiorly with sensory nerves between the trapezius and the SCM muscles to supply the posterior scalp. After giving off the facial and occipital arteries, the external carotid artery divides into its two terminal branches, the superficial temporal artery and

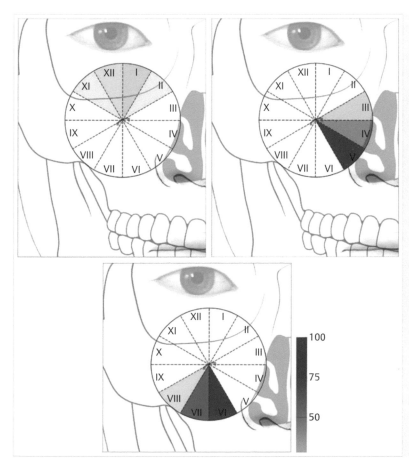

Fig. 1.10 High-risk areas for iatrogenic damage to the infraorbital artery.[49] The infraorbital artery is particularly vulnerable to injury in zones V and VI and in the nasolabial fold.[49] (Reprinted with permission from Kim HS, Lee KL, Gil YC, et al. Topographic anatomy of the infraorbital artery and its clinical implications for nasolabial fold augmentation. Plast Reconstr Surg. 142(3): 273e–280e. Copyright Wolters Kluwer, 2018.)

the internal maxillary artery.[7] The superficial temporal artery supplies a large proportion of the facial skin including the lateral forehead, temple, zygoma, and ear.[47] It arises within the parotid gland approximately 1 cm anterior to the ear.[47] Its branches are numerous and include the frontal and parietal branches and the posterior auricular artery. In one study of 26 adult cadaveric hemifaces, the superficial temporal artery bifurcated into frontal and parietal branches on average 3 cm superior to the tragus.[47] The posterior auricular artery also branches from the superficial temporal artery to supply the posterior auricle and the scalp posterior to the auricle.[6] The posterior auricularis muscle can be used as a topographic landmark for the posterior auricular artery.[6] To avoid direct injury to the frontal branch, Koziej et al suggest performing soft-tissue filler injections of the temporal region from lateral to medial in the superficial subcutaneous plane just below the dermis.[50] Further, it is necessary to remember to stay above the temporoparietal fascia or just above the periosteum so as not to inject filler into the middle temporal vessels.[50]

Additionally, the transverse facial artery branches from the superficial temporal artery and has been described to supply a large region of the lateral malar face, including the SMAS. The SMAS is an organized fibrous network composed of the platysma muscle, parotid fascia, and the fibromuscular layer covering the cheek.[19] It divides the deep and superficial adipose tissue of the face, lies inferior to the zygomatic arch and superior to the muscular belly of the platysma, and integrates with the superficial temporal fascia and frontalis muscle superiorly, and with the platysma muscle inferiorly.[19] The SMAS has been described as a central tendon for coordinated muscular contraction of the face.[19] Because the transverse facial artery runs directly through the SMAS, there is a risk of transection of this vessel during elevation of the SMAS during certain facial procedures.[19] Thus, care must be taken to avoid harming not just the transverse facial artery but also other neurovascular structures that lie in close proximity to the area.[19] Further, the SMAS plays a key role in rhytidectomy, commonly known as the facelift procedure.[19] During face-lifting, the SMAS is surgically manipulated by tightening and suspending the facial muscles through various flap dissections and surgical approaches.[16] Of note, although many neurovascular structures course deep to the SMAS, only sensory branches from the trigeminal nerve course superficial to the SMAS.[19]

The internal maxillary artery branch of the external carotid predominantly runs inside the mouth and nose but supplies terminal vessels that exit the infraorbital and mental foramen with their respective veins and sensory nerves to supply the maxilla region of the face.[7,48]

Although the lateral forehead is supplied by the frontal branch of the superficial temporal artery, branches of the ophthalmic artery, the supraorbital and supratrochlear arteries, perfuse the remainder of the forehead.[47] These vessels exit their foramens and travel deeply in the subcutaneous fat above the frontalis fascia and then over the galea aponeurotica.[7] The supratrochlear artery emerges from the superomedial orbit close to a vertical line at the medial palpebral commissure.[47] It supplies the upper eyelid along with the lacrimal, and supraorbital arteries.[47] The lower eyelid is supplied by the palpebral branch of the infraorbital artery as well as by the lateral and medial palpebral branches from the lacrimal and supratrochlear arteries, respectively.[47]

The main artery of the chin is the mental artery, one of the terminal branches of the inferior alveolar artery.[47] The submental artery extends vertically from around 3 cm below the mandibular border to around 1 cm below the oral commissure, and horizontally from around 1.5 cm posterior to the commissure to around 2 cm anterior of the SCM muscle.[47]

Many veins in the face accompany their corresponding arteries although there are some exceptions to the rule (inferior ophthalmic vein, retromandibular vein).[47]

The facial vein, responsible for the draining of the eyelids, nose, lips, cheek, and mental region, demonstrates a consistently more posterior course relative to the facial artery, traveling on average 15 mm posterior to the facial artery (range: 5–30 mm).[47] The artery and vein also lie in close proximity at the lower border of the mandible until they reach the midface muscles of facial expression where the artery assumes a more tortuous path, while the vein travels in a direct path from the medial canthus to the lower mandible.[47] The venous drainage of the middle forehead and upper eyelid occurs via the angular vein to the ophthalmic veins (superior and inferior) that communicate with the cavernous sinus.[47] Venous drainage of the midface occurs via the infraorbital vein and pterygoid plexus that also has connections to the cavernous sinus.[47] The venous blood from the chin is returned via the mental and inferior alveolar veins to the maxillary vein.[47]

The retromandibular vein is one of the facial veins that does not generally run with its corresponding artery. It has an anterior and an posterior division.[47] The posterior division merges with the posterior auricular vein to form the external jugular vein, whereas the anterior division merges with the facial vein and drains into the internal jugular vein.[47] There has also been a report of an unusual course of the right common facial vein parallel to the course of the external jugular vein, emptying into the ipsilateral subclavian vein in the lateral neck triangle behind the posterior border of the SCM muscle in a 78-year-old male cadaver.[51] Such course may be hazardous for surgical procedures in the region given the high risk of profuse hemorrhage from any injury of the vessel.[51]

Of note, above the zygomatic arch, the neurovascular bundles containing major arteries and veins all course in the deep subcutaneous plane above the fascia or muscles of facial expression.[7] Below the arch, however, the vessels are typically within the mimetic muscles and do not travel with major sensory nerves.[7]

1.2.6 Special Considerations

Aesthetic and reconstructive surgery of the face performed in different races and ethnicities may require special consideration of the variations in anatomy. In the Asian population, for example, orbital and periorbital structures may vary from those in Caucasian patients. Of note, although "Asian" refers to anything related to the continent of Asia and although the Asian population is comprised of various groups such as Chinese, Indian, Middle Eastern, and Southeast Asian, the "Asian eyelid" generally refers to the morphology of eyelids found in native Chinese and those of Chinese descent.[52]

There are generally six types of Asian eyelids that include the single eyelid, the low eyelid crease, and the double eyelid (▶ Fig. 1.11).[52] The double eyelid has a fold, which is formed by the supra-crease of overhanging skin when the eyes are open.[52,53,54] The epicanthal fold is unique to the Asian eyelid and is defined as a skin fold from the upper eyelid that covers the inner angle of the eye. The four types of epicanthal fold according to Johnson's classification are demonstrated in

▶ Fig. 1.12.[52] A study in a Korean cohort found that the prevalence of the epicanthal fold was 86.7%, although the percentage of Asians with a reported epicanthal fold varies from 40 to 90% in the literature.[55] The epicanthal fold is composed of an outer skin lining, a core structure of muscular fibers and fibrotic tissue, and an inner skin lining. Dermatologists should also be aware of the surgical anatomy of this region when performing surgical procedures, such as the epicanthoplasty, or laser procedures on epicanthoplasty scars. When performing surgery involving the epicanthal folds, the muscular and fibrotic tissue should also be removed or reconstructed.[55]

Additionally, variations in measurements of the Asian eyelid compared to the Caucasian eyelid are particularly relevant to blepharoplasties and eyebrow lifts as several studies suggest that the crease height is required to aid the surgeon in the decision of how much extra skin to excise during blepharoplasties.[56,57] The eyelid crease height is 8 to 10 mm in Caucasians and 6.5 ± 0.7 mm in Asians. The upper tarsal height is 11.3 ± 1.7 mm in Caucasians and 9.2 ± 0.8 mm in Asians. The intercanthal distance is

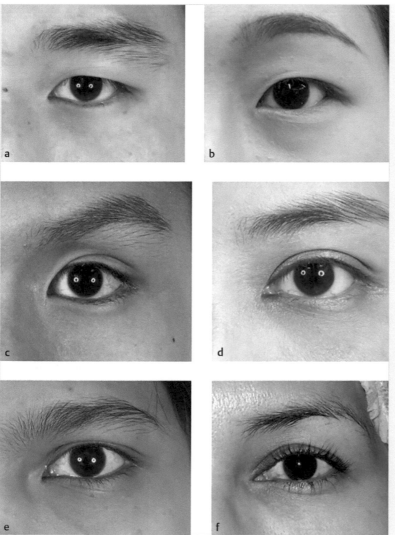

Fig. 1.11 Asian eyelid morphologies are categorized into six types. (a) Single eyelid (no visible lid crease). (b) Low eyelid crease (low-seated, nasally tapered, including hidden fold). (c) Double eyelid crease, in-fold type: the height of the upper lid crease is lower than the epicanthal fold. (d) Double eyelid crease, on-fold type: the height of the crease is right on the epicanthal fold. (e) Double eyelid crease, out-fold type: the height of the crease is higher than the epicanthal fold. (f) Double eyelid crease, out-fold type without an epicanthal fold.[52]

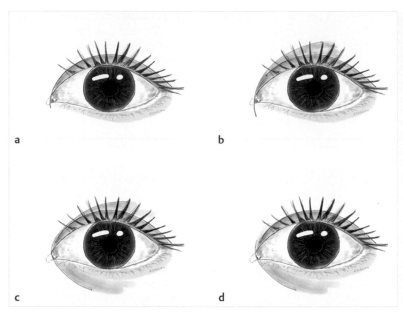

Fig. 1.12 The four types of epicanthal fold according to Johnson's classification. **(a)** Epicanthus tarsalis. **(b)** Epicanthus supraciliaris. **(c)** Epicanthus palpebralis. **(d)** Epicanthus inversus.[52]

25 to 30 mm in Caucasians and 35.55 ± 2.75 mm for Asian females and 37.51 ± 2.92 mm for Asian males.[58]

1.3 Hand

Dermatologic surgery on the hands is performed for extirpation of cutaneous malignancies and in the context of cosmetic procedures. Surgery of the nail bed region is also common, yet complicated. Knowledge of the intricacies of the hand, nail, and superficial anatomy is critical to optimizing patient outcomes following hand surgery.

1.3.1 Innervation

The three major nerves that supply the hand are the ulnar, median, and radial nerves (▶ Fig. 1.13). The median nerve passes through the carpal tunnel to enter the hand.[59] After entering the hand, it gives off four branches: the recurrent, lateral, medial, and palmar cutaneous branches.[59] The recurrent branch of the median nerve runs laterally beyond the flexor retinaculum and dives under the palmar aponeurosis to innervate the thenar muscles (except adductor pollicis and the deep head of flexor pollicis brevis).[59] This nerve is commonly injured during procedures involving structures of the wrist and carpal tunnel.[60,61] Given its role in maintaining a functional hand grip, care should be taken to avoid injury during surgery. The lateral branch of the median nerve innervates the first lumbrical and provides sensation to the thumb and radial half of the second digit.[59] The medial branch of the median nerve runs medially along the second through fourth digits, supplying the second lumbrical and skin of the second through fourth digits.[59] The palmar cutaneous branch of the median nerve is given off proximal to the flexor retinaculum and supplies

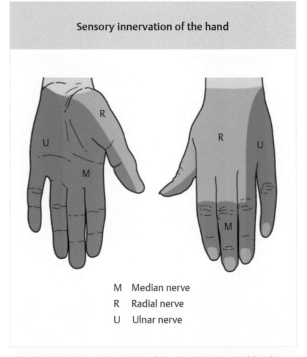

Fig. 1.13 Sensory innervation of the hand is provided by the median, radial, and ulnar nerves. (Reprinted with permission from Bolognia JL, Vandergriff TW. Dermatology. Copyright Elsevier, 2018.)

sensation to the center of the palm.[59] To perform a median nerve block, utilize the palmaris longus tendon, which runs just superior to the median nerve.[62] The palmaris longus tendon can be palpated just lateral to the center of the anterior wrist.[62] Position the needle just medial to palmaris longus (▶ Fig. 1.14).[62]

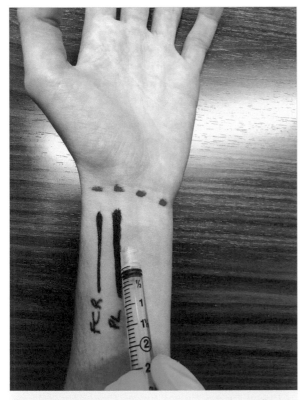

Fig. 1.14 Position for median nerve block. Place the needle just medial to the palmaris longus tendon, approximately 2.5 cm proximal to the wrist crease.

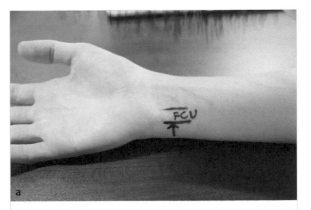

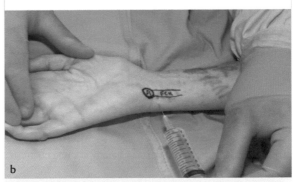

Fig. 1.15 (a, b) Position of the needle for ulnar nerve block. place the needle parallel to the plane of the palm and deep to the flexor carpi ulnaris (FCU).

The ulnar nerve enters the hand through Guyon's canal, alongside the ulnar artery.[59] The ulnar nerve divides into deep and superficial branches as the nerve passes by the hamate and pisiform.[59] The superficial branch of the ulnar nerve divides into two common palmar digital nerves and supplies the palmaris brevis and sensation to the ulnar side of the hand.[59] The deep branch of the ulnar nerve supplies the hypothenar muscles as well as the adductor pollicis and the deep head of the flexor pollicis brevis.[59] The palmar cutaneous branch of the ulnar nerve branches off from the ulnar nerve in the middle of the forearm, pierces the deep fascia, and supplies the skin at the base of the medial palm.[59] The dorsal branch of the ulnar nerve arises in the forearm, passes under the flexor carpi ulnaris, penetrates the deep fascia, and branches off to supply the medial aspect of the dorsum of the hand, the proximal part of the fifth digit, and the medial part of the fourth digit.[59] To perform an ulnar nerve block, utilize the flexor carpi ulnaris tendon, which runs just superior to the ulnar artery and nerve, the ulnar artery being palpable where it crosses the medial anterior wrist.[62] Position the needle parallel to the plane of the palm and deep to the flexor carpi ulnaris (▶ Fig. 1.15).[62]

The radial nerve and its branches supply the extensors of the forearm and hand. The superficial branch of the radial nerve branches off in the cubital fossa and emerges under the brachioradialis, piercing the deep fascia and dividing into two branches.[59] The lateral branch supplies the skin of the radial part of the dorsal thumb, and the medial branch supplies the proximal parts of the dorsum of the second and third digits and the radial half of the fourth digit.[59] There is a risk of radial nerve injury with any type of wrist surgery, including removal of cysts found commonly in the area such as ganglion cysts.[63] To perform a (superficial) radial nerve block at the wrist, place the needle in the subcutaneous tissue just above the radial styloid prior to the bifurcation of the nerve (▶ Fig. 1.16).

1.3.2 Vasculature

The hand is supplied primarily by two arteries: the ulnar and radial arteries. The ulnar artery arises from the brachial artery in the cubital fossa then passes through the Guyon canal to enter the hand and supply the medial aspect of the hand.[59] The radial artery also arises from the brachial artery in the cubital fossa.[59] The artery enters the hand along with the contents of the anatomical snuff box, which include the superficial branch of the radial nerve, cephalic vein, and tendons of extensor carpi radialis longus and brevis.[64] After entering the hand, the ulnar and radial arteries anastomose to form the superficial palmar

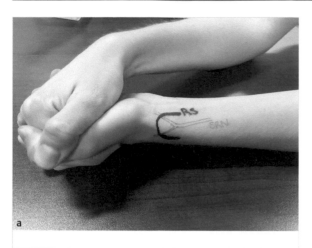

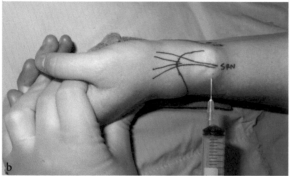

Fig. 1.16 (a, b) Guide for performing a superficial radial nerve block. Place the needle in the subcutaneous tissue just above the radial styloid prior to the bifurcation of the nerve.

arch (dorsal) and the deep palmar arch (ventral), which supply the digits, palm, and dorsum of the hand.[59] The superficial palmar arch is located just deep to the palmar aponeurosis, and the deep palmar arch is located along the metacarpals and interossei muscles.[59]

Given that the majority of cutaneous malignancies occur on the dorsum of the hands, its vasculature becomes particularly relevant.[21] The proximal two-thirds of the dorsal hand is supplied mainly by dorsal metacarpal arteries. These arteries run parallel to the metacarpal bones in the fascia of the dorsal interoessei beneath the extensor tendons.[65,66] All of the dorsal metacarpal arteries give off four to eight cutaneous perforator arteries throughout their length that supply the dorsal skin of the hand.[66] The blood supply to the skin of the distal third of the hand is from the palmar arterial system. The deep palmar arch gives rise to the palmar metacarpal arteries, which also give off perforating arteries to supply the dorsal skin of the distal third of the hand.[67] The perforating arteries to the skin arise 1 cm proximal to the metacarpal head, just distal to the juncture tendium.[67]

The venous drainage of the hand mirrors the arterial supply with both the veins and lymphatics being located superficially in the dorsum of the hand.[68]

1.3.3 Fascia and Soft Tissue

From superficial to deep, the layers of the dorsum of the hand are the epidermis, the dermis, the dorsal superficial lamina, dorsal superficial fascia, dorsal intermediate lamina, dorsal intermediate fascia, dorsal deep lamina, and the dorsal deep fascia.[69] The fascial plane directly beneath the dermis measures 0.3 to 2.2 mm, and the tendinous layer, which is deep to the fascial plane, measures 0.7 to 1.77 mm.[70] Injectable soft-tissue filler for the purposes of hand rejuvenation are typically injected deep to the dermis and superficial fascia and superficial to the deep fascia.[70,71,72] Of note, the deep lamina contains vasculature and tendinous structures susceptible to injury during injections. To identify and protect these structures, they should be separated using skin tenting between the superficial fascial layers and deep lamina.[73] Variations in layer thickness is greatly dependent on age and must be considered when performing injections in order to avoid damaging vital structures. Although the dorsal skin of the hand is very thin, with little subcutaneous fat, the palmar skin is quite thick, contains sensory organs, sweat glands, and many fascial connections.[68] There is significant fibrofatty tissue that sits above the palmar aponeurosis, which provides a cushion for the palm.[68] In addition to the palm, each finger has fibrofatty tissue pads that are separated by flexion creases.[68] These flexion creases are often the ideal location to begin surgical incisions.[68] As a general rule, surgical incisions of the hands should be zigzagged across lines of tension or run longitudinal in neutral zones.[74] This is especially important in the palmar aspect of the hand. The palmar creases are helpful landmarks to locate important structures in the hand. The proximal and transverse creases of the palms overlay the bodies of the metacarpals.[59] The radial longitudinal crease is formed by the thumb muscles and sections off the thumb from the rest of the palm.[59]

1.3.4 Nail Anatomy

Nail biopsies are often performed for a histopathological examination of tissue, in order to provide the patient with a definitive diagnosis of a nail disease. The tip of the digit is known as the pulp.[75] The proximal pulp is the pad of the digit and the distal pulp is the absolute tip of the digit.[75] The pulp is mostly composed of fibrofatty tissue with an extensive nerve network and sweat glands.[75] The matrix is located at the proximal nail fold and can be visualized as the white crescent-shaped area called the lunula (► Fig. 1.17).[76] The nail plate is the actual nail that is made by the matrix and overlays the nail bed.[75] Nail avulsion is the process of removing the nail plate from its attachments and may be diagnostic or therapeutic (► Fig. 1.18).[75]

The major arterial supplies to the nail bed are the proper palmar digital arteries, which arise from the common palmar digital arteries.[59] The dorsal digital arteries arise

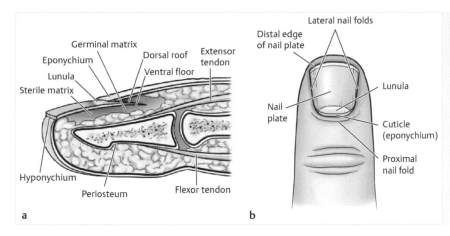

Fig. 1.17 (a, b) Superficial anatomy of the nail unit. (Reproduced from Nail Bed Injuries. In: Janis J, ed. Essentials of Plastic Surgery. 3rd Edition. New York: Thieme; 2022.)

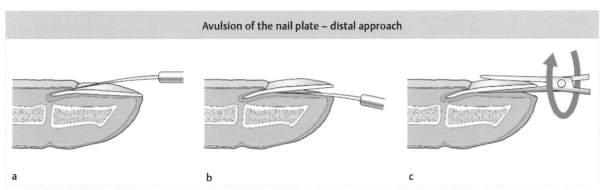

Fig. 1.18 (a–c) Distal approach to nail plate avulsion. (Reprinted with permission from Bolognia J, Schaffer J, Cerroni L. Dermatology. Copyright Elsevier, 2018.)

from the dorsal metacarpal arteries and anastomose with the palmar digital arteries.[77] This creates a network of parallel branches that reach the distal portion of the nail bed. Innervation to the nail bed region is from the dorsal branches of the proper palmar digital nerves (dorsal aspect) and the proper palmar digital nerves (volar aspect), which arise from the common palmar digital nerves near the metacarpal–pharyngeal joint.[59] The dorsal digital nerves arise from radial and ulnar nerves and run along with the dorsal digital arteries.[78]

A common technique for providing local anesthesia during nail surgery is the traditional digital block. To perform this technique, a needle is inserted into the dorsal aspect of the web space on one side of the digit, slightly distal to the knuckle.[79] The needle is then advanced and anesthetic is injected to form a wheal to block the digital nerve.[79] The needle is further advanced toward the palmar surface to block the volar digital nerve.[79] Care must be taken not to inject excessive volumes of local anesthetic as it could potentially compress the digital arteries. A newer approach for delivering anesthetic to the nail region is the transthecal approach. This technique involves a palmar percutaneous injection of lidocaine into the potential space of the flexor tendon sheath at the level of the palmar flexion crease.[80] For this technique, the anesthetic is injected into the flexor digitorum tendon sheath through the volar metacarpophalangeal joint crease.[81] This technique is sometimes preferred, as it attenuates the risk of injuring neurovascular structures.[81] Overall, a thorough understanding of the anatomy of the nail bed region is important when performing dermatologic surgery in this area.

1.4 Lower Extremities

Dermatologists and dermatologic surgeons have an active role in managing cutaneous conditions that manifest on the lower extremities such as skin and soft-tissue tumors, vasculitides, ulcers, and other conditions. As such, knowledge of the surgical anatomy of these regions is critical to successful procedures in the area.

1.4.1 Innervation

To perform dermatologic surgery of the lower extremity, anesthesia of the affected area is typically required. For procedures involving the forefoot, midfoot, or multiple toes, an ankle block is performed.[82] This anesthetizes the posterior tibial nerve, superficial branch of the deep peroneal nerve, sural nerve, saphenous nerve, and superficial peroneal nerve[82] (▶ Fig. 1.19, ▶ Fig. 1.20). The posterior tibial nerve is best found two fingerbreadths proximal to the tip of the medial malleolus.[82] The needle is inserted perpendicular to the shaft of the tibia until it encounters the posterior cortex.[82] The posterior tibial nerve runs in the posterior compartment of the leg along with the posterior tibial artery and terminates under the flexor retinaculum, as it divides into the medial and lateral plantar nerves.[59] The medial and lateral plantar nerves course alongside their respective arteries and supply the intrinsic muscles of the foot.[59] The navicular bone is a useful landmark for injection for the deep peroneal nerve, which can also be identified just lateral to the dorsalis pedis artery.[82] The common peroneal nerve passes around the fibular neck deep to fibularis longus before dividing into the deep and superficial fibular nerves.[59] The

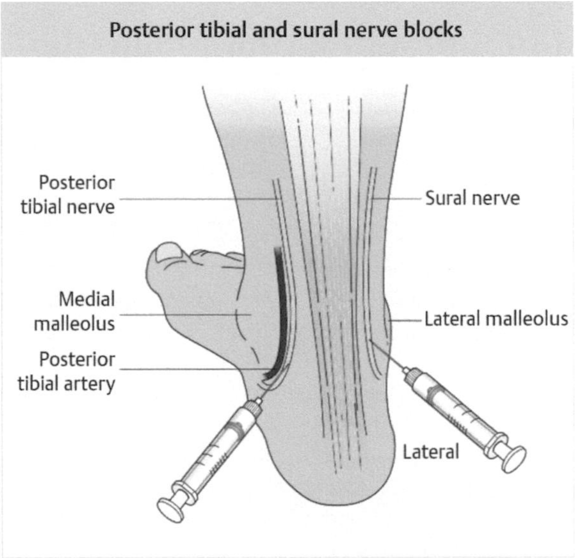

Fig. 1.19 Posterior tibial and sural nerve blocks. The posterior tibial nerve block is performed by palpating the posterior tibial artery and aiming the needle anteriorly and laterally just lateral to the pulse. The anesthetic should be injected into the groove between the medial malleolus and Achilles tendon. The sural nerve is blocked similarly, with the anesthetic injected in the groove between the lateral malleolus and Achilles tendon. (Reprinted with permission from Bolognia J, Jorizzo J, Rapini R. Dermatology, 4th edition. Copyright Elsevier, 2018.)

deep peroneal nerve descends through the leg on the interosseous membrane and enters the dorsum of the foot (▶ Fig. 1.20).[59] The superficial fibular nerve descends in the lateral compartment of the leg and is subcutaneous.[59] The dorsum of the foot is innervated by the superficial fibular nerve except for the space between the first two digits, and the deep fibular nerve provides sensation to this area.[59]

The injection site for the saphenous nerve is one to two fingerbreadths proximal to the tip of the medial malleolus and posterior to the saphenous vein.[82] The saphenous nerve provides innervation to the medial aspect of the foot.[59] The injection site for the sural nerve can be located 1 to 1.5 cm distal to the tip of the lateral malleolus in the subcutaneous fat.[82] The sural nerve passes inferior to the lateral malleolus to provide innervation to the lateral aspect of the foot and some of the heel area.[59] The heel is supplied by the calcaneal nerves, which branch off of the tibial and sural nerves.[59] Both the saphenous and sural nerves can be damaged with sclerotherapy or endovenous thermal ablation for venous insufficiency. Care should be taken to identify these nerves with ultrasound.

The sciatic nerve emerges from the greater sciatic foramen in the gluteal region, where it descends in the posterior thigh deep to the biceps femoris.[59] At the apex of the popliteal fossa, it bifurcates into the tibial and common fibular nerves.[59] A block of the sciatic nerve proximal to the bifurcation in the popliteal fossa is one of the most commonly used proximal nerve blocks for foot and ankle surgery.[83] This block can anesthetize the entire foot except for the saphenous nerve distribution.[83]

The femoral nerve arises from the lumbar plexus in the abdomen and descends through the femoral triangle to supply the anterior thigh muscles.[59] The saphenous branch of this nerve descends to supply the skin of the medial leg and foot. For skin cancers of the leg such as melanoma, an inguinal lymphadenectomy is sometimes performed.[84] Injuries to the femoral neurovasculature have been reported from this procedure.[84] In addition, superficial cutaneous nerves are particularly susceptible to injury during skin cancer surgery of the lower extremity. Sensation to the lateral and anterior aspects of the thigh is provided by the lateral cutaneous nerve of the thigh and the anterior cutaneous branch of the femoral nerve, which course superficially in the upper thigh.[59] The posterior cutaneous nerve of the thigh exits the pelvis, runs under the fascia lata, pierces the deep fascia, and courses along with the small saphenous vein to the middle of the posterior leg.[59] Knowledge of the courses of these structures is important in preventing complications during surgery.

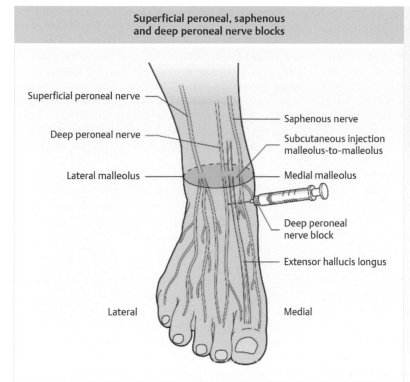

Superficial peroneal, saphenous and deep peroneal nerve blocks

- Superficial peroneal nerve
- Deep peroneal nerve
- Lateral malleolus
- Saphenous nerve
- Subcutaneous injection malleolus-to-malleolus
- Medial malleolus
- Deep peroneal nerve block
- Extensor hallucis longus
- Lateral
- Medial

Fig. 1.20 Superficial peroneal, saphenous, and deep peroneal nerve blocks. The superficial peroneal nerve and saphenous nerves are blocked by injected anesthetic between malleoli across the dorsum of the foot in the subcutaneous tissue. The deep peroneal nerve is blocked by injecting anesthetic lateral to the extensor hallucis longus tendon toward the middle of the foot. (Reprinted with permission from Bolognia J, Jorizzo J, Rapini R. Dermatology, 4th edition. Copyright Elsevier, 2018.)

1.4.2 Vasculature

A sound understanding of the lower extremity vasculature is key to understanding the pathogenesis, management, and prognosis for a number of dermatological conditions such as varicose veins, chronic venous insufficiency, and lower extremity ulcers.

The vasculature of the lower extremity consists of both deep and superficial systems. Since these two are intimately connected, a thorough understanding of both systems is important when performing even superficial surgical procedures. With its origins deep in the pelvis, the femoral artery is the continuation of the external iliac artery distal to the inguinal ligament.[59] It courses through the femoral triangle all the way down to the adductor canal, where it then becomes then popliteal artery.[59] There are several branches of the femoral artery, including the profunda femoris, medial circumflex, and lateral circumflex. The profunda femoris branch enters the posterior region of the thigh as it descends the thigh. The medial and lateral circumflex arteries encircle the upper portion of the femur, anastomosing with each other. The obturator artery arises from the internal iliac artery and divides into anterior and posterior branches in the medial thigh.[59] The popliteal artery begins at the adductor hiatus, where it originates from the femoral artery.[59] It courses laterally through the popliteal fossa and gives off several genicular branches before dividing into the anterior and posterior tibial arteries.[59] The anterior tibial artery passes between the tibia and fibula through the anterior compartment of

the leg.[59] The posterior tibial artery descends in the posterior compartment of the leg before dividing into the medial and lateral plantar arteries distal to the flexor retinaculum.[59]

The dorsalis pedis artery is a continuation of the anterior tibial artery and arises on the anterior aspect of the ankle joint.[59] The posterior tibial artery travels posterior to the medial malleolus, passes through the tarsal tunnel, and divides into the medial and lateral plantar arteries.[59] The dorsalis pedis and posterior tibial arteries are commonly palpated and documented prior to any procedures on the lower extremity or prior to initiation of compression. In the event that pulses are not identified, additional evaluations should include doppler and/or ankle–brachial index studies. The dorsalis pedis artery supplies the dorsum of the foot, while the medial and lateral plantar arteries supply the plantar surface. After passing deep to the abductor hallucis, the medial plantar artery gives off (1) a deep branch that supplies the muscles of the great toe and (2) a superficial branch that supplies the skin on the medial side of the sole and gives off branches that extend to the digits.[59] The lateral plantar artery is located laterally and anteriorly to the medial plantar artery. It dives deep to the abductor hallucis and then courses between the quadratus plantae and the flexor pollicis brevis.[85] As the lateral plantar artery courses medially across the foot, it anastomoses with the deep plantar artery (from dorsalis pedis) to form the deep plantar arch.[85] Occasionally, a superficial plantar arch is formed when the superficial branch of the medial plantar artery anastomoses with the lateral plantar artery or the deep plantar arch.[86] Both of these arteries run with their paired nerves.

Venous drainage of the lower limb is divided into two systems. The deep veins of the lower limb are found beneath the deep muscular fascia and generally run with their respective arteries. The superficial veins are located in the subcutaneous tissue and eventually empty into the deep veins.[87] The superficial veins are more likely to be encountered when performing dermatologic surgery. Venous drainage of the foot is also through deep and superficial venous networks. The deep veins travel with arteries under the deep fascia of the foot and contain many valves and anastomoses.[87] The superficial venous network is located subcutaneously and empties into the dorsal venous arch, which connects the great and small saphenous veins.[85] The origin of the great saphenous vein is the medial side of dorsal venous arch of the foot.[85] This large truncal vein passes anteriorly to the medial malleolus and ascends up the medial side of the leg and joins the deep system at the saphenofemoral junction in the inguinal area.[87] The origin of the small saphenous vein is the lateral side of the dorsal venous arch of the foot.[85] It ascends up the posterolateral aspect of the leg and passes posteriorly to the lateral malleolus.[87] It terminates typically in or just above the popliteal fossa where it drains into the popliteal vein in the saphenopopliteal junction.[87] Further, the venous system has numerous valves to aid in the unidirectional flow of blood back toward the heart. Varicose veins develop when these valves become

incompetent for a number of reasons, such as laxity of the vein wall or cusps.[88] Procedures such as endovenous ablation of the great saphenous and small saphenous veins have been reported to be a successful form of treatment for venous disease, as closure of the abnormal superficial venous system increases the resistance of this system and reroutes blood into the redundant deep venous system whose surrounding musculature helps pump the blood back toward the heart.[89] An overview of veins of the lower extremity is illustrated in ▶ Fig. 1.21.

Dermatologists and dermatologic surgeons have an active role in wound care. On the lower extremities, one of the more common conditions necessitating wound care is ulcers. Venous ulcers are due to chronic venous insufficiency and may be accompanied by significant exudative drainage.[90] Most venous ulcers occurs in the gaiter area, which is the region just above the malleolus, on both the medial and lateral aspects of the leg.[91] The gaiter area is particularly susceptible to ulceration secondary to a dysfunctional calf muscle pump.[92] Ulceration on the medial malleolar area typically correlates with insufficiency of the great saphenous vein, while ulcers on the posterolateral ankle and lower leg point to involvement of the small saphenous vein. Arterial ulcers are typically caused by narrowing of the lumen of vessels secondary to cholesterol plaques and are more commonly found over distal bony prominences.[90] Further, diabetes mellitus affects over 30 million adults in the United States and 1 to 4% of these patients will develop foot ulcers, generally secondary to neuropathy.[93,94] Peripheral arterial disease

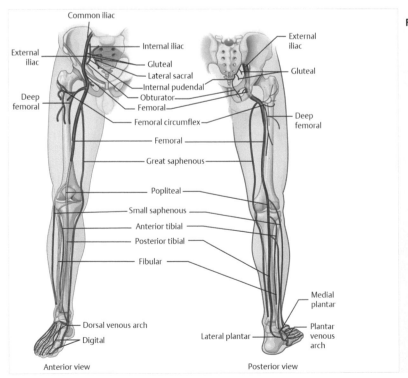

Fig. 1.21 Lower extremity veins.

(PAD) is another condition that is often comorbid with diabetes that predisposes patients to developing foot ulcers.[95] Of note, healing by secondary intention is generally preferred for these ulcers unless they are large enough to necessitate the addition of a graft. In general, secondary intention may be used in many clinical scenarios such as in the case of superficial wounds in concave areas or partial-thickness wounds involving the mucosa of the lip. Areas not appropriate for secondary intention healing include those near a free margin, in which case wound contraction may result in pulling or distortion.

1.4.3 Toe Nails

The toe nail anatomy is very similar to the anatomy of the finger nails (▶ Fig. 1.22). The toe nail consists of four parts: (1) the proximal nail fold, (2) the nail matrix, (3), the nail bed, and (4) the hyponychium.[82] Ingrown toenails are a common cause for dermatologic surgery in this region, and usually involves the lateral or medial nail groove.[82] The ingrown nail typically occurs in the nail bed or hyponychium (▶ Fig. 1.23).[82] The procedure for an ingrown toenail is called the Winograd procedure in which the problematic medial or lateral margin of the nail plate, along with the underlying matrix, is removed.[82] The nail matrix must be removed to prevent the growth of a nail horn, which occurs in 5% of cases.[82] For toe procedures, a digital anesthetic block is typically performed.[82] This involves injection of the agent on the side of the toe within the subcutaneous layer between the skin and the deep fascia.[82] The needle is angled to the plantar side in order to affect the digital nerves.[82] The medial plantar nerve gives off common plantar digital nerves and proper plantar digital nerves that supply the toes.[59] Blood supply to the plantar aspect of toes is from the branches of the plantar arch, the plantar digital arteries, and the plantar metatarsal arteries.[96] The arcuate artery gives off dorsal

metatarsal arteries, which run in the spaces between the toes before dividing into two dorsal digital branches in adjacent toes.[96] The vasculature of the foot runs alongside the nerves; therefore, particular care must be taken to avoid intravascular injection during procedures.

1.5 Genitalia

1.5.1 Female Genital Anatomy

A variety of dermatologic conditions affect the female genital areas such as lichen sclerosis, cancer, and normal aging. Knowledge of the surgical anatomy of the female genital region is necessary for treating patients with these conditions.

Vulva

The vulva is the external component of the female genitalia. The vulvar structures include the mons pubis, the labia majora, labia minora, the clitoris, and glandular vestibular structures.[59] The mons pubis is an area of adipose tissue that sits in front of the pubic symphysis and is covered with hair in the shape of an inverted triangle.[97] The labia majora are two folds of skin that form the lateral portions of the vulva, begin at the mons pubis, and stretch down to the perineum.[97] The labia are filled with loose subcutaneous tissue, fat, and smooth muscle, and are covered with sebaceous glands and pubic hair.[96] There is a rich supply of veins throughout the fat in the labia majora. The thickest part of the labia majora is the anterior portion, where the two folds fuse to form the anterior commissure.[97] The posterior commissure is less defined and represents the point of posterior fusion.[97] It is currently a popular trend to undergo elective vulvar aesthetic surgeries to alter these vaginal structures. For example, the skin of the labia majora may puffy and

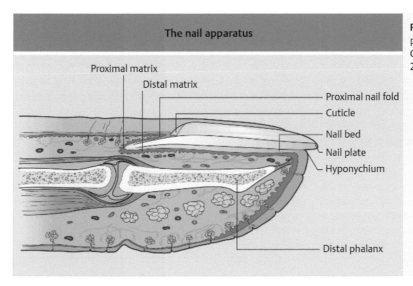

Fig. 1.22 Nail anatomy. (Reprinted with permission from Bolognia J, Schaffer J, Cerroni L. Dermatology. Copyright Elsevier, 2018.)

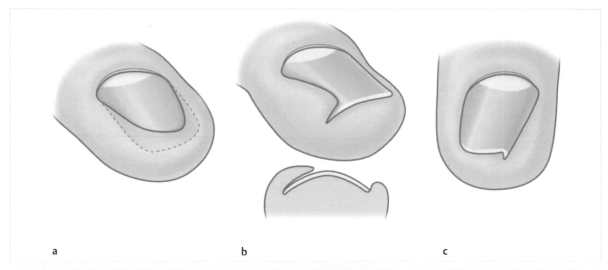

Fig. 1.23 Ingrown toenails of infancy. **(a)** Ingrown toenail of the newborn with the distal and lateral nail walls overlying the corners of the nail. **(b)** Hypertrophic lateral lip overlying the nail surface. **(c)** Congenital misalignment of the great toenail. (Reprinted from Surgery of the Skin. Haneke E. Copyright [2015] with permission from Elsevier.)

prominent or saggy.[98] Cosmetic dissatisfaction with this prompts some women to seek a medical treatment of their labia majora, which may consist of fat injection for augmentation or resection of redundant skin.[98] The labia minora are folds of skin that surround the vestibule of the vagina. The folds are smooth and hairless and contain smooth muscle.[59] The labia minora are important structures with respect to dermatologic and other surgical procedures. Labial hypertrophy, or a labia minora width that in enlarged, is also a condition for which care is sought due to functional or cosmetic concerns.[99] When appropriate, labial hypertrophy is treated with a labioplasty, in which a physician reshapes the labia minora. The trim technique involves excising excess labial tissue along the outer edge of the inner labia, and the wedge technique involves removing a v-shaped wedge of tissue from both sides of the labia and suturing the remaining edges.[100] Anteriorly, the labia fuse to form the prepuce of the clitoris and posteriorly to form the frenulum.[97] The clitoris is an erectile organ that is formed by the anterior fusion of the labia minora. The corpus clitoridis is the erectile body and contains the crura clitoridis and glans clitidoris.[100] The crura of the clitoris are below the ischiocavernosus muscles and superiorly fuse to form the glans.[97] Knowledge of the clitoral anatomy is important to preserve its structure during surgical procedures.

Lymphatic drainage from the vulva is to the superficial subinguinal lymph nodes or to the deep inguinal lymph node.[59] The arterial supply of the vulvar area is mainly from the internal pudendal artery, which arises from the internal iliac artery.[59] The internal pudendal artery gives off branches including the dorsal and deep arteries of the clitoris.[97] The vulva has a rich venous plexus, which ultimately drains into the internal pudendal vein.[59] Varicosities in this region are often associated with central pelvic venous insufficiency and may warrant additional workup and imaging. Innervation to the vulva is from the anterior labial nerves (anteriorly), which are branches of the ilioinguinal nerve.[59] Posteriorly, the innervation is from the posterior labial nerves, which are branches of the superficial perineal nerve.[59] Injury to this nerve is not uncommon, and occurs through episiotomies, impact injuries, and vulvar surgeries.[101]

Vagina

Dermatologists and dermatologic surgeons may perform a variety of procedures involving the vagina, necessitating thorough knowledge of the vaginal anatomy. The vagina is a musculomembranous organ and is compressed by several muscles and sphincters including the external urethral sphincter, urethrovaginal sphincter, pubovaginalis muscle, and bulbospongiosus muscle.[59] The inferior opening of the vagina is the vaginal orifice. The vaginal orifice opens into the vestibule of the vagina, which is the space between the two labia minora.[59] The vagina is a collapsed tube and extends from the vestibule to the middle of the cervix.

Procedures such as vaginal rejuvenation aim to decrease the diameter of the vaginal canal and opening.[67] This may be done by incising the opening of the vagina, removing excess tissue, and suturing the remaining tissue.[67] The mucosa is a site of potential laser application for vaginal rejuvenation, which delivers energy to the area to stimulate collagen and elastin contraction, neocollagenesis, and neovascularization. Laser treatment is thought to ultimately work to increase the thickness of the tissue and decrease the diameter of the vaginal opening.[102] Although more robust studies are needed, laser technology has thus far been shown to be a potential option for vaginal rejuvenation procedures.[103]

1.5.2 Male Genital Anatomy

Procedures in dermatology involving the male genitals most commonly involve surgical excision of a malignancy of the penis, the most common being squamous cell carcinoma (SCC), although excisions are performed for basaloid carcinoma and verrucous carcinoma of the penis as well.[104]

Penis

Although SCC of the penis is rare in the United States, the majority of cutaneous malignancies presenting on the penis will be SCCs.[105,106,107,108] As 78% tumors are located on the glans or prepuce, organ-sparing procedures have emerged that are both curative and allow preservation of penile function.[109] In the case of urethral involvement or larger tumors, these options include a glansectomy.[110] Other cancers of the penis, such as melanoma or basal cell carcinoma, may present in any location on the penis. Cancers located in other areas of the penis may also require surgical intervention, more often in the form of partial penile resection.[109]

The penis is composed of three parts: the root, the body, and the glans.[59] The most superior portion of the penis is the root, which is composed of the crura, the bulb, the ischiocavernosus, and the bulbospongiosus.[59] The body of the penis is an extension of the root of the penis and contains no additional muscles.[59] The glans of the penis is an extension of the corpus spongiosum erectile body.[59] The corona of the glans is the rim of tissue that covers the neck of the glans, which separates the glans penis from the body of the penis.[59] In an uncircumcised male, the skin and fascia of the penis form the prepuce, which is also called the foreskin.

The corpora cavernosa are paired structures on the dorsal side of the penis that are the main erectile bodies of the penis.[85] They are covered by a thick outer layer, the tunica albuginea, and sinusoidal tissue that expands with blood during an erection. The single erectile body on the ventral aspect of the penis is the corpora spongiosum, which is continuous with the glans.[85] Superficial to the tunica albuginea lies the deep penile (Buck) fascia, which is deep to the dartos fascia, which is just beneath the penile skin.[85] The glansectomy begins by using the plane between the deep penile fascia and the deep surface of the penis in order to expose the corpora cavernosa.[110] The glans is excised from the corpora cavernosa and the dartos and skin are sutured along, generally with a split skin graft, to construct a new glans.[110] Neurovascular bundles and the urethra are distally sectioned and then fixed to the distal corpora cavernosa.[110]

There are three components to the male urethra: (1) the prostatic portion, (2) the membranous portion, and (3) the spongy portion.[59] It is critical to understand the urethral anatomy, as many procedures involve reconstruction of some component of the urethra. The prostatic portion of the urethra is the most proximal portion and begins at the neck of the bladder.[59] This portion of the urethra is bordered by the prostate and empties into the membranous portion. The membranous portion of the urethra begins at the apex of the prostate and runs through the deep perineal pouch.[59] This portion is surrounded by the external urethral sphincter and opens to the spongy portion of the urethra.[59] The spongy portion of the urethra runs from the distal part of the membranous urethra and terminates at the external urethral orifice.[59] The spongy urethral lumen is expanded to form the intrabulbar fossa in the bulb of the penis, and the navicular fossa in the glans of the penis.[59] There are small openings for secretions of the bulbourethral and urethral glands throughout the spongy urethra.[59]

The penis is richly supplied by many arteries and nerves. The neurovasculature is sometimes separated out during surgical procedures in order to avoid injuring these structures.[110] The dorsal aspect of the penis is supplied by the dorsal arteries of the penis, which run along the dorsum of the penis between the dorsal artery and deep dorsal vein.[59] The corpora cavernosa are supplied by the deep arteries of the penis, which run along the shaft and give off helicine arteries to supply the erectile tissue.[59] The bulbous part of the corpus spongiosum and the bulbourethral glands are supplied by the arteries of the bulb of the penis.[59] The branches of the external pudendal arteries supply the skin of the penis.[59]

There are multiple levels of venous drainage of the penis. The superficial veins are located throughout the dartos fascia, which is likely to be encountered during reconstructive procedures such as the glansectomy.[85] The deep dorsal vein of the penis drains blood from the cavernous space and courses in the deep fascia.[59]

Sensory and sympathetic innervation to the penis is through the dorsal nerve of the penis, a branch of the pudendal nerve.[59] Parasympathetic innervation to the erectile tissue is through the cavernous nerves.[59] The pudendal nerve is particularly vulnerable to injury during surgery, and consequences of injury are devastating. Pudendal nerve injury is known to cause erectile dysfunction, voiding dysfunction, and pain.[111] The dorsal nerve of the penis is the branch of the pudendal nerve that is particularly susceptible to injury during dermatologic surgery. To avoid injuring this structure during surgery, one must recognize the variations of this nerve, including the different branching patterns throughout the penis. The branches within the glans are well documented; however, there are variations as to how far branches may extend out laterally on the shaft, which must be kept in mind during surgical procedures.[23]

1.6 Conclusion

An ever-expanding number of dermatologic procedures are performed on the head and neck, extremities, and genitalia. A sound understanding of the neurovascular and other clinically relevant anatomy is imperative to optimizing patient outcomes and mitigating procedural risk.

References

[1] Salasche SJ, Mandy SH. Anatomy. In: Rohrer TE, Cook JL, Kaufman AJ, eds. Flaps and Grafts, in Dermatologic Surgery. Philadelphia, PA: Elsevier; 2007:1–14

[2] Robinson J. Anatomy for procedural dermatology. In: Robinson J, Hanke WC, Siegel D, Fratila A, Bhatia A, Rohrer T, eds. Surgery of the Skin. New York, NY: Saunders; 2015:1–27

[3] Schenck TL, Koban KC, Schlattau A, et al. The functional anatomy of the superficial fat compartments of the face: a detailed imaging study. Plast Reconstr Surg. 2018; 141(6):1351–1359

[4] Wysong A, Kim D, Joseph T, MacFarlane DF, Tang JY, Gladstone HB. Quantifying soft tissue loss in the aging male face using magnetic resonance imaging. Dermatol Surg. 2014; 40(7):786–793

[5] Wysong A, Joseph T, Kim D, Tang JY, Gladstone HB. Quantifying soft tissue loss in facial aging: a study in women using magnetic resonance imaging. Dermatol Surg. 2013; 39(12):1895–1902

[6] Pessa JE, Rohrich RJ. Facial Topography: Clinical Anatomy of the Face. St. Louis, MO: Quality Medical Publishing, Inc.; 2012

[7] Salasche SJ. Anatomy. In: Rohrer TE, Cook JL, Nguyen T, eds. Flaps and Grafts in Dermatologic Surgery. Philadelphia, PA: Saunders, Elsevier; 2008

[8] Kazkayasi M, Ergin A, Ersoy M, Bengi O, Tekdemir I, Elhan A. Certain anatomical relations and the precise morphometry of the infraorbital foramen: canal and groove: an anatomical and cephalometric study. Laryngoscope. 2001; 111(4, Pt 1):609–614

[9] Tubbs RS, Johnson PC, Loukas M, Shoja MM, Cohen-Gadol AA. Anatomical landmarks for localizing the buccal branch of the trigeminal nerve on the face. Surg Radiol Anat. 2010; 32(10):933–935

[10] Allen S, Sengelmann R. Nerve injury. In: Gloster HM, ed. Complications in Cutaneous Surgery. New York, NY: Springer; 2008:21–35

[11] Moore KL, Dalley AF. Clinically Oriented Anatomy. 4th ed. New York, NY: Lippincott Williams & Wilkins; 1999

[12] Standring S. Gray's Anatomy: The Anatomical Basis of Clinical Practice. 39th ed. New York, NY: Churchill Livingstone; 2005

[13] Baker DC, Conley J. Avoiding facial nerve injuries in rhytidectomy. Anatomical variations and pitfalls. Plast Reconstr Surg. 1979; 64(6):781–795

[14] Pessa JE. SMAS fusion zones determine the subfascial and subcutaneous anatomy of the human face: fascial spaces, fat compartments, and models of facial aging. Aesthet Surg J. 2016; 36(5):515–526

[15] Borle RM, Jadhav A, Bhola N, Hingnikar P, Gaikwad P. Borle's triangle: a reliable anatomical landmark for ease of identification of facial nerve trunk during parotidectomy. J Oral Biol Craniofac Res. 2019; 9(1):33–36

[16] von Arx T, Nakashima MJ, Lozanoff S. The face: a musculoskeletal perspective. A literature review. Swiss Dent J. 2018; 128(9):678–688

[17] Joseph ST, Sharankumar S, Sandya CJ, et al. Easy and safe method for facial nerve identification in parotid surgery. J Neurol Surg B Skull Base. 2015; 76(6):426–431

[18] Curtin HD, Wolfe P, Snyderman N. The facial nerve between the stylomastoid foramen and the parotid: computed tomographic imaging. Radiology. 1983; 149(1):165–169

[19] Whitney ZB, Zito PM. Anatomy, Skin, Superficial Musculoaponeurotic System (SMAS) Fascia. Treasure Island, FL: StatPearls Publishing; 2018

[20] Pitanguy I, Ramos AS. The frontal branch of the facial nerve: the importance of its variations in face lifting. Plast Reconstr Surg. 1966; 38(4):352–356

[21] Maciburko SJ, Townley WA, Hollowood K, Giele HP. Skin cancers of the hand: a series of 541 malignancies. Plast Reconstr Surg. 2012; 129(6):1329–1336

[22] Brown H, Burns S, Kaiser CW. The spinal accessory nerve plexus, the trapezius muscle, and shoulder stabilization after radical neck cancer surgery. Ann Surg. 1988; 208(5):654–661

[23] Kozacioglu Z, Kiray A, Ergur I, Zeybek G, Degirmenci T, Gunlusoy B. Anatomy of the dorsal nerve of the penis, clinical implications. Urology. 2014; 83(1):121–124

[24] Schwember G, Rodríguez A. Anatomic surgical dissection of the extraparotid portion of the facial nerve. Plast Reconstr Surg. 1988; 81(2):183–188

[25] Gosain AK, Sewall SR, Yousif NJ. The temporal branch of the facial nerve: how reliably can we predict its path? Plast Reconstr Surg. 1997; 99(5):1224–1233, discussion 1234–1236

[26] Ammirati M, Spallone A, Ma J, Cheatham M, Becker D. An anatomicosurgical study of the temporal branch of the facial nerve. Neurosurgery. 1993; 33(6):1038–1043, discussion 1044

[27] Al-Kayat A, Bramley P. A modified pre-auricular approach to the temporomandibular joint and malar arch. Br J Oral Surg. 1979; 17(2):91–103

[28] Hwang K, Kim YJ, Chung IH. Innervation of the corrugator supercilii muscle. Ann Plast Surg. 2004; 52(2):140–143

[29] Owsley JQ, Agarwal CA. Safely navigating around the facial nerve in three dimensions. Clin Plast Surg. 2008; 35(4):469–477, v

[30] Salas E, Ziyal IM, Bejjani GK, Sekhar LN. Anatomy of the frontotemporal branch of the facial nerve and indications for interfascial dissection. Neurosurgery. 1998; 43(3):563–568, discussion 568–569

[31] Kim DI, Nam SH, Nam YS, Lee KS, Chung RH, Han SH. The marginal mandibular branch of the facial nerve in Koreans. Clin Anat. 2009; 22(2):207–214

[32] Drake R. Gray's Anatomy of Students. Philadelphia, PA: Elsevier/Churchill Livingstone; 2010:855–866

[33] Wang TM, Lin CL, Kuo KJ, Shih C. Surgical anatomy of the mandibular ramus of the facial nerve in Chinese adults. Acta Anat (Basel). 1991; 142(2):126–131

[34] Basar R, Sargon MF, Tekdemir Y, Elhan A. The marginal mandibular branch of the facial nerve. Surg Radiol Anat. 1997; 19(5):311–314

[35] Savary V, Robert R, Rogez JM, Armstrong O, Leborgne J. The mandibular marginal ramus of the facial nerve: an anatomic and clinical study. Surg Radiol Anat. 1997; 19(2):69–72

[36] Al-Hayani A. Anatomical localisation of the marginal mandibular branch of the facial nerve. Folia Morphol (Warsz). 2007; 66(4):307–313

[37] Hazani R, Chowdhry S, Mowlavi A, Wilhelmi BJ. Bony anatomic landmarks to avoid injury to the marginal mandibular nerve. Aesthet Surg J. 2011; 31(3):286–289

[38] Batra AP, Mahajan A, Gupta K. Marginal mandibular branch of the facial nerve: an anatomical study. Indian J Plast Surg. 2010; 43(1):60–64

[39] Bindra S, Choudhary K, Sharma P, Sheorain A, Sharma CB. Management of mandibular sub condylar and condylar fractures using retromandibular approach and assessment of associated surgical complications. J Maxillofac Oral Surg. 2010; 9(4):355–362

[40] Valtonen EJ, Lilius HG. Late sequelae of iatrogenic spinal accessory nerve injury. Acta Chir Scand. 1974; 140(6):453–455

[41] Nason RW, Abdulrauf BM, Stranc MF. The anatomy of the accessory nerve and cervical lymph node biopsy. Am J Surg. 2000; 180(3):241–243

[42] Brown SM, Oliphant T, Langtry J. Motor nerves of the head and neck that are susceptible to damage during dermatological surgery. Clin Exp Dermatol. 2014; 39(6):677–682, quiz 681–682

[43] Overland J, Hodge JC, Breik O, Krishnan S. Surgical anatomy of the spinal accessory nerve: review of the literature and case report of a rare anatomical variant. J Laryngol Otol. 2016; 130(10):969–972

[44] Durazzo MD, Furlan JC, Teixeira GV, et al. Anatomic landmarks for localization of the spinal accessory nerve. Clin Anat. 2009; 22(4): 471–475

[45] Salgarelli AC, Landini B, Bellini P, Multinu A, Consolo U, Collini M. A simple method of identifying the spinal accessory nerve in modified radical neck dissection: anatomic study and clinical implications for resident training. Oral Maxillofac Surg. 2009; 13(2):69–72

[46] Anderson BW, Al Kharazi KA. Anatomy, Head and Neck, Skull. Treasure Island, FL: StatPearls Publishing; 2018

[47] von Arx T, Tamura K, Yukiya O, Lozanoff S. The face: a vascular perspective. A literature review. Swiss Dent J. 2018; 128(5):382–392

[48] Westbrook KE, Varacallo M. Anatomy, Head and Neck, Facial Muscles. Treasure Island, FL: StatPearls Publishing; 2018

[49] Kim HS, Lee KL, Gil YC, Hu KS, Tansatit T, Kim HJ. Topographic anatomy of the infraorbital artery and its clinical implications for nasolabial fold augmentation. Plast Reconstr Surg. 2018; 142(3): 273e–280e

[50] Koziej M, Trybus M, Hold M, et al. The superficial temporal artery: anatomical map for facial reconstruction and aesthetic procedures. Aesthet Surg J. 2019; 39(8):815–823

[51] Umek N, Cvetko E. Unusual course and termination of common facial vein: a case report. Surg Radiol Anat. 2019; 41(2):239–241

[52] Kiranantawat K, Suhk JH, Nguyen AH. The Asian eyelid: relevant anatomy. Semin Plast Surg. 2015; 29(3):158–164

[53] Kim DW, Bhatki AM. Upper blepharoplasty in the Asian eyelid. Facial Plast Surg Clin North Am. 2005; 13(4):525–532, vi

[54] Doxanas MT, Anderson RL. Oriental eyelids. An anatomic study. Arch Ophthalmol. 1984; 102(8):1232–1235

[55] Park JW, Hwang K. Anatomy and histology of an epicanthal fold. J Craniofac Surg. 2016; 27(4):1101–1103

[56] Watanabe K. Measurement method of upper blepharoplasty for Orientals. Aesthetic Plast Surg. 1993; 17(1):1–8

[57] Flowers RS. Upper blepharoplasty by eyelid invagination. Anchor blepharoplasty. Clin Plast Surg. 1993; 20(2):193–207

[58] Saonanon P. Update on Asian eyelid anatomy and clinical relevance. Curr Opin Ophthalmol. 2014; 25(5):436–442

[59] Moore KL, Dalley A, Agur AMR, Clinically Oriented Anatomy. 7th ed. Philadelphia, PA: Wolters Kluwer; 2014

[60] MacDonald RI, Lichtman DM, Hanlon JJ, Wilson JN. Complications of surgical release for carpal tunnel syndrome. J Hand Surg Am. 1978; 3(1):70–76

[61] Bland JD. Treatment of carpal tunnel syndrome. Muscle Nerve. 2007; 36(2):167–171

[62] Lifchez SD, Kelamis JA. Surgery of the hand and wrist. In: Brunicardi F, Andersen D, Billiar TR, et al, eds. Schwartz's Principles of Surgery. New York, NY: McGraw-Hill; 2015

[63] Gündeş H, Cirpici Y, Sarlak A, Müezzinoglu S. Prognosis of wrist ganglion operations. Acta Orthop Belg. 2000; 66(4):363–367

[64] Hallett P, Ashurst JV. Anatomy, Shoulder and Upper Limb, Hand Anatomical Snuff Box. Treasure Island, FL: StatPearls Publishing; 2018

[65] Vuppalapati G, Oberlin C, Balakrishnan G. "Distally based dorsal hand flaps": clinical experience, cadaveric studies and an update. Br J Plast Surg. 2004; 57(7):653–667

[66] Omokawa S, Tanaka Y, Ryu J, Kish VL. The anatomical basis for reverse first to fifth dorsal metacarpal arterial flaps. J Hand Surg [Br]. 2005; 30(1):40–44

[67] Sobanko JF, Fischer J, Etzkorn JR, Miller CJ. Local fasciocutaneous sliding flaps for soft-tissue defects of the dorsum of the hand. JAMA Dermatol. 2014; 150(11):1187–1191

[68] Rohrer TE, Leslie B, Grande DJ. Dermatologic surgery of the hand. General principles and avoiding complications. J Dermatol Surg Oncol. 1994; 20(1):19–34, quiz 36–37

[69] Bidic SM, Hatef DA, Rohrich RJ. Dorsal hand anatomy relevant to volumetric rejuvenation. Plast Reconstr Surg. 2010; 126(1):163–168

[70] Lefebvre-Vilardebo M, Trevidic P, Moradi A, Busso M, Sutton AB, Bucay VW. Hand: clinical anatomy and regional approaches with injectable fillers. Plast Reconstr Surg. 2015; 136(5) Suppl:258S–275S

[71] Bertucci V, Solish N, Wong M, Howell M. Evaluation of the Merz hand grading scale after calcium hydroxylapatite hand treatment. Dermatol Surg. 2015; 41 Suppl 1:S389–S396

[72] Gargasz SS, Carbone MC. Hand rejuvenation using Radiesse. Plast Reconstr Surg. 2010; 125(2):259e–260e

[73] Fathi R, Cohen JL. Challenges, considerations, and strategies in hand rejuvenation. J Drugs Dermatol. 2016; 15(7):809–815

[74] Young DM, Hansen SL, Doherty GM. Hand surgery. In: Doherty GM, ed. Current Diagnosis & Treatment: Surgery. New York, NY: McGraw-Hill; 2014

[75] Robinson JK, Hanke C, Rohrer TE, Siegel DM, Fratila A, Bhatia AC. Surgery of the Skin: Procedural Dermatology. 2nd ed. London: Mosby, Elsevier; 2015

[76] Ashish Bhatia TR. Nail surgery. In: Robinson JK, Hanke WC, Siegel D, Fratila A, Bhatia A, Rohrer T, eds. Surgery of the Skin: Procedural Dermatology. Philadelphia, PA: Mosby, Elsevier; 2010:755–780

[77] Yang D, Morris SF. Vascular basis of dorsal digital and metacarpal skin flaps. J Hand Surg Am. 2001; 26(1):142–146

[78] Yun MJ, Park JU, Kwon ST. Surgical options for malignant skin tumors of the hand. Arch Plast Surg. 2013; 40(3):238–243

[79] Napier A, Taylor A. Digital Nerve Block. Treasure Island, FL: StatPearls Publishing; 2018

[80] Chiu DT. Transthecal digital block: flexor tendon sheath used for anesthetic infusion. J Hand Surg Am. 1990; 15(3):471–477

[81] Hart RG, Fernandas FA, Kutz JE. Transthecal digital block: an underutilized technique in the ED. Am J Emerg Med. 2005; 23(3): 340–342

[82] Mann JA, Chou L, Ross SDK. Foot and ankle surgery. In: Skinner HB, McMahon P, eds. Current Diagnosis & Treatment in Orthopedics. New York, NY: McGraw-Hill; 2014

[83] Fraser TW, Doty JF. Peripheral nerve blocks in foot and ankle surgery. Orthop Clin North Am. 2017; 48(4):507–515

[84] Joyce KM. Surgical management of melanoma. In: Ward WH, Farma J, eds. Cutaneous Melanoma: Etiology and Therapy. Brisbane, Australia: Codon Publications; 2017

[85] Morton DA, Foreman KB, Albertine KH. The Big Picture Gross Anatomy. 2nd ed. New York, NY: McGraw-Hill Medical; 2011

[86] Ozer MA, Govsa F, Bilge O. Anatomic study of the deep plantar arch. Clin Anat. 2005; 18(6):434–442

[87] Creager MA, Loscalzo J. Chronic venous disease and lymphedema. In: Longo DL, Fauci AS, Kasper DL, Hauser SL, Jameson JL, Loscalzo J, eds. Harrison's Principles of Internal Medicine. 20th ed. New York, NY: McGraw-Hill; 2011

[88] Goel RR, Abidia A, Hardy SC. Surgery for deep venous incompetence. Cochrane Database Syst Rev. 2015(2):CD001097

[89] Deatrick KB, Wakefield TW, Henke PK. Chronic venous insufficiency: current management of varicose vein disease. Am Surg. 2010; 76(2): 125–132

[90] Foman N. Leg ulcers. In: Soutor C, Hordinsky MK, eds. Clinical Dermatology. New York, NY: McGraw-Hill; 2012

[91] Grey JE, Harding KG, Enoch S. Venous and arterial leg ulcers. BMJ. 2006; 332(7537):347–350

[92] London NJ, Donnelly R. ABC of arterial and venous disease. Ulcerated lower limb. BMJ. 2000; 320(7249):1589–1591

[93] Bartus CL, Margolis DJ. Reducing the incidence of foot ulceration and amputation in diabetes. Curr Diab Rep. 2004; 4(6):413–418

[94] National Diabetes Statistics Report. Estimates of Diabetes and Its Burden in the United States. 2017 [cited 2019 January 12, 2019]. Available from: https://www.cdc.gov/diabetes/pdfs/data/statistics/national-diabetes-statistics-report.pdf

[95] Armstrong DG, Cohen K, Courric S, Bharara M, Marston W. Diabetic foot ulcers and vascular insufficiency: our population has changed, but our methods have not. J Diabetes Sci Technol. 2011; 5(6):1591–1595

[96] Williams PL, Warwick R, Dyson M, Bannister LH. Gray's Anatomy. 37th ed. New York, NY: Churchill Livingstone; 1989

[97] Owen CM, Heitmann R. Anatomy of the female reproductive system. In: Nathan L, DeCherney AH, Laufer N, Roman AS, eds. Current Diagnosis & Treatment: Obstetrics & Gynecology. New York, NY: McGraw-Hill; 2013: 1–37

[98] Hunter JG. Labia minora, labia majora, and clitoral hood alteration: experience-based recommendations. Aesthet Surg J. 2016; 36(1): 71–79

[99] Westermann LB, Oakley SH, Mazloomdoost D, et al. Attitudes regarding labial hypertrophy and labiaplasty: a survey of members of the Society of Gynecologic Surgeons and the North American Society for Pediatric and Adolescent Gynecology. Female Pelvic Med Reconstr Surg. 2016; 22(3):175–179

[100] Wong Cp, Bhimji Sp. Labiaplasty, Labia Minora Reduction. Treasure Island, FL: StatPearls Publishing; 2018

[101] Wan EL, Goldstein AT, Tolson H, Dellon AL. Injury to perineal branch of pudendal nerve in women: outcome from resection of the perineal branches. J Reconstr Microsurg. 2017; 33(6):395–401

[102] Barbara G, Facchin F, Buggio L, Alberico D, Frattaruolo MP, Kustermann A. Vaginal rejuvenation: current perspectives. Int J Womens Health. 2017; 9:513–519

[103] Karcher C, Sadick N. Vaginal rejuvenation using energy-based devices. Int J Womens Dermatol. 2016; 2(3):85–88

[104] Higgins S, Nazemi A, Chow M, Wysong A. Review of nonmelanoma skin cancer in African Americans, Hispanics, and Asians. Dermatol Surg. 2018; 44(7):903–910

[105] Pow-Sang MR, Ferreira U, Pow-Sang JM, Nardi AC, Destefano V. Epidemiology and natural history of penile cancer. Urology. 2010; 76(2) Suppl 1:S2–S6

[106] Barnholtz-Sloan JS, Maldonado JL, Pow-sang J, Giuliano AR. Incidence trends in primary malignant penile cancer. Urol Oncol. 2007; 25(5):361–367

[107] Brady KL, Mercurio MG, Brown MD. Malignant tumors of the penis. Dermatol Surg. 2013; 39(4):527–547

[108] Burt LM, Shrieve DC, Tward JD. Stage presentation, care patterns, and treatment outcomes for squamous cell carcinoma of the penis. Int J Radiat Oncol Biol Phys. 2014; 88(1):94–100

[109] Brown CT, Minhas S, Ralph DJ. Conservative surgery for penile cancer: subtotal glans excision without grafting. BJU Int. 2005; 96 (6):911–912

[110] Morelli G, Pagni R, Mariani C, et al. Glansectomy with split-thickness skin graft for the treatment of penile carcinoma. Int J Impot Res. 2009; 21(5):311–314

[111] Possover M, Forman A. Voiding dysfunction associated with pudendal nerve entrapment. Curr Bladder Dysfunct Rep. 2012; 7(4): 281–285

2 Reconstruction of the Forehead Unit

Ardeshir Edward Nadimi, Sonal A. Parikh, and Vishal Anil Patel

Summary

The forehead is one of the more unpredictable anatomic units of the head and neck due to the variance in mobility and topography within the forehead itself and between individuals. It has a rich vascular supply and predictable innervation. Each subunit has unique features that influence closure choice. Closure options include secondary intention healing, primary closure, local and regional flaps, split thickness and partial thickness skin grafts, free tissue transfers, and a few specialized flaps. Given its proximity to the eyebrow and hairline, careful consideration is given to maintaining the natural relationship between the hair-bearing and non–hair-bearing regions of the forehead, in addition to reasonable maintenance of the natural location of and distance between the eyebrows. Eyebrow elevation and ptosis are two of the more undesirable outcomes of forehead surgery. The main parameters influencing closure choice include defect size, forehead subunit(s) involved, and patient factors including desire for a simple closure and overall aesthetic orientation. The largest forehead defects, which may extend to the scalp superiorly or cheek inferolaterally, can be closed with a combination of multiple repair options, intraoperative tissue expansion, and/or internal/external tissue expanders. Though reconstruction choice requires keeping in mind many defect- and patient-specific factors, we present a general algorithm based on the parameters above.

Keywords: forehead, mid forehead, paramedian forehead, lateral forehead, reconstruction, flaps, Mohs defect, tissue expansion

2.1 Introduction

When approaching the surgical reconstruction of forehead defects, a few general principles should be kept in mind. The forehead is divided into four subunits—central, lateral, temple, and eyebrow—with the former being divided into midline and paramedian components (▶ Fig. 2.1). The forehead unit is deceptive in its limited mobility, despite undermining, and it is one of the most unpredictable units of the head and neck. As with any anatomical unit, reconstructive goals should include preserving motor and sensory function, maintaining the aesthetic subunit boundaries of the forehead, which include the frontal hairline, temporal hairline, and the eyebrows, and optimizing scar camouflage within aesthetic boundaries or relaxed skin tensions lines (RSTLs).[1,2] Complications can occur during forehead reconstruction but can be avoided with care and advanced planning.

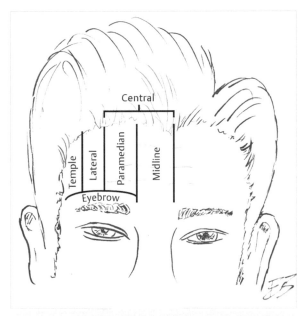

Fig. 2.1 The forehead is divided into four aesthetic subunits – central, lateral, temple, and eyebrow – and the central subunit is subdivided into mid and paramedian components. (Image courtesy of Edward Bae, MD, and Hannah Singer, MD.)

Complications unique to surgery of the forehead include eyebrow ptosis/paralysis, oblique mid-forehead scars, iatrogenic alopecia in an eyebrow, and an asymmetric hairline; in the hands of a skilled surgeon, these can be avoided.

Reconstruction of the forehead requires noting each patient's unique anatomy, including forehead height, the sebaceous quality of the skin and how it changes with the topography of the forehead, the presence of rhytids in which to hide scars, the tightness of the forehead and scalp skin, and the presence of redundant skin that can be used to provide tension, amongst other factors.

2.1.1 Anatomy

The layers of the forehead closely mirror the layers of the scalp, with one major difference. From external to internal, the basic layers of the scalp are: the skin (S), consisting of epidermis and dermis; the subcutaneous tissue (C), containing the subdermal vascular plexus; the galea aponeurosis (A); loose connective tissue (L); and the periosteum (P). The acronym "SCALP" can be used to remember these basic layers of the scalp.[3] The forehead contains the same layers with the major difference in that the aponeurosis is replaced by the frontalis muscle.

There is considerable variation in the vertical height of the forehead, which is primarily a function of the height of the frontal hairline. In addition, the distance and amount of non–hair-bearing skin between the lateral eyebrow and the frontal hairline/sideburn varies between people and increases with aging, especially in men with male-pattern balding. These factors play a role in the reconstruction of surgical wounds in this region.

Forehead Musculature

The main muscle of the forehead is the occipitofrontalis muscle. The vertically oriented skeletal fibers are responsible for the horizontal orientation of the RSTLs as well as the horizontal direction of rhytids with aging skin. The nearly inevitable development of horizontal rhytids of the forehead with aging makes the cosmetic outcome of a forehead repair likely to improve over time, especially with horizontal repairs that will eventually be obscured within a soon-to-develop crease.[1] The galeal median raphe, located in the mid forehead, is devoid of muscular fibers, and thus reconstruction of a defect overlying it often has a great cosmetic outcome (▶ Fig. 2.2). The galea is a tough and inelastic layer of connective tissue, also known as the epicranial aponeurosis, that joins with the frontalis muscle anteriorly and with the occipitalis muscle posteriorly, whereas laterally it connects with and ultimately becomes the temporoparietal fascia.[3] Other muscles that contribute to forehead movement include the orbicularis oculi, the procerus, and the corrugator supercilii.[2] Of all the muscles contributing to forehead movement, the greatest consequence results from transection of the occipitofrontalis muscle, which could result in local palsies and prolonged recovery from reconstruction.[2]

Blood Supply and Lymphatics of the Forehead

The forehead is supplied mainly by the supratrochlear and supraorbital arteries, both of which are branches off the internal carotid system (▶ Fig. 2.3).[3,4] Both arteries are located in the subcutaneous plane and are relatively easy to locate; the former pierces the orbital septum medially, whereas the latter exits through the supraorbital foramen or notch, eventually anastomosing with each other and the arteries of the lateral forehead. These vessels are often transected when operating medial to the midpoint of the eyebrow, though transection of vessels in the forehead generally should not have major consequences for blood flow, as there is ample collateral circulation.[2] The lateral forehead and temple are supplied by the superficial temporal artery, which is a branch of the external carotid system and is also easily identifiable visually and by palpation.

There are no lymph nodes in the forehead or scalp; lymphatic drainage is via lymphatic channels directly feeding the parotid glands, anterior and posterior auricular chains, and occipital regions.[3]

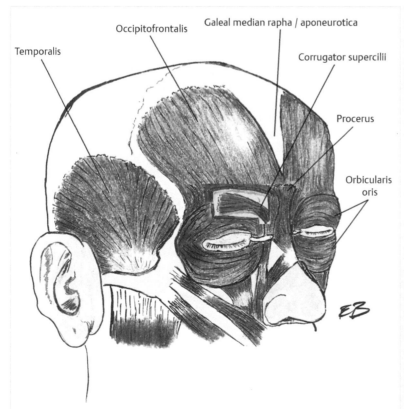

Temporalis

Occipitofrontalis

Galeal median rapha / aponeurotica

Corrugator supercilii

Procerus

Orbicularis oris

Fig. 2.2 The main muscle of the forehead is the occipitofrontalis muscle. The lack of muscle fibers at the midline—the galeal midline raphe—improves cosmesis of vertical midline closures. (Image courtesy of Edward Bae, MD, and Hannah Singer, MD.)

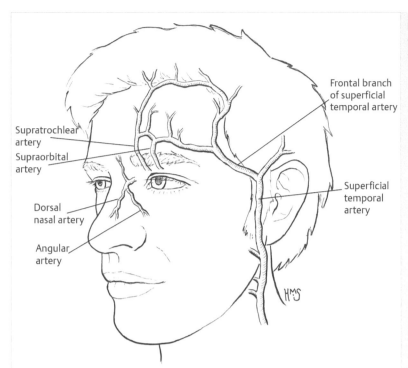

Fig. 2.3 Forehead vasculature. (Image courtesy of Edward Bae, MD, and Hannah Singer, MD.)

Frontal branch of superficial temporal artery

Supratrochlear artery

Supraorbital artery

Superficial temporal artery

Dorsal nasal artery

Angular artery

Innervation of the Forehead

Sensory innervation of the forehead comes from the supraorbital and supratrochlear nerves, both of which arise from the first branch of the trigeminal nerve and follow the path of their named arteries (▶ Fig. 2.4).[2,3] The supraorbital and supratrochlear nerves exit the orbit approximately 2.5 and 1 cm lateral from midline, respectively, and traverse superiorly beneath the corrugator supercilii muscle, innervating the conjunctiva, upper eyelid, and medial forehead.[3] The supraorbital nerve exits the supraorbital foramen (or notch), also traveling superiorly but in a more lateral direction and eventually extending over the frontalis muscle to innervate the central forehead; a deep branch of this nerve travels deep to the frontalis between the periosteum and galea, innervating the rest of the anterior scalp and vertex.[3] Transection of these nerves is not always avoidable and can result in anesthesia distal to the point of injury, possibly extending to the parietal scalp; for this reason, careful undermining in the superficial subcutaneous plane when dissecting flaps in this unit is required. Alternatively, when creating a larger flap below the muscle, incisions can be made peripherally to these nerves' expected paths to preserve function. The paresthesia and numbness typically self-resolve within 5 to 7 months, though regrowth of sensory nerves can take up to a year or longer.[1,2] Anticipatory guidance is key to help patients prepare for and tolerate this consequence. Local anesthesia for the forehead is relatively easily achieved with local infiltration of anesthetics. If complete forehead anesthesia is desired, bilateral nerve blocks can be used, injecting a 2-mL dose of 1% lidocaine with epinephrine at a 1:100,000 concentration bilaterally beneath the brow, just above the frontal bone, near the supraorbital foramen.[5]

The temporal branch of the facial nerve (CN VII) is responsible for motor function of the frontalis muscle (▶ Fig. 2.4). It is important to note that this nerve is most vulnerable to injury in the temporal area—where the skin and subcutaneous tissue is thin—especially during flap elevation from the temple and/or zygomatic arch.[2] The nerve becomes superficial here and because of its small size is difficult to identify and thus easy to transect. It emerges from the parotid gland below the zygomatic arch, is conveyed via the temporoparietal fascia over the zygomatic arch, and pierces the frontalis muscle from its deep surface.[2,6] Some surgeons use the Pitanguy line to help predict the location of this nerve (▶ Fig. 2.5). It is drawn from two points: one point is 0.5 cm inferior to the tragus and the other point is made approximately 1.5 cm superior to the lateral aspect of the supraorbital rim; the line connecting these two dots is the Pitanguy line.[3] Transection results in palsy of or complete paralysis of the ipsilateral eyebrow, leading to either the unilateral expression of surprise (on the contralateral side of the affected nerve) or eyebrow ptosis, respectively.[1,2,3] Injury to the nerve may lead to prolonged temporary paralysis or paresis of the eyebrow.

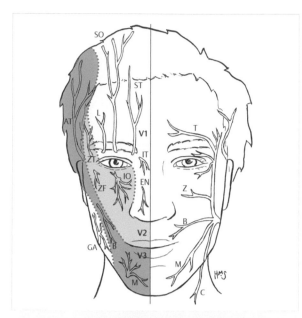

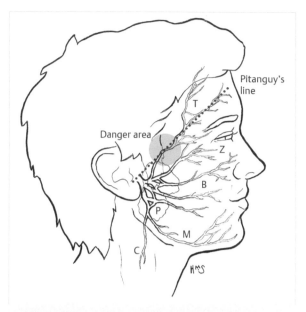

Fig. 2.4 Sensory (*left*) and motor (*right*) innervation of forehead. AT, auriculotemporal nerve; B, buccal nerve; B, Buccal branch of facial nerve; C, cervical branch of facial nerve; EN, external nasal nerve; GA, great auricular nerve; IO, infraorbital nerve; IT, infratrochlear nerve; L, lacrimal nerve; M, marginal mandibular branch of facial nerve; M, mental nerve; SO, supraorbital nerve; ST, supratrochlear nerve; T, temporal branch of facial nerve; V1, ophthalmic nerve branch of trigeminal nerve; V2, maxillary nerve branch of trigeminal nerve; V3, mandibular nerve branch of trigeminal nerve; Z, zygomatic branch of facial nerve; ZF, zygomaticofacial nerve; ZT, zygomaticotemporal nerve. (Image courtesy of Edward Bae, MD, and Hannah Singer, MD.)

Fig. 2.5 Pitanguy Line/Danger Zone. B, buccal branch of facial nerve; C, cervical branch of facial nerve; M, marginal mandibular branch of facial nerve; P, parotid gland; T, temporal branch of facial nerve; Z, zygomatic branch of facial nerve. (Image courtesy of Edward Bae, MD, and Hannah Singer, MD.)

2.2 Aesthetic Subunits

The forehead has both a perceived and actual boundary,[2] making it unique amongst facial aesthetic subunits (▶ Fig. 2.1); it is bordered superiorly by the anterior hairline, laterally by the temporal fossae/sideburn, and inferiorly by the eyebrows and glabella, along with the supraorbital rim. It is important while crafting reconstructions to respect these boundaries, maintain position and symmetry of the eyebrows and hairline, and to preserve facial expression. Scars in this region are ideally hidden in the hairline or eyebrows, the direction is preferably horizontal (except for at the mid forehead, in which case vertical scars result in a more ideal cosmetic outcome), and diagonal scars are generally avoided (with a few exceptions, discussed below).[2] In women, smaller defects located at the hairline can be covered with small alterations in hairstyle, whereas men with male-pattern androgenic alopecia may lose skin elasticity, making reconstruction more difficult.[1] It is also important to note that the thickness and sebaceous gland content of the forehead decreases as one moves superiorly from the eyebrows to the anterior hairline.[5]

Though not specifically tailored to the unique features of the forehead discussed herein, a size-based algorithm for repair of scalp defects has been proposed that may help guide the decision making process with regard to approaching repair of forehead surgical defects as well.[7] Overall, linear closures are the most common type of repair on the forehead.[8] Defects smaller than 5 cm^2 in size or less than 2.5 cm in diameter can usually be closed primarily; moderate-sized defects of 5 to 20 cm^2 typically close with local or regional flaps but may require split thickness or full thickness skin grafts; and larger defects greater than 20 cm^2 may require free tissue transfer. Local flaps, which include rotation, advancement, and transposition flaps, offer the advantage of replacing the surgical defect with similar-appearing tissue. We also present a unique subunit- and size-based algorithm for forehead repair (▶ Fig. 2.6). As a general principle, transposition flaps play a lesser role in reconstruction of the forehead than other regions of the face. This is because these flaps create visible scars that are difficult to camouflage and often result in a contour abnormality. Skin grafts generally play a lesser role in forehead reconstruction, largely because they usually offer a poor color and texture match in most aesthetic subunits of the forehead. Skin grafts may play a role in tumor surveillance, however, especially if a patient is at high risk for recurrence and moving tissue locally with a flap may not be an option. Common donor sites for skin grafts include the supraclavicular fossa and periauricular areas.[3] As with a graft for any site, the surgeon should assess the status of the wound bed, namely the vascularity of the wound bed; where dermis, fascia, fat and muscle all accept skin grafts readily, devascularized tissue such as exposed bone or cartilage without

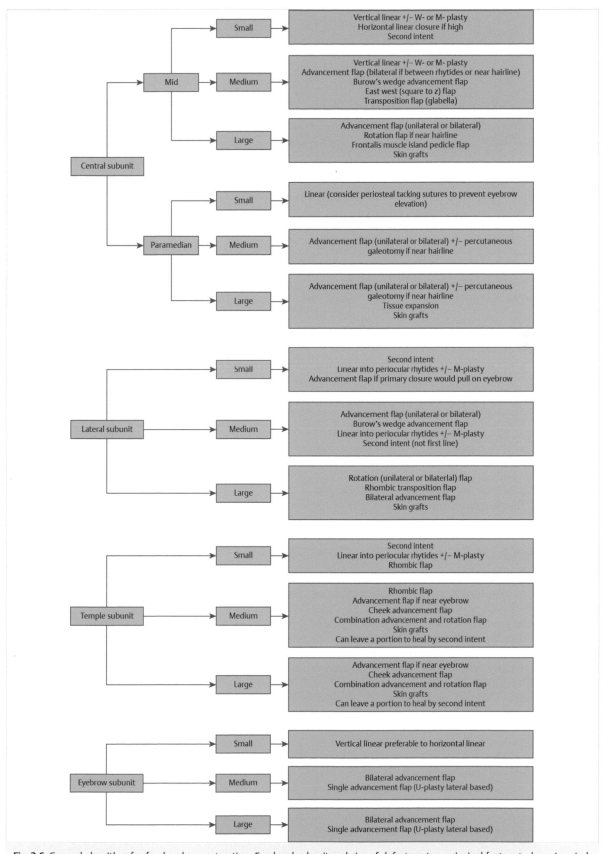

Fig. 2.6 General algorithm for forehead reconstruction. Forehead subunit and size of defect are two principal factors to keep in mind, though patient-specific parameters and the patient's overall aesthetic orientation play a role in choosing the final closure method.

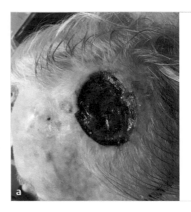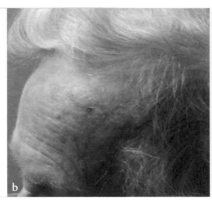

Fig. 2.7 (a,b) Even large defects > 1 cm on forehead have been shown to heal well by second intention, particularly on nonsebaceous skin. (Photograph courtesy of Dr. David H. Ciocon.)

perichondrium will not accept grafts. Patient factors to evaluate for include arterial insufficiency, history of radiation to the site,[3] and smoking status. For massive forehead defects, larger flaps, including myocutaneous flaps, or multiple repair options may be required for sufficient and functional repair.

2.2.1 Central Subunit

The central forehead is supplied by the right and left supratrochlear and supraorbital arteries.[2] The central subunit of the forehead can be further subdivided into the midline or mid forehead and the paramedian forehead subunits (▶ Fig. 2.1). These subunits are important to recognize, as the topography varies, which affects reconstruction options. The mid forehead refers to the central midline forehead, while the paramedian forehead refers to the tissue spanning from midline to midbrow or mid pupillary line, which involves the convexity of the forehead.[2,5]

Mid Forehead

Unique to the mid forehead is the lack of any underlying muscle fibers, as instead, only the extension of the galea exists in this location (▶ Fig. 2.3). The minimal muscular movement here helps to create a very thin, at times barely perceptible, fine white line as the final scar when a mid-forehead closure is oriented vertically. The local reservoir for tissue in this region includes the central forehead and the glabella, as there is greater laxity of the skin in this region.[1] The convex nature of the forehead often results in accentuated dog-ears or standing cones and in some cases can make it difficult to get an incision to lie flat. Techniques that can be employed include converting a linear closure into an A to T or M-plasty.[9]

Generally adequate cosmetic outcomes can be achieved for small defects (< 1 cm) in the mid forehead that are allowed to heal by secondary intention (▶ Fig. 2.7).[2] Defects that are amenable to primary closure in this area may do better oriented vertically rather than horizontally, for reasons noted above, with the inferior limb potentially

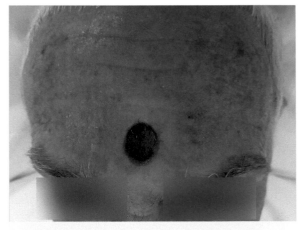

Fig. 2.8 Mid forehead wound closed vertically hiding the ends in glabellar line (*before*).

hidden within creases of the glabella using a W- or M-plasty or the superior limb in the anterior hairline (▶ Fig. 2.8, ▶ Fig. 2.9).[1,2] Vertical orientation of the primary closure will also decrease the risk of transecting neurovascular bundles. One risk involved in a vertical closure is the appearance of a *coup de sabre*-type depressed scar if only the dermis—and not the deeper structures like the fascia and muscle—is well approximated during closure.[9] Some surgeons prefer to break up the single vertical scar into multiple Z-plasties to minimize this scar inversion and avoid the sharp line of a single repair, though the risk involved in utilizing this technique is a "zig-zag" across the forehead, which is far from ideal and may require revision.[9] The surgeon should also discuss preoperatively the medial displacement of the eyebrows that may result from vertically oriented scars. This can be corrected postoperatively with laser hair removal of the medial aspect of each.[5]

If the wound is small and high enough on the forehead to not significantly pull upward on the eyebrow upon closure, a horizontal primary closure can be performed (▶ Fig. 2.10, ▶ Fig. 2.11). Larger defects in the central forehead do well with primary closures or M-plasties that can

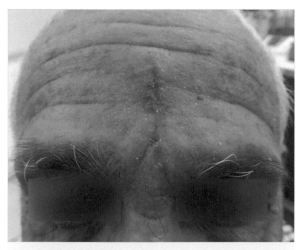

Fig. 2.9 Mid forehead wound closed vertically hiding the ends in glabellar line (*after*).

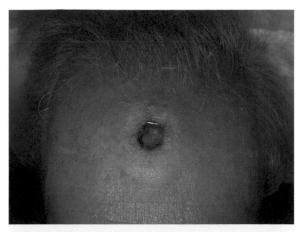

Fig. 2.10 Mid high forehead horizontal primary closure (*before*).

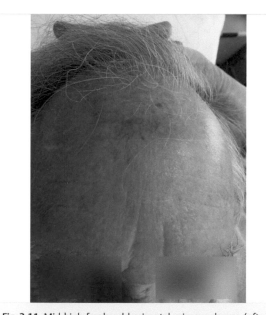

Fig. 2.11 Mid high forehead horizontal primary closure (*after*).

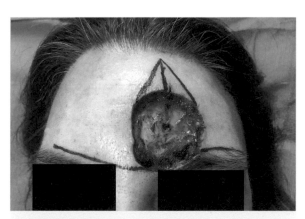

Fig. 2.12 Double advancement flap near eyebrow (*before*). (Image courtesy of Sailesh Konda, MD.)

be hidden in the natural horizontal creases of the forehead.[1] The larger the vertical component of the defect, the greater the risk of elevating the medial eyebrow margin to an unacceptable degree. If tissue does not move, tissue expansion may be an option to assist with primary closure (see section 2.4).

Flaps are a common mode of reconstruction in forehead defects including the mid forehead; laxity is often brought in from the glabella, temples, or forehead.[1] Flaps can be cutaneous or musculocutaneous, which differ in their plane of undermining. Cutaneous flaps are dissected in the subcutaneous plane, preserving the subdermal plexus. There is typically more bleeding with preparation

of the cutaneous flap compared to a musculocutaneous flap, though once the flap is prepared and set into the defect, recovery is generally rapid. Musculocutaneous flaps are often reserved for larger defects and require dissection beneath the frontalis muscle, with undermining in the avascular plane beneath the fascia. While the field may have less bleeding, these flaps tend to be limited in their mobility as they are fixed to the underlying frontal bone, thus causing excessive tension.[3]

Single or double advancement flaps are reasonable options to close a defect in this region, with the goal of aiming the vertical component of the scar toward midline (▶ Fig. 2.12, ▶ Fig. 2.13). Advancement flaps are the most commonly used flaps in forehead reconstruction. They allow for optimal scar placement in a natural crease and provide a good source of skin movement for reconstruction. Advancement flaps should generally be designed with a 4:1 ratio of length to width[2] to prevent vascular compromise because they are placed under high tension. This is one of the downsides of using advancement flaps

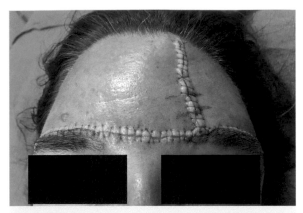

Fig. 2.13 Double advancement flap near eyebrow (*after*). (Image courtesy of Sailesh Konda, MD.)

on the forehead, given the sometimes unpredictable amount of tension present on forehead skin, with some patients having very taut, almost "drum-like" skin on the forehead. Cutaneous flap dissection should remain in the mid-subcutaneous plane, superficial to the neuromuscular bundles, though deep enough to avoid a too thin flap.[2] In the mid forehead, standing cones can easily be hidden in the hairline superiorly and the glabella inferiorly. A Burow's wedge advancement flap can produce good cosmetic results for wounds of the mid forehead, by removing a triangular cone of tissue from the glabella; this can be achieved by creating a vertical linear closure on the forehead and connecting it to a triangular Burow's flap in the glabella via an incision strategically placed just above the superior margin of the ipsilateral eyebrow for camouflage.[9]

A to T advancement flaps do best in the upper central forehead by the hairline, with the Burow's triangles hidden in the hairline, and only the vertical component remains visible.[1] Implementing bilateral advancement flaps may help to minimize tension on the closure. A variation of the O to Z flap, known as a square to Z flap, can also be useful in the central forehead.[1] In this flap, the tumor is excised as a square, and two incision lines are made at opposite sides of the square and into the patient's natural wrinkles; this results in two less scar lines compared to a bilateral advancement flap. After wide undermining, the flap is slightly rotated and advanced to create a Z-shaped scar. Once healed, only the central, diagonal portion of the scar should be slightly noticeable.[1] One disadvantage to advancement flaps is the large area of undermining required for successful closure.

A rotation flap may be a viable option for the central upper forehead, where the defect naturally extends into or can be extended into the hairline for better camouflage.[2,5] Oftentimes this requires the flap to be based inferolaterally,[2] including a camouflaged "back-cut" into the sideburn area for large lesions to bring in more laxity.[1] These flaps offer a pivoting movement, which works well with the

inelastic skin of the forehead and allows for greater coverage of a defect.[3,5] They are often larger flaps, and thus have a greater associated vascularity, as opposed to the classic single or double advancement flaps used on the forehead with a relatively short stalk and thus vascular supply. For larger midline tumors, bilateral flaps may be best to maintain the natural symmetry of the hairline, which oftentimes may be lowered during the repair process.[2] The curvilinear length of a rotation flap should generally be 6 times longer than the defect.[10] Larger defects of the forehead will likely require undermining in the subfascial plane, thus resulting in transection of the sensory nerves and causing numbness of the anterior scalp, which again requires preoperative patient counseling.[2,9]

Skin grafts are generally avoided in the midline forehead, as this results in generally unsatisfactory cosmetic outcomes. One unique repair option for large defects of the lower mid forehead is an island pedicle flap brought down from the anterior scalp, using the supratrochlear artery and a sling of the frontalis muscle; the involvement of the muscle is critical in bringing enough laxity downward to cover the defect.[9] This helps to avoid the less aesthetically pleasing outcome that would result from a full thickness skin graft in this location, and obviates the need for medially displacing the eyebrows with a large vertical side-to-side closure.

Moving downward in the mid forehead, for defects involving the region closer to the glabella, transposition flaps are an appropriate repair choice with good cosmetic outcomes. These include a rhombic flap, bringing the laxity of the glabellar skin upward, and resulting in only one vertically oriented midline scar and two horizontal scars ideally hidden in RSTLs.[1]

Paramedian Forehead

Compared to the mid forehead, the paramedian forehead has fewer good options for repair, as it is generally a convex surface when compared to the midline.[2] Primary closures hidden in the horizontal creases are the best and most simple options when amenable; however, this option is restricted by the degree of eyebrow elevation, which can vary depending on patient age and degree of forehead skin mobility and redundancy.

In an older individual, the presence of rhytids and increased skin laxity may allow for an eyebrow elevation up to 1 cm above the opposite eyebrow, as gravity will likely cause it to settle down over the course of several weeks postoperatively, though this process can take up to 6 months.[1,2] This skin laxity is often lacking in a younger patient. A technique to prevent excessive eyebrow elevation includes suturing the dermis and muscle of the eyebrow to the periosteum of the superior orbital rim; this will limit the upward movement of the eyebrow during advancement of the skin.[2]

Advancement flaps are useful in this region, especially for defects that are large or have a greater vertical component.[2] Bipedicle advancement flaps do well for defects near the anterior hairline that may be difficult to close primarily, hiding the secondary defect in the hair-bearing scalp parallel to the upper border of the defect and carrying it full thickness through galea (percutaneous galeotomy) (▶ Fig. 2.14).[1] This is achieved by making an incision through the galea 2.0 to 3.0 cm into the hair-bearing scalp, making sure to incise parallel to the direction of the hair follicles and parallel to the long axis of the primary defect; subsequently, the secondary defect is undermined through to the primary defect, allowing much easier closure of the primary defect as the galea has been released above it.[1] Of note, the galea is left open, but the secondary skin defect above the galea is closed, owing to the elastic nature of the skin (whereas the galea is inelastic).[1] This type of closure can result in lowering the hairline, and the length of lowering the hairline is directly proportional to the vertical component of the defect.[2] Rectangular advancement flaps can again be useful in the paramedian forehead defect, as they allow for mobility of adjacent skin and maximize scar camouflage by hiding incisions in the natural RSTLs, but again

with the downside of a relatively short vascular stalk with which to work. Any resultant standing cone on the lateral side can be removed either parallel to or in the periocular rhytids.[2]

Tissue expansion can also be a viable option in the paramedian forehead (see section 2.4).

2.2.2 Lateral Subunit

The lateral forehead is defined as the forehead from the mid pupillary line to the lateral eyebrow just as it joins the temple (▶ Fig. 2.1). It is supplied by the anterior branch of the temporal arteries (▶ Fig. 2.6). This area is unique in that the topography changes from the convex surface of the paramedian forehead to the concave surface of the temple—the transition point as the hallmark of the lateral subunit.[2]

Primary closure is always one of the simplest and least burdensome options for patients; asking the patient to squint or raise her/his eyebrows may reveal subtle radial wrinkles from sleep or curving horizontal creases, which would be ideal locations to camouflage the scar (▶ Fig. 2.15, ▶ Fig. 2.16). Standing cones should be removed following the RSTL so that the final scar may be

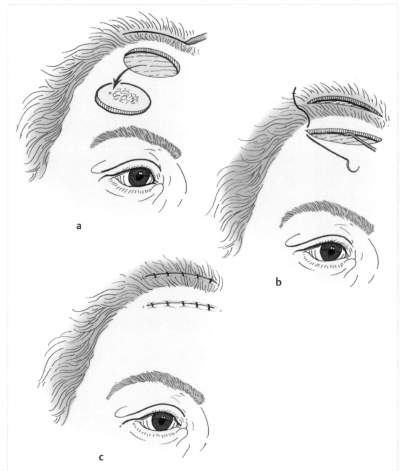

Fig. 2.14 (a–c) Bipedicle advancement flap with large vertical component and near hairline, using galeotomy. (Reprinted with permission from Reconstruction of the Forehead. In Baker SR. Local Flaps in Facial Reconstruction. Copyright Elsevier, 2014.)

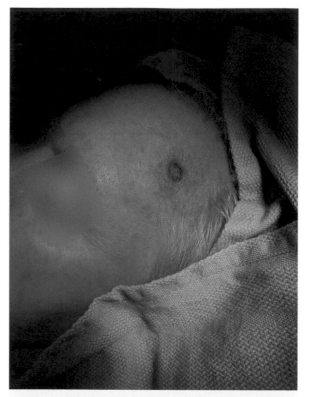

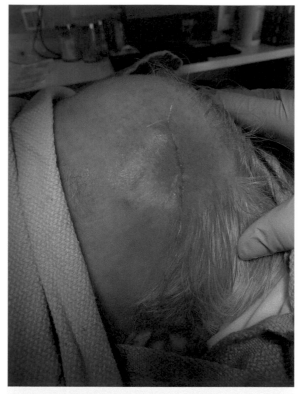

Fig. 2.15 Lateral subunit primary closure hidden in curved relaxed skin tensions lines (RSTLs) (*before*).

Fig. 2.16 Lateral subunit primary closure hidden in curved relaxed skin tensions lines (RSTLs) (*after*).

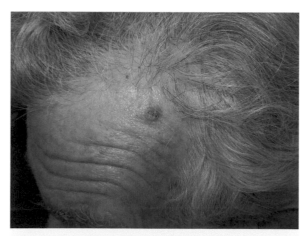

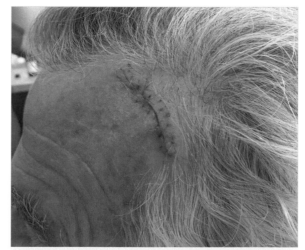

Fig. 2.17 Curvilinear hairline closure (*before*).

Fig. 2.18 Curvilinear hairline closure (*after*).

curvilinear to avoid disrupting the normal symmetry of the eyebrows, the lateral canthus, or the hairline (▶ Fig. 2.17, ▶ Fig. 2.18). Repairs extending into the hairline may be closed more easily and with a better cosmetic outcome with a bevel–antibevel approach following the direction of hair growth to avoid cutting through hairs.[9] An M-plasty is another option in this region, allowing the surgeon to hide one of the limbs of the primary closure around the lateral canthus and its associated periocular rhytids.

A variety of flaps can be employed in this region of the forehead, with the main tissue reservoir coming laterally from the temporal fossa and cheek. Great caution should be taken to avoid injury to the temporal branch of CN VII while harvesting any flap from this region, as this nerve runs through the superficial fascia over the zygomatic arch.[2] Dissection should be blunt and should remain in the mid subcutaneous fat, superficial to the temporoparietal fascia. A guiding principle in the lateral forehead is that taller defects with less of a horizontal component do better closed with an advancement flap, whereas defects with a larger horizontal component close best with transposition.[9]

Unilateral advancement flaps work well for small defects that may not be reconstructed well with primary closures, such as proximal to the eyebrow where primary closure may pull on and/or distort the contour of the eyebrow; in this situation, it may be beneficial to extend the wound to hide it within the superior margin of the lateral eyebrow (▶ Fig. 2.19, ▶ Fig. 2.20).[2] The Burow's wedge advancement flap, which has both advancement and rotation components, is a great choice in the lateral forehead; an arcing incision created from the inferior aspect of the defect is continued laterally and inferiorly to the temple, with the Burow's triangle excised within the periocular rhytids (▶ Fig. 2.21, ▶ Fig. 2.22). This flap may be a purely advancing flap if the incision is terminated prior to reaching the temple.[5] Bilateral advancement flaps are also a great option and do especially well in the lateral forehead adjacent to the eyebrow; O to T and A to T variations allow for only a single incision at the superior border of the eyebrow, camouflaging all but the central vertical closure line.[2] The galeal relaxing bipedicle advancement flap technique discussed earlier is a viable option for the lateral forehead.[1]

Wounds of the lateral forehead may at times involve the temple, bringing in skin laxity from the temporal fossae and thus an increased number of repair options, as discussed below and in section 2.2.3. Rotation flaps may

be a better option for larger defects in the lateral forehead. They utilize the tissue reservoir in the temporal fossa and are often rotated medially so that the curvilinear incision can be made parallel to or hidden in the hairline, often removing a Burow's triangle from the periocular rhytids, above the ear, or in the sideburn. O to Z repairs can be useful in this subunit to reduce the size of the flap needed to close a defect and to minimize tension, resulting in an oblique scar that may be acceptable in those who have more curvilinear RSTLs of the lateral forehead.[2]

While transposition flaps such as rhombic flaps may not be very versatile or helpful in other subunits of the forehead due to the contour abnormalities and dog-ears they tend to leave behind, they can be less noticeable in the concave surface of the lateral forehead, thus making them a reasonable reconstructive option, especially in the setting of a receded or naturally high hairline. Bringing up loose skin of the temple will not significantly alter the eyebrow or hairline, and the scars are relatively short and within a confined space. Rhombic flaps and 30 degree angled flaps are commonly used in this area.[2,3,9]

2.2.3 Temple Subunit

The temple is defined by the sideburn laterally, the zygomatic process of the temporal bone inferiorly, the zygoma medially, and superiorly by the change in topography from the concave temporal fossae to the convex frontal bone, which can be appreciated by palpation (▶ Fig. 2.1). This change in topography allows for greater skin elasticity, thus allowing for more closure options. However, this region also poses unique challenges, including the short distance between the lateral eyebrow and the temporal hair; the fact that it overlies the temporal branch of

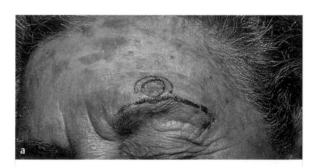

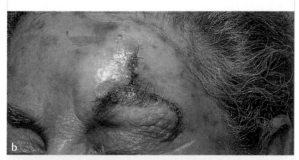

Fig. 2.19 (a,b) Advancement flap at lateral subunit near eyebrow (*before*). (Reprinted from Advancement Flaps. In: Papel I, Frodel J, Holt R, Larrabee Jr W, Nachlas N, Park S, Sykes J, Toriumi D, ed. Facial Plastic and Reconstructive Surgery. 4th Edition. New York: Thieme; 2016.)

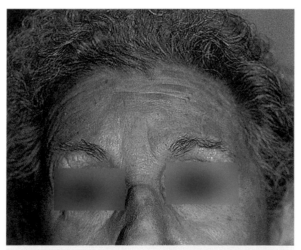

Fig. 2.20 Advancement flap at lateral subunit near eyebrow (*after*). (Reprinted from Advancement Flaps. In: Papel I, Frodel J, Holt R, Larrabee Jr W, Nachlas N, Park S, Sykes J, Toriumi D, ed. Facial Plastic and Reconstructive Surgery. 4th Edition. New York: Thieme; 2016.)

Burow's advancement flap

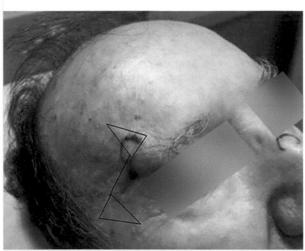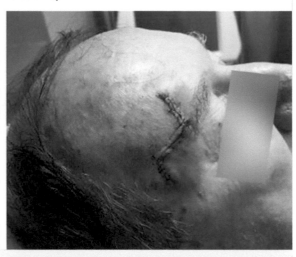

Fig. 2.21 Burow's wedge advancement flap near eyebrow (*before*). (Photograph courtesy of Dr. David H. Ciocon.)

Burow's advancement flap

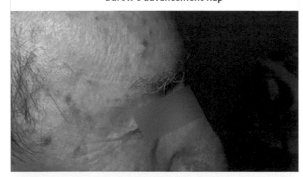

Fig. 2.22 Burow's wedge advancement flap near eyebrow (*after*). (Photograph courtesy of Dr. David H. Ciocon.)

CN VII; and the relatively abrupt transition from the thin skin overlying the lateral periorbital area to the thickened hair-bearing skin of the temple.[1] Avoiding displacement of hair from the sideburn, temple, and frontal hairline onto non–hair-bearing areas is of paramount concern in this subunit, as it can cause a negative cosmetic outcome; at times, this necessitates modifications to the planned closure. The temple is supplied by branches of the superficial temporal artery, which run in the superficial fascia and should be avoided during surgery (▶ Fig. 2.6). The auriculotemporal nerve runs just anterior to the ear, providing sensory innervation to the upper ear; it is at risk of transection during repairs involving the lateral temple, which is a common cause of neuritic pain (▶ Fig. 2.2).[9] The deepest structures of the temple include the strong temporal fascia, to which anchoring sutures can be placed, and the temporalis muscle.

As discussed in section 2.2.2, wounds of the concave surface of the lateral forehead subunit and extending into the temple can be allowed to heal by secondary intention if reasonably small, and linear closures work well placed strategically in the periocular radial RSTLs. Rhombic flaps, though not often used on other subunits of the forehead, work well for repair of wounds involving the temporal fossae.

For wounds that would otherwise be closed linearly but lie proximal to or within the horizontal line extending from the eyebrow, an advancement flap to inferiorly displace the medial dog-ear works well and avoids impinging on the eyebrow itself.[9] Larger temple wounds can be closed with a good cosmetic outcome by combining advancement and rotation flaps, bringing laxity from the cheek and lower temple and hiding scars in front of the ear, behind the ear, and in the hairline (▶ Fig. 2.23, ▶ Fig. 2.24). The cheek advancement flap removes a horizontal dog-ear lateral to the canthus and a dog-ear behind the ear. The cheek is advanced upward and outward, with the majority of the incision hidden in front of the ear in a strictly vertical fashion. At times it may be necessary to add a component of rotation to close a larger wound of the temple and avoid a graft. This is achieved by bringing in laxity from just beneath the jawline or the neck and adding a rotational element to an otherwise advancing type of flap in front of the ear using the cheek.

For large wounds of the lateral forehead subunit and temple, multiple repair options may be considered, including a local or distant skin graft. Tumors of the temple may be quite large by the time they are recognized, thus leaving the potential for similarly large surgical defects. One option is to close as much of the wound as possible with local flap repair and allow the remaining portion of the wound to heal—albeit very slowly—by secondary intention; an alter-

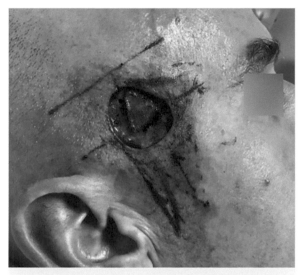

Fig. 2.23 Moderately large temple subunit defect repaired with advancement flap, recruiting laxity from cheek, and hiding incision in side burn (*before*). (Image courtesy of Dr. Ardeshir Edward Nadimi.)

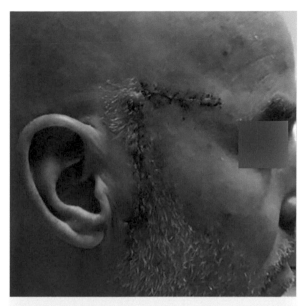

Fig. 2.24 Moderately large temple subunit defect repaired with advancement flap, recruiting laxity from cheek, and hiding incision in sideburn, 7 days postoperative. (Image courtesy of Dr. Ardeshir Edward Nadimi.)

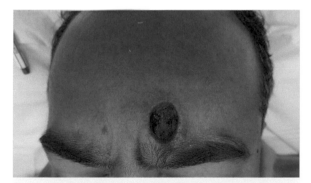

Fig. 2.25 Vertical primary closure of small defect near eyebrow (*before*).

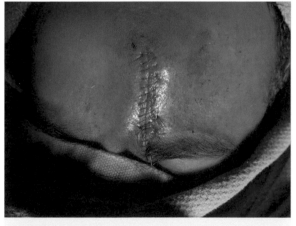

Fig. 2.26 Vertical primary closure of small defect near eyebrow (*after*).

native approach is to use a dog-ear from the local flap repair as a full-thickness skin graft (FTSG).[9]

2.2.4 Eyebrow Subunit

The eyebrows are cosmetically one of the most important features of the forehead, and maintaining position, continuity, and symmetry of the eyebrows is vital for patient satisfaction. When closing wounds on the forehead and near the eyebrow, it is imperative to ensure the tension on the closure does not distort the eyebrow—noticeable eyebrow asymmetry is a negative cosmetic outcome, even if the scar is well-hidden. Small tumors on/around the eyebrow that are being closed primarily should ideally be closed vertically, as horizontal closure reduces the height of the eyebrow, which is significantly more

noticeable (▶ Fig. 2.25, ▶ Fig. 2.26). Another consideration is the natural convexity of the supraorbital rim, which naturally creates dog-ears that can cause a small mound or elevation which persists for a long time, primarily at the superior pole of a vertical closure (since the inferior pole's dog-ear can at least partially hide in the redundancy of the superior eyelid).[9] If a defect involves the hair-bearing region of the eyebrow, any incision for flaps should be made parallel to the hair shafts with a bevel-antibevel technique as discussed before, so as to minimize risk of transecting hair bulbs, which could later result in alopecia, ingrown hairs, or milia.[2] Additionally, undermining too superficially may cause injury to hair bulbs, resulting in subsequent alopecia. For defects within the eyebrow, one option is a bilateral advancement flap (H-plasty), where the upper and lower incisions are created to be hidden within the respective margin of the eyebrow; again, ensuring that the incisions are parallel to hair shafts.[2] A laterally based single advancement flap (U-plasty) is also an option for this area and may provide better cosmetic outcomes. As a general rule of thumb for the brow, most of the laxity is present laterally, and in general, moving the brow slightly laterally is more cosmetically acceptable than moving the medial brow further medially.[9] A surgical defect of the far lateral brow may not require brow reconstruction to provide a positive cosmetic outcome. Given that the lateral brows thin as patients age, it may be acceptable to perform a tissue rearrangement of a far lateral brow defect without consideration of replacing hair-bearing skin to the lateral brow; a hair transplant for the lateral brow could be performed if the surgery results in obvious asymmetry or an otherwise unacceptable cosmetic outcome for the patient.[9]

2.3 Massive Forehead Defects

For very large defects in which cutaneous forehead flaps alone would result in excess tension, deeper musculocutaneous flaps can be used, often in single or bilateral advancement fashion. These flaps are dissected under the frontalis muscle at the level of the periosteum, and undermined at the level of the fascial plane.[2,5] A few specialized flaps become useful in the setting of massive forehead defects. Temporoparietal and extended deep-plane cervicofacial flaps require extensive inferolateral dissection to the level of the zygoma, which puts structures such as the temporal branch of CN VII and the temporal artery at risk. They are more often used in defects on the lateral forehead or temple.[10] The Orticochea flap is most often used in defects of the parietal or occipital regions. Classically a 3-pedicle flap, the Orticochea flap can also be achieved by forming a bipedicle flap from the tissue on either side of the defect. Scoring of the galea on the flap can enhance the laxity of the scalp. This flap requires extensive flap mobilization and often results in secondary defects that require subsequent surgeries to repair.[10]

The frontalis myocutaneous transposition flap has been described as an alternative closure option for large defects of the forehead/frontal scalp that involve part of the frontalis muscle or its fascia, extending to the periosteum. It is a lobulated flap with an inferiorly-based pedicle, designed lateral to the defect and placed perpendicular to the anterior hair line. Incisions are made down to the frontalis muscle or its fascia, and the flap is then placed into the primary defect. Unlike other transposition flaps, the donor site is closed first as this can help determine

the flap's maximum width. The flap is then sewn into place. Utilization of the muscle in the flap allows enough blood supply that the base of the flap can be narrower.[11] Other common options for large and deep forehead defects extending to the periosteum include local flaps, subgaleal-subperiosteal flaps with split-thickness skin grafts, tissue expansion (see section 2.4), or microvascular free tissue transfers.[4,11]

Where a flap is not sufficient to close a massive forehead defect, a FTSG may be necessary. Given that massive forehead/scalp defects may extend down to bone, which is poorly vascularized, a FTSG in this location is at risk of failure. Hinge flaps that are harvested from tissues underlying advancement flaps are an option to create a favorable wound bed for a FTSG (▶ Fig. 2.27, ▶ Fig. 2.28). Though adipomuscular hinge flaps, such as the paramedian forehead flap, are more commonly used in nasal reconstruction, a frontalis muscle hinge flap can be used for a massive defect of the forehead/scalp if this muscle is not resected during tumor removal; it provides vasculature for graft survival and transfers tissue volume into the broad/deep defect for improved cosmesis of the overlying FTSG.[10] For tumor surveillance, a FTSG can be sutured overlying the areas of deepest tumor invasion without incorporating any underlying hinge flap, to allow for

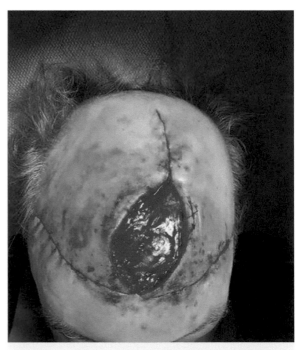

Fig. 2.27 Bilateral O to T advancement flap with galeal hinge flap and Burow's FTSG after advancement of both limbs and creation of hinge flap (*center*), before placement of Burow's FTSG. (Reprinted with permission from Singer HM, Patel VA. Forehead reconstruction after resection of squamous cell carcinoma. Dermatol Surg. 44(7):1018–1022. Copyright Wolters Kluwer, 2018.)

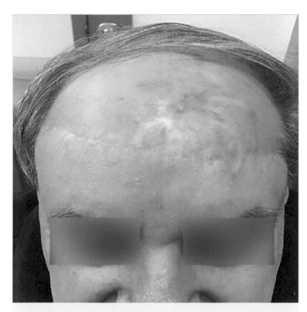

Fig. 2.28 Bilateral O to T advancement flap with galeal hinge flap and Burow's FTSG (*after*). (Reprinted with permission from Singer HM, Patel VA. Forehead reconstruction after resection of squamous cell carcinoma. Dermatol Surg. 44(7):1018–1022. Copyright Wolters Kluwer, 2018.)

palpation of tumor recurrence through only the FTSG; a Burow's triangle can be used to create this FTSG. If a muscular reservoir is not available (e.g., the frontalis is resected during the tumor removal), another option to provide a vascularized wound bed is a galeal hinge flap. The galea of the scalp has a rich microvascular network and a flap of 1 to 2 cm can be formed to support a skin graft. This technique is performed by taking a partial thickness plane of galea and folding it over, like the page of a book, onto the exposed underlying bone. Multiple galeal hinge flaps may be necessary to fully cover the exposed defect.[10] This technique lacks the volumizing effect of a muscular flap but may be the only option in massive forehead defects without a muscular reservoir and when a single-stage operation is desired.

2.4 Tissue Expansion

2.4.1 Introduction

Tissue expansion is a technique that can be used in multiple repair scenarios, including primary closures under significant tension and when local flaps are insufficient on their own to close a defect.[4] The main advantage tissue expansion provides is its ability to mobilize nearby tissue. This technique is governed by the concepts of biological and mechanical creep; the former dictates that the mitotic activity of tissue increases when it is stretched for a certain amount of time, while the latter states that skin

elongates with a constant load over time beyond its intrinsic extensibility by way of displacing water from collagen and partially fragmenting elastic fibers.[4,5] In turn, these mechanisms drive thickening of the epidermis, temporary dermal thinning, and increased blood flow during the expansion period.[4] Skin that has been previously radiated or infected may not be good candidates for tissue expansion due to inherent weakness, which may result in tissue expansion failure.[3,4]

There are various methods to induce tissue expansion; the principal difference amongst them is whether they are designed to assist in closure during the initial surgery (intraoperative tissue expansion), or whether the tissue expander will be stretched serially over time (days to weeks, rarely up to months[3]) to allow a more ideal closure at a future date.

2.4.2 Intraoperative Tissue Expansion

One intraoperative tissue expansion technique that can assist in high-tension closures of the forehead involves tunneling a 30-mL Foley catheter beneath the frontalis muscle beyond the supraorbital nerve to the lateral forehead and temple. The catheter balloon is inflated with saline until the skin blanches, maintained at this volume for three minutes, then decompressed for three minutes; this cycle is repeated twice more, as each expansion helps to stretch the tissue.[5] This technique is often sufficient to close midline defects under high tension with primary closure.

2.4.3 Internal and External Tissue Expanders

When tissue expansion is planned over the course of several weeks or longer, internal and external tissue expansion devices can be employed. This type of tissue expansion is often used in an effort to avoid a larger reconstruction, multiple incisions, or local grafts for patients in whom these techniques may be otherwise unsuitable.[3] Internal expanders are placed in the subgaleal layer and expanded slowly over time, necessitating frequent visits for intraoffice inflation of the device, approximately every 48 to 72 hours[3]; typically, up to 10% of the expander capacity may be added weekly, as patient discomfort and tissue perfusion are limiting factors.[4] There is a risk of infection or extrusion of the internal expander. The subgaleal placement of the expander in a site remote from the defect helps to decrease the risk of extrusion into the wound.[4] The labor-intensive nature and prolonged time period required for closure are the main disadvantages of this type of tissue expansion,[3] while the temporary deformity the patient will experience requires counseling.[4]

External expanders have also been developed to aide in primary closure of larger defects (usually involving the scalp and/or the forehead) by placing constant mechanical pressure to the wound edges—typically over the course of 1 to 2 weeks—while decreasing the tension on the primary skin closure.[3] These devices also require multiple visits, typically a few times a week, for advancement of the device.[3]

2.5 Conclusion

Knowledge of the unique topography of the aesthetic subunits of the forehead, its vasculature and innervation, and potential complications, allows the surgeon to weigh multiple repair options, provide appropriate preoperative counseling, and ultimately choose an appropriate closure based on the surgical defect. Recognizing patient-specific factors, including individual anatomic variance and overall aesthetic orientation, also plays a role in determining the most ideal method to close each defect and assure an optimal surgical outcome in forehead reconstruction.

References

[1] Tromovitch TA, Stegman SJ, Glogau RG. Forehead. In: Flaps and Grafts in Dermatologic Surgery. Chicago, IL: Year Book Medical Publishers, Inc.; 1989

[2] Baker S. Local Flaps in Facial Reconstruction. 2nd ed. St. Louis, MO: Mosby; 2007

[3] Olson MD, Hamilton GS, III. Scalp and forehead defects in the post-Mohs surgery patient. Facial Plast Surg Clin North Am. 2017; 25(3): 365–375

[4] Sokoya M, Inman J, Ducic Y. Scalp and forehead reconstruction. Semin Plast Surg. 2018; 32(2):90–94

[5] Seline PC, Siegle RJ. Forehead reconstruction. Dermatol Clin. 2005; 23 (1):1–11, v

[6] Babakurban ST, Cakmak O, Kendir S, Elhan A, Quatela VC. Temporal branch of the facial nerve and its relationship to fascial layers. Arch Facial Plast Surg. 2010; 12(1):16–23

[7] Cherubino M, Taibi D, Scamoni S, et al. A new algorithm for the surgical management of defects of the scalp. ISRN Plast Surg. 2013; 2013:1–5.n

[8] Ibrahim AM, Rabie AN, Borud L, Tobias AM, Lee BT, Lin SJ. Common patterns of reconstruction for Mohs defects in the head and neck. J Craniofac Surg. 2014; 25(1):87–92

[9] Goldman GD, Dzubow LM, Yelverton CB. Facial Flap Surgery. 2nd ed. New York, NY: McGraw-Hill; 2013

[10] Singer HM, Patel VA. Forehead reconstruction after resection of squamous cell carcinoma. Dermatol Surg. 2018; 44(7):1018–1022

[11] Tomás-Velázquez A, Redondo P. Assessment of frontalis myocutaneous transposition flap for forehead reconstruction after Mohs surgery. JAMA Dermatol. 2018; 154(6):708–711

3 Reconstruction of the Nasal Unit

Ian Maher, Jamie L. Hanson, and Gabriel Amon

Summary

The nose has important functional and aesthetic purposes. As an anatomic landmark in the center of the face, the nose serves an integral role in the perception of appearance.[1] With a complex architecture comprising convex and concave surfaces, the nose poses a significant challenge to dermatologic surgeons attempting to preserve the aesthetics of this facial unit. To do so successfully, understanding its key structural and anatomic features is fundamental.

Keywords: nasal reconstruction, bilobed flaps, trilobed flap, paramedian flap, crescenteric advancement flap, dorsal rotation flap

3.1 Structure and Function

The structural support system of the nose consists of the nasal bone proximally, which transitions to a distal cartilaginous skeleton. The cartilaginous portion of the nose can be further subdivided into three parts: the nasal septum and the paired upper and the lower lateral cartilages.[2] Above this structural support system lies the nasalis muscle, which is overlaid by skin. With regard to the nasal airway, there are two key anatomic structures of functional importance: the internal and external nasal valves. The external nasal valve serves as the gateway to the nasal passage and is formed by the nasal septum, the nasal floor, the caudal edge of the upper lateral cartilage, and the nasal ala.[3] The internal nasal valve is a narrow passage found at the level of the pyriform aperture and is the site of maximum air resistance; its boundaries are formed by the upper lateral cartilage, the nasal septum, the nasal floor, and the inferior turbinate.[4] Because collapse of these valves can obstruct inspiratory airflow, their preservation is vital to all nasal reconstruction.

3.2 Skin Characteristics

The characteristics of the skin overlying the nose vary markedly by location. There are three primary zones, each with unique features.[5] Zone I (proximal) involves the nasal dorsum and proximal nasal sidewalls; the overlying skin in this region is thin, mobile, and elastic. Zone II (distal) corresponds to the distal half of the nose and contains thick, sebaceous skin that is stiff and less mobile. Zone III extends to the infratip lobule and consists of thinner skin, but it is tightly affixed to underlying tissue and therefore less mobile.[5]

3.3 Nasal Subunits

The concept of facial aesthetic units described by Gonzalez-Ulloa[6] in 1954 introduced the concept of restoring regions of skin to achieve optimal aesthetic results. Burget and Menick[7] subsequently introduced the nasal subunit theory, applying similar principles on a smaller scale again in an attempt to achieve improved aesthetic outcomes. Using this approach, incisions and scars are designed to fall between subunits where natural shadows and transitions help disguise their appearance. These concepts have remained a common approach to facial reconstructive surgery in today's practice. There are nine nasal subunits in total, which include the tip, columella, right and left alar lobules, right and left soft triangles, nasal dorsum, and right and left dorsal sidewalls. The nasal dorsum and dorsal sidewalls are mobile subunits in the majority of patients, as they are composed of elastic, nonsebaceous skin, are largely planar, and overlie the bony nasal skeleton. In contrast, the remaining subunits are considered immobile. The nasal tip and alar lobules are highly sebaceous and located on convex surfaces; in these locations, volume replenishment is key in preventing indent deformities. The columella and soft triangles are nonsebaceous and flat.

3.4 Keys to Success

When planning an operative repair of the nose, preserving proper function and cosmetic structure are important components that often go hand in hand. There are a few key principles that will assist in achieving these goals. In general, maintaining horizontal tension vectors when planning operative closures on the nose is best; this schematic prevents vertical forces that can distort the free margin at the alar rim. Additionally, repairs should be planned so as to minimize horizontal tension over the compressible cartilaginous nasal skeleton, as this can lead to saddle nose deformity. The next key point when executing a repair is to undermine within the correct tissue plane. In general, undermining should be performed within the subnasalis tissue plane, which is a relatively bloodless plane, since the nasalis provides relative structural stability for the sebaceous and fragile distal nasal skin.[8] Meticulous attention to suture placement and technique will also ensure ideal cosmetic outcomes. By placing emphasis on precise deep sutures that incorporate the nasalis muscle, the overall integrity of the closure will be optimized, thus preventing scar spreading, scar depression, as well as other contour deformities such as trapdoor deformity. When planning a flap repair on the nose, it is advisable to always deepen the primary defect to the subnasalis plane to avoid "overfilling" of the defect, which is another cause of trapdoor deformity. Finally, gentle handling of the tissue throughout the repair will serve well in achieving even closures with well-disguised surgical scars.

3.5 Local Reconstruction of Subunits

The unique characteristics of each subunit with regard to skin characteristics and tissue mobility will guide the reconstructive choices in each location. Many approaches can be employed successfully; herein we will review our "go-to" choices. Notably, the size of the operative defect relative to the total nasal surface area and the corresponding tissue mobility is the most important determinant regarding the feasibility of a closure as opposed to a hard and fast rule. This section discusses closure options for defects in the 8- to 15-mm range. Our algorithm for reconstruction of nasal defects can be found in this figure.

3.5.1 Mobile Subunits

Nasal Dorsum/Bridge

Primary Closure

In this location with a largely planar surface and thin mobile tissue, small defects can often be closed primarily with a direct linear closure, particularly if the wound is smaller and in the horizontal rather than vertical dimension. Some surgeons believe a primary closure is best used for midline nasal defects, as the tension is then spread symmetrically across both sides of the nose.[9] Closures in this area should generally be vertically oriented and widely undermined to insure a tension-free closure. Excess tension across the dorsum will result in a saddle nose deformity, which can be appreciated on the lateral view. Other tips to prevent these deformities from a primary closure include designing an ellipse with a ratio of greater than 3:1 in the vertical domain and planning elongated standing cones.[9,10] These strategies will result in a longer surgical scar, but the overall profile of the nose will be preserved without tenting at the edges of the incision.

Full-Thickness Skin Grafts

The most important consideration when using a full-thickness skin graft (FTSG) is selecting an appropriate color and texture match of the graft to the donor site. The skin of the nasal dorsum is thin, nonsebaceous, and on a sun-exposed area. Previously reported donor sites with similar texture and color qualities include preauricular, postauricular, lateral forehead, and melolabial skin.[11,12,13,14] There are inherent risks with use of an FTSG leading to poor cosmetic outcomes; these include wound contraction and graft ischemia.[4,10] Precise sizing of the graft will minimize contour deformity that results from wound contraction.[4] Limiting the size of the graft to smaller defects will reduce vascular demands and subsequent risk of tissue ischemia and potential necrosis; however, 90% of grafts with a good vascular bed should survive.[10] Finally, although there is no substitute for meticulous suturing of the graft to the recipient base with good apposition to achieve an even closure, the texture match between donor and graft site can still be improved with postoperative dermabrasion or laser resurfacing.[14]

Transposition Flaps

The thin, mobile tissue of the nasal dorsum allows for closure with a single-lobed transposition flap such as the rhombic or banner flap (► Fig. 3.1).[15,16,17] Again, in order to maintain an ideal tension vector, the flap should be designed vertically.[18] A vertically designed flap will also ensure that you are drawing from the most generous tissue reservoir located cephalad to the defect.

Nasal Sidewalls

Proximal

Transposition Flap

The nasal sidewall contains skin from zone I, similar to the nasal dorsum. Again, the thin and elastic nature of the skin from this region allows for adequate closure with a single-lobed transposition flap such as the rhombic or banner flap. The glabellar tissue reservoir is ideal for tissue defects on the nasal sidewall, as it allows for a vertical tension vector, and the donor site scar can easily be disguised into preexisting glabellar frown lines. One drawback to the glabellar donor site is that closure of the secondary defect may lead to narrowing of the interbrow distance.[19] Careful planning of the flap and avoiding a broad base can mitigate this undesired outcome.

Rotation Flap

A rotation-based flap, again using the proximally based glabellar tissue reservoir, can also be utilized for closure of defects involving the proximal nasal sidewall.

Burow's Graft

A Burow's graft is another option that can be utilized for nasal sidewall repair. The schematic of a Burow's graft is to harvest an FTSG from an excess tissue "dog-ear," which would have been removed in a traditional linear repair, to aid in closing the remainder of the defect.[20,21,22] This technique is particularly useful if the defect also involves the medial cheek. In these cases, a cheek advancement flap combined with a melolabial Burow's graft to close the nasal sidewall defect can be employed.[11]

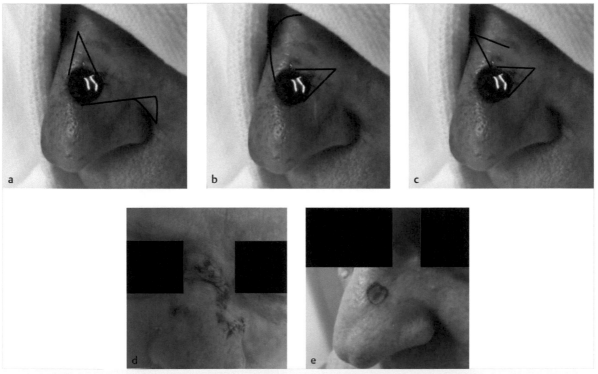

Fig. 3.1 (a) Dorsum option 1. Crescentic cheek flap illustrated to repair the defect of the left lateral nasal sidewall. Flap is designed with a standing cutaneous defect (SCD) superior to the primary defect sulcus and a second SCD in the left nasolabial fold extended laterally from the defect. Undermining must transition from the subnasalis plane on the nose to the subcutaneous plane on the cheek. This option allows for horizontal tension vectors and for scars to be hidden partially in the nasolabial fold. (b) Dorsum option 2. Rotation flap illustrated to repair the defect of the left lateral nasal sidewall. Flap is designed to provide a good tissue match by using similar skin superior to the defect via a curved incision extending along the nasal ridge and back to the left lateral sidewall to recruit proximal nasal and glabellar laxity. (c) Dorsum option 3. This is the option we chose. Rhombic flap illustrated to repair the defect of the left lateral nasal sidewall. Flap is designed to incorporate tissue from an SCD in the nasal root and another SCD in the sidewall. When incising the flap overlying the procerus complex, the flap is elevated in the subcutaneous plane with transition of undermining to the subnasalis plane at the nasion. (d) Sutured. (e) Follow-up at 12 weeks.

Distal

In general, advancement flaps are favored for closure of nasal sidewall defects, particularly when the skin is sebaceous. Sebaceous skin tends to be more rigid, less mobile, and poorly vascularized, which predisposes it to poorer healing.[23] The lines of advancement flaps on the distal nasal sidewall conform more readily to natural boundaries and this favorable placement is advantageous when optimal healing may not occur even with the most fastidious surgical technique.

Crescentic Cheek Advancement Flap

The crescentic cheek advancement flap was introduced by Webster[24] and has subsequently been modified as an excellent repair option for surgical defects involving the lateral nasal sidewall.[25,26] The crescentic cheek advancement flap allows for the donor site scar to be hidden within the nasolabial fold and the scar from the primary defect can then be disguised within the shadows of the nasofacial sulcus. This technique can be thought of as a

modification of Burow's advancement flap with a crescent-shaped standing cone along the nasolabial fold as opposed to the traditional triangular design used in other locations.[27] The redundant tissue superior to the primary defect along the nasofacial sulcus can be removed as a traditional triangular standing cone. To ensure adequate tissue mobility and to minimize tension upon closure, the flap along the nasolabial sulcus should be designed so that the curvilinear outer edge of the flap is made to be as long as the shorter inner edge plus the length of the primary defect.[27] Minimizing horizontal tension of the primary defect is particularly important in the region of the internal nasal valve so as not to impair function with inspiratory airflow.

3.5.2 Immobile Subunits

Sebaceous and Convex

The skin in these locations will have zone II characteristics, meaning it will be thicker, more sebaceous, and less mobile. In general, volume replenishment will be key in achieving optimal cosmetic results with minimal contour deformity.

Nasal Tip

For small (< 4 mm) midline defects involving the nasal tip, a vertically oriented primary closure can be utilized. If the defect is small but slightly displaced from midline, then an east–west advancement flap may be considered. This closure technique is best used in patients with relatively flexible skin with a broad nasal tip.

East–West Advancement Flap

Traditionally the east–west advancement flap has been advocated for patients with particularly sebaceous skin.[23] Ideally, this closure should be reserved for defects that are taller than they are wide. The overall design is a linear closure with a larger standing cone taken superior to the defect and displacement of the inferior standing cone medially over the columella.[28] Key design concepts include elongation of the superior standing cone to avoid a saddle nose deformity with closure, wide undermining in the subnasalis plane, and careful attention to tension vectors when advancing the skin horizontally to avoid any upward pull on the alar free margin.[29] Particular attention should be placed on meticulous deep sutures to reduce tension on the overlying sebaceous epidermis.

Bilobed and Trilobed Transposition Flaps

Our favored repair in this location is a bilobed or trilobed transposition flap (▶ Fig. 3.2, ▶ Fig. 3.3), both of which have been extensively described in the literature.[30,31,32,33,34,35,36] These flaps recruit from tissue reservoirs located more proximally in zone I, reducing tension and anatomic distortion, which would result from a single-lobed flap in this location. Some authors believe that transposition flaps (including bilobed and trilobed flaps) also induce Z-plasty-like lengthening—although this is debated by others.[34] The bilobed flap is designed with a total arc of rotation of approximately 90 degrees,[30] which allows for redirection of the terminal tension bearing defect vertically over the bony nasal skeleton and away from the alar free margin. In general, it is recommended to remove the standing cutaneous defect (SCD) first.[31,32] The standing cone should be oriented so as to avoid encroachment on any neighboring cosmetic subunits. In most cases, the length of the SCD should approach, if not exceed, one primary defect diameter in order to minimize tissue redundancy at its apex, which may result in inward push on the nasal aperture or downward push of the ipsilateral alar rim.[18,31,37] As originally described by Zitelli,[30] the lobes would be of equal size with equal rotational angles, although this can be modified based on local tissue characteristics. Lobes situated in mobile skin can be expected to stretch and rotate more; thus, undersizing of the secondary lobe would be possible. If interlobe angles are unequal, it is crucial that more acute

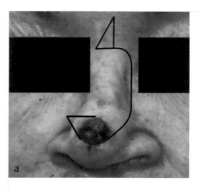
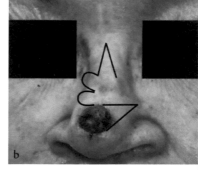
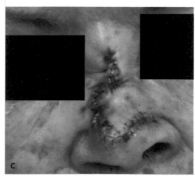
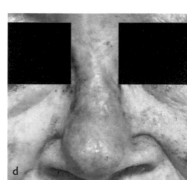

Fig. 3.2 (a) Nasal tip option 1. Dorsal nasal rotation flap illustrated to repair the defect of the nasal tip. Flap is designed to provide a good tissue match by using similar skin lateral to the defect, whereas a second standing cone defect with extension to the glabella is required due to the amount of repair tissue required. (b) Nasal tip option 2. This is the option we chose. Trilobed flap illustrated to repair the defect of the nasal tip. Flap recruits zone 1 tissue and with vertical orientation of the tertiary lobe allows horizontal tension vectors to maintain alar symmetry. (c) Sutured. (d) Follow-up at 8 weeks.

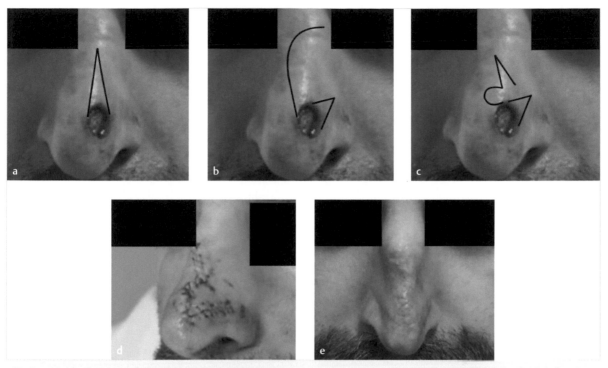

Fig. 3.3 (a) Supratip option 1. Nasalis sling island pedicle flap illustrated to repair the defect of the nasal dorsum and tip. This flap uses biplanar undermining to create a laterally based muscle-only pedicle. This is a wonderful repair option for "wider than tall" defects on the nasal tip. (b) Supratip option 2. Rotation flap illustrated to repair the defect of the nasal dorsum and tip. Flap is designed to provide a good tissue match and mobility via a curved incision extending superiorly from the defect along the dorsum to the left lateral sidewall. (c) Supratip option 3. This is the option we chose. Bilobed flap illustrated to repair the defect of the nasal dorsum and tip. Flap is designed so that the standing cone does not encroach on the alar crease and the tension bearing tertiary defect is oriented vertically or perpendicular to the ipsilateral alar margin. (d) Sutured. (e) Follow-up at 2 weeks.

angles be seated in stiffer skin proximate to the primary defect and more obtuse angles be located in more mobile skin nearer the tension bearing defect.[18]

Some authors have advocated for oversized primary lobes to overcome rotational shortening, but this only seems to occur in patients with particularly stiff, sebaceous skin.[38,39] As always, meticulous suturing in combination with wide undermining will limit contour defects such as pin cushioning or trapdoor deformities. Additionally, as with all nongraft nasal closures, defects should always be deepened to the subnasalis plane as opposed to thinning of the flap.

The trilobed flap follows similar tissue mechanics, but allows for even greater movement with the ability to recruit more distant tissue reservoirs and further reduce tension of the closure.[18,33,40] The arc of rotation in a trilobed flap is increased to 120 to 150 degrees,[33] which provides additional advantages. The wider rotational arc creates a wider flap pedicle, which provides more flexibility for design and placement of the SCD.[40] Additionally, it optimizes the ability to create a crucial horizontal tension vector over the bony nasal skeleton.[41] These authors have found that this can be achieved more readily with a slight modification of the traditional trilobed flap in which the external angle is made more acute between the primary defect and the primary lobe with increasingly more obtuse external angles for each subsequent lobe.[42] This technique reduces rotational shortening of the primary lobe and pushes the tension vector proximally into zone I skin where there is greater tissue laxity.

The dorsal nasal rotation flap, also known as the Rieger flap, is another closure technique that can be utilized for distal nasal defects. In its original design, the dorsal nasal flap is a random pattern flap that recruits mobile tissue from the glabella and nasal dorsum and rotates this tissue down into the more distal surgical defect. Traditionally, this closure technique is best for defects less than 2 cm in size and at least 5 mm from the alar rim.[43] Attempting to use this flap to cover larger defects or pulling the flap too inferior can result in undesirable tip elevation or alar retraction. Notably, various design modifications have been proposed to broaden the scope of this flap,[44] particularly in patients who desire a one-stage surgery that might otherwise be better suited by an interpolation flap.

Ala

The ala is a functionally critical structure to the nasal airway via the external nasal valve, and extra attention should be placed on repairs in this location.[45,46,47] In general, if there is any concern for compromise of the alar free margin or patency of the external nasal valve, there should be a low threshold to select a cheek interpolation flap for repair. Although these are two-stage procedures, the long-term structural and functional consequences of under-repair in this location can be severe; thus, it is worthwhile to spend the necessary time and attention in planning the repair upfront.

The nasal ala is anatomically unique among the nasal subunits in that there is no bony or cartilaginous component.[48] The ala maintains its patency due to the structural integrity of the stiff curved sebaceous alar skin—much like an arch bridge. Therefore, cartilage grafting is typically not necessary unless there is compromise of the nasal valves after tumor excision. Prior to planning repair, we close the contralateral nostril and have the patient inhale and exhale to monitor for valvular collapse. When collapse occurs and structural grafting is deemed necessary, a free cartilage batten graft can be utilized. These are most often harvested from the antihelix or conchal bowl, because they are comprised of elastic cartilage, which provides desired strength and shaping properties. Grafts may also be harvested from the nasal septum or rib; however, these sites are comprised of hyaline cartilage, which is weaker and less moldable.[49,50,51,52]

For defects involving the ala with or without involvement of the nasal sidewall, a single-stage cheek transposition flap, such as the nasolabial transposition flap, may be considered. However, this type of closure can lead to blunting of the alar crease and the nasofacial sulcus. Although tacking sutures can help preserve the natural concavities, we tend to eschew this option as more reliable closure techniques are available.

Small Defects (< 7 mm in width) on the Superior Alar Crease

For flaps that rely on rearrangement of alar skin, the horizontal width of the primary defect is the key determinate. If excess horizontal tension is placed on the ala, it will result in inward collapse of the ala and obstruction of the nasal valves.

Alar rotation flap: This flap uses the nasal ala lateral to the surgical defect as a tissue donor, providing an excellent skin texture match and allowing for scars to be easily disguised in the shadow of the alar groove. However, its use should be limited to small defects (< 6–7 mm) on the anterior two-thirds of the ala in proximity to the alar groove.[45,53] These limitations are intended primarily to avoid distortion of the alar free rim and to ensure availability of an adequate tissue reservoir lateral to the defect. There are a few key design steps to ensure a successful repair with the alar rotation flap. First, the SCD should be taken from the inferior aspect of the defect and perpendicular to the alar-free margin. The SCD should be removed first, to allow for easier transfer of the flap into

the defect. Next, any intervening skin between the defect and the alar groove should be excised. The incision can then be extended in an arcuate fashion along the alar groove to the alar base. The secondary defect can then be closed in a layered fashion. In general, a second standing cone is not necessary if the defect is closed carefully using the "rule of halves."[4]

Spiral flap: The spiral flap is alternative local rotation flap that allows for recreation of the alar groove while maintaining the convex structure of the ala when the primary defect spans the alar crease to involve both the nasal sidewall and the ala. The design of the spiral flap as outlined by Mahlberg et al is a rotation flap with a tip extension.[54] The origination point for the spiral flap is at the inferomedial portion of the defect and should then extend superiorly in an arcuate fashion. Next, the width of the flap's tip extension should be equal to the vertical height of the alar portion of the primary defect. The length of the tip extension should be equal to the horizontal dimension of the primary defect. The key suture connects the distal portion of the tip extension to the lateral portion of the alar primary defect, hinging the tip extension 90 degrees laterally, and beginning the spiral design of the flap. The second deep suture is then used to bring the body of the rotation flap down to the desired height of the alar crease. The remainder of the flap can then be sutured in place.

Island pedicle flap: Also known as a V-Y advancement flap, this is a myocutaneous flap that maintains a superior nasalis muscle pedicle providing a rich vascular supply.[45,55] Similar to the alar rotation flap, the island pedicle flap is ideal for small defects on the anterior aspect of the ala and maintains an excellent tissue match.[4,45] The overall design involves transfer of a laterally based triangular flap into the primary defect, followed by linear closure of the secondary defect. However, there are limitations to the island pedicle flap and precautions should be taken to avoid cosmetic distortion. The zone II alar tissue is stiff and less mobile; therefore, overall movement of the flap is limited. Additionally, closure of the horizontal secondary defect inherently causes some vertically oriented tension with risk of distorting the alar free margin. Proper selection of a small defect (< 7 mm in width), located relatively near the alar crease and at least 5 mm from the alar margin, will mitigate these risks.[55] Design of an elongated tapered triangular flap will also limit the vertically oriented tension vector created upon closure of the secondary defect.[4] It is inevitable that some elevation of the lateral ala will occur with closure of this secondary defect, and we advise counseling the patient to this fact preoperatively.

Defects of the Anterior Ala

Medially based multilobed transposition flaps: Medially based multilobed transposition flaps allow for recruitment of tissue reservoirs remote from the alar margins—thus preserving alar symmetry—and allow the primary lobe to transpose over the deeper, more lateral portions of the alar crease, avoiding disturbance of a key aesthetic landmark. Our choice between bilobed and trilobed flaps depends on the ability to place the tension-bearing terminal defect in an area of relative tissue mobility.

The principles of a bilobed flap have previously been discussed; herein, we will address the key aspects to success when executing this repair on the nasal ala. In general, medially based transposition flaps are preferable on the ala as they allow the lobes to be transposed over the alar groove, preserving this anatomic structure. Additionally, the standing cone should be designed horizontally to the defect. This ensures that the tension vector of the tertiary defect is oriented vertically and also aligns the long axis of the primary lobe to run parallel

with the alar free margin.[4] Both of these design features minimize distortion of the alar rim (► Fig. 3.4).

In many patients, a medially based trilobed may be more effective in recruiting the more forgiving zone I nasal skin reservoir.[42] The addition of a third lobe adds approximately one primary defect diameter to the height of the flap. The superior movement of the flap's terminal defect reduces the tension of closure and allows for more effortless preservation of alar symmetry.

Defects of the Middle to Posterior Ala: Large or Involving the Alar Rim

Large defects (>1.5 cm) in this location are often best repaired with interpolation flaps. There are a few different flap choices in such a case, each with a particular niche for which it is best suited. The melolabial interpolation flap

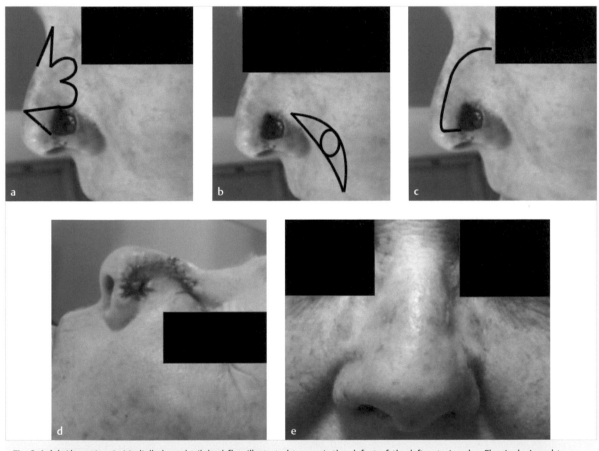

Fig. 3.4 (a) Ala option 1. Medially based trilobed flap illustrated to repair the defect of the left anterior alar. Flap is designed to incorporate the tension bearing quaternary defect in zone 1 where tissue is more easily mobile, and allow for horizontal tension vectors. **(b)** Ala option 2. Melolabial interpolation flap illustrated to repair the defect of the left anterior alar crease. Flap is designed to be a good tissue match while concealing the donor scar in the melolabial fold. This is a reliable option, but does require a secondary procedure and ~4 weeks of wound care. **(c)** Ala option 3. This is the option we chose. Spiral flap illustrated to repair the defect of the left anterior nasal alar crease. The body of the flap repairs the nasal sidewall portion of the defect, whereas the tip extension hinges 90 degrees laterally to resurface the alar portion of the defect. A small area was allowed to granulate to reform the alar crease. Incision extends from the primary defect to the superior aspect of the nasofacial sulcus. **(d)** Sutured. **(e)** Follow-up at 8 weeks.

(MLIF) is our preferred option and the most widely used repair option for the ala.[4,45,56,57,58]

Melolabial interpolation flap: By definition, the MLIF is a two-stage repair that is more labor intensive for the patient, requiring more wound care and multiple office visits. However, there are several notable advantages. Drawing from tissue residing along the melolabial fold, the MLIF provides an excellent tissue match for the nasal ala. Additionally, the melolabial fold provides a convenient location to disguise a surgical scar. The MLIF is a random pattern flap drawing its vascular supply from perforators of the angular artery.[59] The flap can be designed with either a myocutaneous (including skin in the pedicle) or myosubcutaneous pedicle (an "islanded" pedicle), each with different caveats.[56] Although the myocutaneous flap is easier to harvest in the first stage of the repair, it has greater metabolic demands[56] and may cause rotational shortening due to the stiffer pedicle base.[4] When designing the flap, the contralateral nasal ala can be used as a template if the surgeon is attempting subunit repair. Overall the flap should be precisely sized to the primary defect.[56,60] The medial border of the flap should align just lateral to the ipsilateral melolabial fold, and the alar template located at or above the level of the oral commissure.[56,61] Once mobilized, the flap is generally advanced medially and should overlie the defect without tension. The pedicle is typically divided after 3 weeks. The residual alar subunit is then excised, with the exception of 1 to 2 mm of alar base lateral to the defect. This remaining alar base will serve as the attachment point for the flap, allowing preservation of the native alar groove.[4] The donor site can then be closed primarily.

Although the MLIF is the preferred repair for this location, it is not plausible in all patients. For example, male patients often have terminal beard hair within the melolabial donor region. Although laser hair removal can be considered, this option is not permanent and has limitations—especially in those with gray or white hair. For these patients, it may be preferable to select a different repair such as the paranasal interpolation flap (PIF) or the paramedian forehead flap (PMFF).

Paranasal interpolation flap: The PIF is an inferiorly based random pattern flap that draws from a tissue reservoir along the nasofacial sulcus. Apart from the advantage of providing a hairless donor site, the PIF has an axis of rotation less than 90 degrees, which also allows for a shorter flap design.[62] Careful consideration should be paid to the mobility of the medial cheek as well as the position and laxity of the lower eyelid to ensure adequate closure of the donor site.[62] Key design principles include ensuring the flap width is equal to the height of the primary defect and tapering the end of the flap to 30 degrees to achieve ideal linear closure of the donor site.[62] The medial border of the flap is typically kept just lateral to the nasofacial sulcus, but if a wider flap is deemed necessary, the flap should instead straddle the nasofacial sulcus.[62] Once complete, the flap is again left in place for 3 weeks prior to takedown.

Nonsebaceous and Flat

Soft Triangle

For repair of the soft triangles that are composed of zone III skin and adherent to underlying structures, recruiting tissue from more distant donor sites is often necessary. In this location, there is a low threshold for interpolation flaps, the details of which have been reviewed in previous sections. We favor the use of the paranasal flap or MLIF for repairs in this location, as opposed to the PMFF. If a two-staged repair is declined by the patient, there are a few preferred options for local repair of the soft triangles. The first option is the trilobed flap, as discussed in more detail in previous sections. The third lobe allows for recruitment of more remote and mobile tissue from zone I. The second option for local repair is the nasalis sling flap (NSF).

The NSF has been described in the literature as an excellent option for repair of full-thickness defects of the nasal tip[63] and more recently has been described for repair of defects involving the soft triangles.[64] The NSF is a myocutaneous island pedicle flap from the nasal dorsum. This repair option has several advantages. Drawing from a nearby tissue donor site in zone II, the NSF provides an excellent color and texture match to the nasal tip and avoids distortion of the alar free margin by maintaining a horizontal tension vector.[64] The key to soft triangle repair lies within the rotational reach of the NSF, which is attributed to the flexible nasalis pedicle. The intrinsic movement and reach of the NSF allow for the excess skin from the leading edge of the flap to be in-folded onto itself, thus recreating the lining and structure of the soft triangles.[64]

Columella

Surgical defects of the columella are rare.[65] Fortunately, this region of the nose is not highly visible and therefore defects not involving the alar free margin are often amenable to a more simple repair. Allowing small defects of the columella to heal by secondary intention is a reasonable option but does require significant wound care on behalf of the patient. If patients desire a formal closure of the wound, the split-thickness skin graft (STSG) from the postauricular skin is another practical repair option.

3.5.3 Large or Multisubunit Defects

Paramedian Forehead Flap

The PMFF has been extensively described in the literature and is well established as the gold standard closure technique for large defects involving multiple subunits of the nose (▶ Fig. 3.5).[60,66,67,68] The PMFF is an axial pattern flap

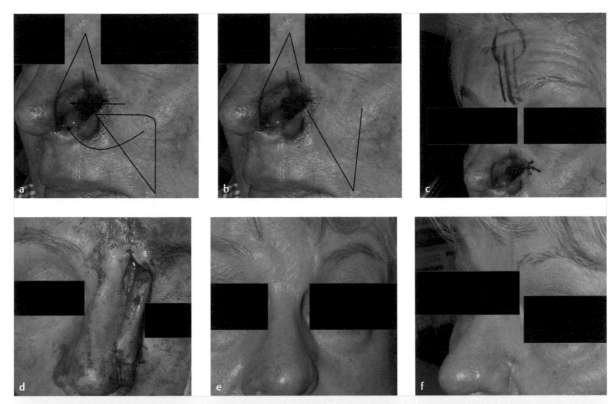

Fig. 3.5 (a) Full-thickness ala option 1. Combination of the melolabial interpolation flap (MLIF) with the crescentic cheek advancement flap illustrated to repair the defect of the left nasal ala. The melolabial standing cutaneous defect (SCD) is islanded and used as an MLIF to repair the ala, whereas the cheek is advanced to resurface the nasal sidewall. This option is preferred for patients with good cheek laxity, which was not present in our patient. **(b)** Full-thickness ala option 2. Single-stage cheek transposition flap illustrated to repair the defect of the left nasal ala. Flap is designed to use the medial cheek skin to resurface the nasal sidewall and the ala. Tacking sutures are used to recreate the alar crease and the nasofacial sulcus. Due to the involvement of the alar rim and lining as well as the cheek in this case, this option was not chosen. **(c)** Full-thickness ala option 3. This is the option we chose. The paramedian forehead flap (PMFF) illustrated to repair the defect of the left nasal ala. Flap is optimal for large, full-thickness defects affecting multiple nasal subunits. **(d)** Sutured. **(e)** Front view of the PMFF at 2 months of follow-up. **(f)** A 2-month follow-up L ¾ view.

drawing its blood supply from the supratrochlear artery; it can be performed in two or three stages depending on the extent of the defect. Skin-only defects or those involving fewer nasal subunits are often amenable to the two-stage PMFF. However, more extensive defects requiring fold over flaps for nasal lining repair or recreation of multiple subunit transitions may benefit from the three-stage repair, which allows for establishment of a more robust vascular supply.[66,69]

Successful execution of the PMFF requires meticulous planning with careful design of the template in order to ensure adequate reach. Doppler can be used to identify the supratrochlear artery and define the pedicle base. Alternatively, the glabellar frown line and 6 mm of skin immediately lateral to it serves as a reliable landmark for the supratrochlear artery.[70] Therefore, a thinner 1-cm pedicle base can be safely planned to incorporate this region.

In a two-stage repair, the distal "paddle" of the flap will be elevated in the subcutaneous tissue plane until the

juncture with the "stalk," where the dissection should move into the subfrontalis/supraperiosteal plane in order to preserve the neurovascular bundle. Alternatively, in a three-stage repair, the flap will be elevated entirely from the subfrontalis plane. Each stage of the repair is separated by a period of 3 weeks. In the three-stage repair, the intermediate operation allows for thinning of the flap, removal of excess subcutis/muscle, and placement of any cartilage grafts. The flap is then sewn into what will be the final configuration. The final stage is the same for both approaches and involves division of the pedicle and inset and closure of the flap and donor site.

Although the PMFF serves as an excellent repair option for large, full-thickness defects, there are several drawbacks. Overall, the number of operations and necessary wound care is labor and time intensive for the patient. Additionally, patients with vascular compromise due to extremely heavy smoking, underlying medical comorbidities, or previous forehead surgeries may not be ideal candidates due to risk of flap necrosis. Generally, the PMFFs, particularly the three-stage PMFFs, are quite safe even in smokers and flap loss is incredibly rare. Finally, some patients find that the resultant forehead scar is unappealing; however, in most cases, the forehead heals well—even with granulation—and emphasis should be placed on restoration of the aesthetically and functionally critical nose.

Combination of MLIF and Local Flaps

Although the PMFF has historically been the repair of choice for large multisubunit nasal repairs, there are several drawbacks that may deter patients. The bandaging required for the PMFF is bulky, which is more noticeable and socially stigmatizing for patients; it also interferes with activities of daily living such as driving or wearing eyeglasses. These disadvantages have been shown to impair quality of life for many patients[71] and may lead many to prefer other repair options. In these cases, the combination of an MLIF with an additional local flap provides an excellent alternative.[72] The overall approach utilizes the MLIF to reconstruct the nasal tip or alar portion of the defect, whereas a local flap such as the crescentic cheek advancement or a V-Y advancement flap will repair the nasal sidewall. In general, it is recommended to perform the local flap for nasal sidewall repair first, followed by inset of the MLIF into the distal portion of the defect.[72]

MLIF + V-Y advancement

This repair option is ideal for defects of the nasal sidewall that are wider than tall or in patients with sufficient vertical laxity. The V-Y advancement in this setting is designed as a myocutaneous flap from the vertical side of the defect, drawing its blood supply from a laterally based nasalis pedicle. In order to achieve this design, a bilevel undermining technique is used—undermining the subnasalis medially and above the nasalis laterally.[72] Once the V-Y advancement is sewn into place, the MLIF can be designed in a standard manner to close the distal defect, the details of which have been reviewed in previous sections. Advantages of the V-Y advancement in combination with the MLIF include two separate robust blood supplies for each flap. Additionally, the V-Y flap on is muscular pedicle is able to move independently from the MLIF, without creating undue restraint from the overlying skin.[72]

MLIF + Crescentic Cheek Advancement

This combination is ideal for defects whose sidewall components are taller than wide, or in patients with significant horizontal laxity. Again, the local flap—the crescentic advancement flap—will be performed first. The SCD will be taken superior to the primary defect and should be excised to the subnasalis plane. The cheek advancement flap should also be undermined in the subnasalis plane until the juncture with the nasofacial sulcus, at which point undermining should move to the superficial subcutaneous plane in order to preserve the pedicle of the MLIF.[72] The MLIF can once again be designed and inset to the distal defect in a standard manner as described in previous sections.

3.6 Conclusion

The nose is a complex anatomic and functional structure. Successful reconstruction of the nose requires precise planning and individualization of the repair to the characteristics of the defect, the local anatomy, and the patient (▶ Fig. 3.6).

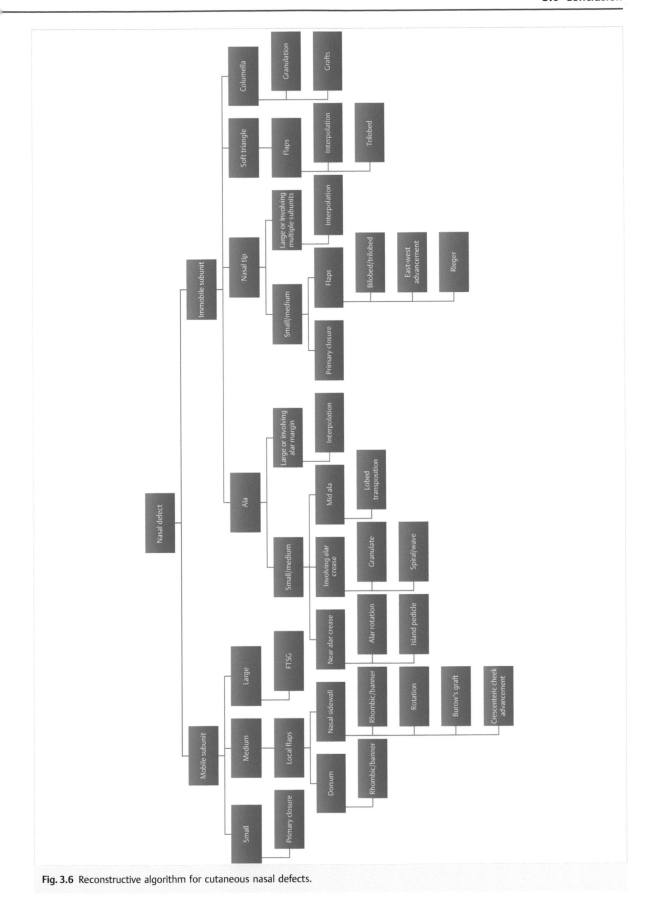

Fig. 3.6 Reconstructive algorithm for cutaneous nasal defects.

References

[1] Heppt WJ, Vent J. The facial profile in the context of facial aesthetics. Facial Plast Surg. 2015; 31(5):421–430

[2] Bruintjes TD, van Olphen AF, Hillen B, Huizing EH. A functional anatomic study of the relationship of the nasal cartilages and muscles to the nasal valve area. Laryngoscope. 1998; 108(7):1025–1032

[3] Hamilton GS, III. The external nasal valve. Facial Plast Surg Clin North Am. 2017; 25(2):179–194

[4] Maher I, Bordeaux J. Post-skin cancer alar reconstruction. Facial Plast Surg. 2013; 29(5):351–364

[5] Menick F. Nasal Reconstruction: Art and Practice. 1st ed. New York, NY: Saunders; 2008

[6] Gonzalez-Ulloa M, Castillo A, Stevens E, Alvarez Fuertes G, Leonelli F, Ubaldo F. Preliminary study of the total restoration of the facial skin. Plast Reconstr Surg (1946). 1954; 13(3):151–161

[7] Burget GC, Menick FJ. The subunit principle in nasal reconstruction. Plast Reconstr Surg. 1985; 76(2):239–247

[8] Oneal RM, Beil RJ. Surgical anatomy of the nose. Clin Plast Surg. 2010; 37(2):191–211

[9] Cook J, Zitelli JA. Primary closure for midline defects of the nose: a simple approach for reconstruction. J Am Acad Dermatol. 2000; 43(3):508–510

[10] Wolfswinkel EM, Weathers WM, Cheng D, Thornton JF. Reconstruction of small soft tissue nasal defects. Semin Plast Surg. 2013; 27(2):110–116

[11] Kim KH, Gross VL, Jaffe AT, Herbst AM. The use of the melolabial Burow's graft in the reconstruction of combination nasal sidewall-cheek defects. Dermatol Surg. 2004; 30(2, Pt 1):205–207

[12] McCluskey PD, Constantine FC, Thornton JF. Lower third nasal reconstruction: when is skin grafting an appropriate option? Plast Reconstr Surg. 2009; 124(3):826–835

[13] Gloster HM, Jr. The use of full-thickness skin grafts to repair nonperforating nasal defects. J Am Acad Dermatol. 2000; 42(6):1041–1050

[14] Rohrich RJ, Griffin JR, Ansari M, Beran SJ, Potter JK. Nasal reconstruction: beyond aesthetic subunits: a 15-year review of 1334 cases. Plast Reconstr Surg. 2004; 114(6):1405–1416, discussion 1417–1419

[15] Elliott RA, Jr. Rotation flaps of the nose. Plast Reconstr Surg. 1969; 44(2):147–149

[16] Zitelli JA, Fazio MJ. Reconstruction of the nose with local flaps. J Dermatol Surg Oncol. 1991; 17(2):184–189

[17] Field LM. The glabellar transposition "banner" flap. J Dermatol Surg Oncol. 1988; 14(4):376–379

[18] Blake BP, Simonetta CJ, Maher IA. Transposition flaps: principles and locations. Dermatol Surg. 2015; 41 Suppl 10:S255–S264

[19] Turgut G, Ozcan A, Yeşiloğlu N, Baş L. A new glabellar flap modification for the reconstruction of medial canthal and nasal dorsal defects: "flap in flap" technique. J Craniofac Surg. 2009; 20(1):198–200

[20] Chester EC, Jr. Surgical gem. The use of dog-ears as grafts. J Dermatol Surg Oncol. 1981; 7(12):956–959

[21] Zitelli JA. Burow's grafts. J Am Acad Dermatol. 1987; 17(2, Pt 1):271–279

[22] Eliezri YD. Variations on Burow's grafts. J Am Acad Dermatol. 1988; 18(5, Pt 1):1143–1145. United States

[23] Dzubow LM. Repair of defects on nasal sebaceous skin. Dermatol Surg. 2005; 31(8, Pt 2):1053–1054

[24] Webster JP. Crescentic peri-alar cheek excision for upper lip flap advancement with a short history of upper lip repair. Plast Reconstr Surg (1946). 1955; 16(6):434–464

[25] Mellette JR, Jr, Harrington AC. Applications of the crescentic advancement flap. J Dermatol Surg Oncol. 1991; 17(5):447–454

[26] Jackson I. Local Flaps in Head and Neck Reconstruction. St. Louis, MO: Mosby; 1985:245–249

[27] Yoo SS, Miller SJ. The crescentic advancement flap revisited. Dermatol Surg. 2003; 29(8):856–858

[28] Lambert RW, Dzubow LM. A dorsal nasal advancement flap for off-midline defects. J Am Acad Dermatol. 2004; 50(3):380–383

[29] Geist DE, Maloney ME. The "east-west" advancement flap for nasal defects: reexamined and extended. Dermatol Surg. 2012; 38(9):1529–1534

[30] Zitelli JA. The bilobed flap for nasal reconstruction. Arch Dermatol. 1989; 125(7):957–959

[31] Cook JL. A review of the bilobed flap's design with particular emphasis on the minimization of alar displacement. Dermatol Surg. 2000; 26(4):354–362

[32] Cook JL. Reconstructive utility of the bilobed flap: lessons from flap successes and failures. Dermatol Surg. 2005; 31(8, Pt 2):1024–1033

[33] Albertini JG, Hansen JP. Trilobed flap reconstruction for distal nasal skin defects. Dermatol Surg. 2010; 36(11):1726–1735

[34] Steiger JD. Bilobed flaps in nasal reconstruction. Facial Plast Surg Clin North Am. 2011; 19(1):107–111

[35] Mobley S. Bilobed flap design in nasal reconstruction. Ear Nose Throat J. 2004; 83(1):26–27

[36] Zitelli JA. Design aspect of the bilobed flap. Arch Facial Plast Surg. 2008; 10(3):186

[37] Zitelli J. Commentary on the trilobed flap for inferior-medial alar defect. Dermatol Surg. 2014; 40(7):799–800

[38] Xue CY, Li L, Guo LL, Li JH, Xing X. The bilobed flap for reconstruction of distal nasal defect in Asians. Aesthetic Plast Surg. 2009; 33(4):600–604

[39] Zoumalan RA, Hazan C, Levine VJ, Shah AR. Analysis of vector alignment with the Zitelli bilobed flap for nasal defect repair: a comparison of flap dynamics in human cadavers. Arch Facial Plast Surg. 2008; 10(3):181–185

[40] Miller CJ. Design principles for transposition flaps: the rhombic (single-lobed), bilobed, and trilobed flaps. Dermatol Surg. 2014; 40 Suppl 9:S43–S52

[41] Zitelli JA. Comments on a modified bilobed flap. Arch Facial Plast Surg. 2018; 8(6):410

[42] Wang CY, Armbrecht ES, Burkemper NM, Glaser DA, Maher IA. Bending the arc of the trilobed flap through external interlobe angle inequality. Dermatol Surg. 2018; 44(5):621–629

[43] Rieger RA. A local flap for repair of the nasal tip. Plast Reconstr Surg. 1967; 40(2):147–149

[44] Redondo P, Bernad I, Moreno E, Ivars M. Elongated dorsal nasal flap to reconstruct large defects of the nose. Dermatol Surg. 2017; 43(8):1036–1041

[45] Bloom JD, Ransom ER, Miller CJ. Reconstruction of alar defects. Facial Plast Surg Clin North Am. 2011; 19(1):63–83

[46] Gruber RP, Melkun ET, Strawn JB. External valve deformity: correction by composite flap elevation and mattress sutures. Aesthetic Plast Surg. 2011; 35(6):960–964

[47] Weber SM, Baker SR. Management of cutaneous nasal defects. Facial Plast Surg Clin North Am. 2009; 17(3):395–417

[48] Ali-Salaam P, Kashgarian M, Davila J, Persing J. Anatomy of the Caucasian alar groove. Plast Reconstr Surg. 2002; 110(1):261–266, discussion 267–271

[49] Immerman S, White WM, Constantinides M. Cartilage grafting in nasal reconstruction. Facial Plast Surg Clin North Am. 2011; 19(1):175–182

[50] Campbell T, Eisen DB. Free cartilage grafts for alar defects coupled with secondary-intention healing. Dermatol Surg. 2011; 37(4):510–513

[51] van der Eerden PA, Verdam FJ, Dennis SCR, Vuyk H. Free cartilage grafts and healing by secondary intention: a viable reconstructive combination after excision of nonmelanoma skin cancer in the nasal alar region. Arch Facial Plast Surg. 2009; 11(1):18–23

[52] Cervelli V, Spallone D, Bottini JD, et al. Alar batten cartilage graft: treatment of internal and external nasal valve collapse. Aesthetic Plast Surg. 2009; 33(4):625–634

[53] Neltner SA, Papa CA, Ramsey ML, Marks VJ. Alar rotation flap for small defects of the ala. Dermatol Surg. 2000; 26(6):543–546

[54] Mahlberg MJ, Leach BC, Cook J. The spiral flap for nasal alar reconstruction: our experience with 63 patients. Dermatol Surg. 2012; 38(3):373–380

[55] Asgari M, Odland P. Nasalis island pedicle flap in nasal ala reconstruction. Dermatol Surg. 2005; 31(4):448–452

[56] Nguyen TH. Staged cheek-to-nose and auricular interpolation flaps. Dermatol Surg. 2005; 31(8, Pt 2):1034–1045

[57] Smith H, Elliot T, Vinciullo C. Repair of nasal tip and alar defects using cheek-based 2-stage flaps: an alternative to the median forehead flap. Arch Dermatol. 2003; 139(8):1033–1036

[58] Barlow RJ, Swanson NA. The nasofacial interpolated flap in reconstruction of the nasal ala. J Am Acad Dermatol. 1997; 36(6, Pt 1):965–969

[59] Oneal RM, Beil RJ, Jr, Schlesinger J. Surgical anatomy of the nose. Clin Plast Surg. 1996; 23(2):195–222

[60] Mellette JR, Ho DQ. Interpolation flaps. Dermatol Clin. 2005; 23(1):87–112, vi

[61] Jewett BS. Interpolated forehead and melolabial flaps. Facial Plast Surg Clin North Am. 2009; 17(3):361–377

[62] Fisher GH, Cook JW. The interpolated paranasal flap: a novel and advantageous option for nasal-alar reconstruction. Dermatol Surg. 2009; 35(4):656–661

[63] Willey A, Papadopoulos DJ, Swanson NA, Lee KK. Modified single-sling myocutaneous island pedicle flap: series of 61 reconstructions. Dermatol Surg. 2008; 34(11):1527–1535

[64] Piontek JE, Mattox AR, Maher IA. Reconstruction of a defect of the infratip and soft triangle. Dermatol Surg. 2018; 44(12):1603–1606

[65] Goldman GD. Reconstruction of the nasal infratip, columella, and soft triangle. Dermatol Surg. 2014; 40 Suppl 9:S53–S61

[66] Menick FJ. A 10-year experience in nasal reconstruction with the three-stage forehead flap. Plast Reconstr Surg. 2002; 109(6):1839–1855, discussion 1856–1861

[67] Menick FJ. Nasal reconstruction with a forehead flap. Clin Plast Surg. 2009; 36(3):443–459

[68] Brodland DG. Paramedian forehead flap reconstruction for nasal defects. Dermatol Surg. 2005; 31(8, Pt 2):1046–1052

[69] Jellinek NJ, Nguyen TH, Albertini JG. Paramedian forehead flap: advances, procedural nuances, and variations in technique. Dermatol Surg. 2014; 40 Suppl 9:S30–S42

[70] Vural E, Batay F, Key JM. Glabellar frown lines as a reliable landmark for the supratrochlear artery. Otolaryngol Head Neck Surg. 2000; 123(5):543–546

[71] Somoano B, Kampp J, Gladstone HB. Accelerated takedown of the paramedian forehead flap at 1 week: indications, technique, and improving patient quality of life. J Am Acad Dermatol. 2011; 65(1):97–105

[72] Patel PM, Greenberg JN, Kreicher KL, Burkemper NM, Bordeaux JS, Maher IA. Combination of melolabial interpolation flap and nasal sidewall and cheek advancement flaps allows for repair of complex compound defects. Dermatol Surg. 2018; 44(6):785–795

4 Reconstruction of the Eyelid Units

Anne Barmettler

Summary

Eyelid reconstruction requires an in-depth knowledge of anatomy and careful attention to structures, specifically the eye and tear drainage system. Damage to these areas can be irreversible and are better prevented than treated. As these vital adjacent structures can be easily damaged, thorough preparation and collaboration with your local ophthalmic plastic and reconstructive surgeon can improve outcomes. This chapter provides an approach to reconstruction, based on location, depth, and size of defect. Location is broken into the following eyelid units: lower, upper, lateral, and medial. Identification of the location allows the surgeon to better prepare equipment for surgery. For example, medially, the tear drainage system can be involved and requires stents and special instrumentation for reconstruction. The second method of categorization is determining the defect's depth; whether the defect is a skin-only defect or a full-thickness defect (skin and tarsus) will dictate the type and extent of reconstruction. A full-thickness defect cannot be addressed by replacing only the skin; it also requires replacement of the tarsus and conjunctiva. Without tarsus and conjunctiva, the surface of the eye can be damaged directly (with the irregular margins causing a corneal abrasion) and indirectly (through eyelid margin instability, causing entropion or ectropion). Finally, the horizontal size of a full-thickness defect guides the type of reconstruction possible for the upper and lower lids. The options for reconstructive surgery are based on classification of the defect in relation to the total horizontal eyelid margin length: less than 33%, 33 to 50%, and greater than 50%.

Keywords: eyelid, reconstruction, Hughes, Cutler–Beard, Tenzel, tarsus, conjunctiva, orbicularis, tear drainage, canaliculus

4.1 Eyelid Reconstruction

At first glance, reconstruction of the eyelid appears complex and daunting, but facility can be achieved with an understanding of the anatomy and application of four foundational principles. Due to the delicate nature of the eye, collaboration with an ophthalmic plastic and reconstructive (aka oculoplastics) surgeon can improve outcomes. Optimally, this is coordinated in advance to allow for the best patient care, but in cases of unexpected defects, place ophthalmic ointment on the defect and consult your ophthalmology colleague immediately.

The four foundational principles are the following:

- *The eye is extremely delicate and must be protected.* If uncovered, even for moments, this can result in extreme pain, scarring to the cornea, vision loss, and even loss of the eye itself. While operating, ophthalmic ointment and/or a protective shell should be placed onto the surface of the eye. Needles, blades, and other sharp instruments should always be pointed away from the eye. For example, when injecting local anesthesia into the eyelid, the needle must be kept parallel to the surface of the eye, so if the patient moves or the needle/syringe malfunctions, the needle does not risk entry into the eye. In terms of reconstruction concepts, the eye requires a smooth surface with no exposed sutures or suture tails. This smooth surface typically comes in the form of conjunctiva or tarsus and conjunctiva. Additionally, reconstruction should avoid vertical tension on the eyelid margin and result in the ability to close the eye. Inability of the eye to close is called lagophthalmos and must be avoided, as this, too, can cause pain and damage to the eye.

- *Replace like with like.* The minimal requirements for eyelid reconstruction can be broken down into skin and muscle, called anterior lamella, and the tarsoconjunctival layer, called the posterior lamella. When reconstructing a skin-only defect, only the skin needs to be replaced, whereas a full-thickness defect (both skin and tarsus are missing) requires both the skin and the tarsoconjunctival layer to be replaced.

  o *Skin*: When replacing skin, prioritize utilizing skin replacements that are similar to the eyelid skin, which is the thinnest in the body and has extremely fine vellus hairs. Skin sources that are ideal include the following, in order of preference: eyelid (whether as a flap or taken as a full-thickness skin graft from an upper eyelid), postauricular (less sun damaged), preauricular, and supraclavicular. Other skin sources, such as the ventral surface of the upper arm and the lower abdomen, can be considered when the preferred sources are not possible.

  o *Tarsus*: Reconstructive replacements for the tarsus should be carefully chosen due to the delicate nature of the cornea. Rough surfaces over the cornea can result in corneal abrasion and permanent scarring, so it should be avoided. Recommended sources include, in order of preference, the following: tarsus as a flap from the opposite eyelid (e.g., if reconstructing the lower eyelid, a tarsoconjunctival flap from the upper eyelid); a tarsal graft from the contralateral upper lid; and hard palate. If using a tarsal replacement without a natural mucosal layer, such as ear cartilage, a conjunctival flap advancement from the fornix can be considered to protect the cornea. The tarsoconjunctival layer should always be reconstructed prior to the skin layer.

- *Protect and reconstruct the canaliculi immediately.* Once damaged, it is extremely difficult to reconstruct the canaliculi, so the best management is preventative. The tear drainage system consists of a punctum (the drainage hole located in the medial upper and lower lid), which is connected by the canaliculi (drainage pipes) to the lacrimal sac (a dilated area of the nasolacrimal duct), which then drains through the nasolacrimal duct into the nose under the inferior turbinate (▶ Fig. 4.1).
  If the punctum or canaliculi are damaged or endangered, place stenting to prevent scarring, which occurs within days. Once the canaliculi are scarred down, management options are limited, usually requiring implantation of a glass tube. On the other hand, treatment for damage to the lower portion of the tear drainage system, the lacrimal sac and the nasolacrimal duct, is best done at a later date. Excellent outcomes to this portion of the nasolacrimal system can be achieved with delayed treatment and this allows confirmation of tumor-free margins prior to connection of the orbit to the nose.
- *Categorize the defect in terms of location, depth, and size.* This includes identification of the eyelid margin, canthal tendon, underlying muscle, and the nasolacrimal system involvement. Prior to reconstruction, take several in-focus, well-lit photographs of the defect.

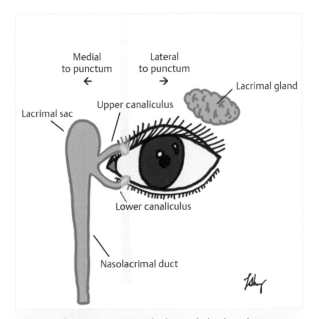

Fig. 4.1 The tearing system: the lacrimal gland produces tears, which flow onto the surface of the eye and into punctum medially. This then passes through the canaliculi, the lacrimal sac, the nasolacrimal duct, and into the nose. Damage or defects medial to the punctum (medial to the *yellow line*) should be explored for tear drainage damage, which can be irreversible if not addressed promptly. (Figure courtesy of Tiffany Cheng.)

4.1.1 Location

In addition to categorizing the location of defects to upper versus lower lid or medial versus lateral canthus, categorize the location of the defect into the following: medial to the punctum or including the punctum versus lateral to the punctum (▶ Fig. 4.1).

Medial to the punctum or including the punctum indicates a high likelihood of tear drainage system. If the canaliculus or punctum is involved, stents must be used to prevent epiphora postoperatively.

Lateral to the punctum, the area directly over the cornea requires careful partial-thickness suturing through the posterior lamella (the layer of conjunctiva and tarsus directly anterior to the cornea). This prevents damage to the underlying cornea, which is easily abraded and scarred by rough borders or exposed sutures, which can cause permanent vision loss.

4.1.2 Depth

Determine the depth of defect. Is only skin missing? Are both skin and tarsus missing, leaving a full-thickness defect and exposing the eye (▶ Fig. 4.2)? This vital information is the first step to choosing the right type of reconstructive surgery as the surface of the eye requires a smooth adjacent surface with complete coverage to avoid damage, which can lead to permanent vision loss.

4.1.3 Size

Full-thickness defects of the eyelid, meaning both the skin and the tarsus are absent, can be reconstructed using an algorithm based on the horizontal size of the defect. The reconstructive options differ based on the location of the defect, whether in the upper or the lower eyelid.[1]

4.2 Lower Lid Unit

Examine the defect for depth of involvement: skin only versus both skin and tarsus. Take note of the location medial to or involving the punctum, as this may require additional reconstruction in the form of a stent (see section "Medial Canthal Subunit").

4.2.1 Skin-Only Defects

For small, skin-only defects, primary skin closure can be attempted. Primary closure can be done with or without undermining of the surrounding skin. This is typically the better option over healing by granulation, which should be limited to small areas away from important landmarks. A 6–0 plain gut suture can be used to reapproximate the skin under little or no tension. Although closure should normally be done along skin relaxing lines (the lines in which wrinkles typically form), this should be avoided in the lower eyelid, where this can lead to a

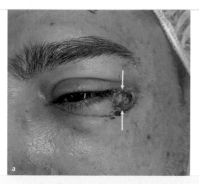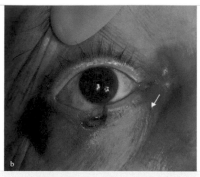

Fig. 4.2 Demonstration of skin only and full-thickness defects. **(a)** In this lateral canthal skin-only defect, closure can be made following the skin relaxing lines. If the defect was more medial, this type of closure (leaving a surgical scar parallel to the eyelid margin) would put the eyelid at risk of ectropion and should be avoided. Instead, a closure that would be perpendicular to the lower eyelid would be more appropriate to allow the tension to lie horizontally. **(b)** In this example of a full-thickness defect, the eyelid anatomy is clearly seen. The tarsus is adjacent to the eye and the orbicularis oculi muscle lays anterior. Along the eyelid margin, the orbicularis oculi muscle is visible as the "gray line" (*white arrow*).

cicatricial ectropion (outward turning eyelid margin, which causes exposure to the eye). Instead, defects in the lower lid should be closed so that the surgical scar is perpendicular to the eyelid margin and tension lies in the horizontal plane (▶ Fig. 4.3). Caution should be taken in areas of nerves, such as the supra- and infraorbital nerves in the areas where they exit the skull superior and inferior to the orbit, respectively, as well as the facial nerve, where it crosses over the zygomatic arch.

If primary skin closure will change the contour or height of the lower eyelid margin, a skin flap (myocutaneous advancement flap) or full-thickness skin graft can be considered. The amount and quality of the adjacent tissue will vary depending on age, genetics, and sun damage. A 6–0 plain gut suture can be used to reapproximate the skin. For full-thickness skin grafts, prioritize using similar skin (thin with fine vellus hairs only) and consider using a cotton bolster tied with 4–0 silk sutures to the surrounding skin. This gentle pressure promotes vascular growth into the graft. Should the skin reconstruction be along the eyelid margin, be sure to keep the skin exactly level with the tarsus. Skin that is too superior may rotate in (posteriorly) and cause an entropion, abrading the cornea. Tarsus that is too superior is less dangerous to the surface of the eye, but typically is not cosmetically acceptable. Sutures placed at the eyelid margin to affix the graft must be partial thickness (full-thickness sutures through the tarsus and conjunctiva can damage the cornea). Sutures along the eyelid margin should also be tied in a buried, interrupted fashion to ensure that the knot and the suture do not come in contact with the surface of the eye.

4.2.2 Full-Thickness Defects (Skin and Tarsal Defects)

In a full-thickness defect, the horizontal width determines the type of closure. The horizontal length of the

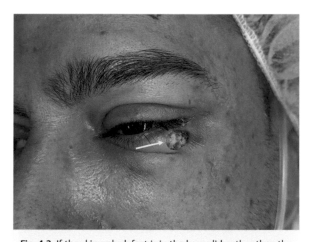

Fig. 4.3 If the skin-only defect is in the lower lid, rather than the lateral canthus as in ▶ Fig. 4.2a, closure should not be along a skin relaxing line. In the lower lid, this puts tension vertically and can result in ectropion. To avoid this, the tension should lie horizontally and closure should result in a scar that is perpendicular to the eyelid margin.

average palpebral fissure is about 30 mm and the defect size is examined in relation to this and separated into three groups: small (< 33% of the horizontal eyelid margin), moderate (33–50% of the horizontal eyelid margin), and large (> 50% of the horizontal eyelid margin).

Small Defect

A small defect (consisting of < 33% of the horizontal eyelid margin) can be reconstructed with direct closure with or without lateral canthotomy and cantholysis. Direct closure can be considered if the margins of the defect come together easily with little force. One way to check is to bring the edges together as far as they can stretch. If they can overlap by at least several millimeters, there is likely sufficient tissue to continue. If they are not able to overlap or cause the lower lid to retract, consider additional procedures, such as a lateral canthotomy and cantholysis to allow more laxity or alternative procedures, such as a Tenzel flap procedure.

Direct Closure

Direct closure commences with freshening up the margins to create tarsal edges that are straight and at 90 degrees to the eyelid margin. The next step is a vertical mattress suture along the eyelid margin. One arm of a double-armed, 6–0 polyglactin suture (Vicryl, Ethicon, New Brunswick, New Jersey, United States) is passed through the defect, 1 mm from the eyelid margin through the anterior portion of the tarsus, out through the gray line 1 mm from the eyelid margin, into the gray line 1 mm from the prior exit point and out through the anterior portion of the tarsus, keeping the sutures in the same plane throughout. This is repeated with the other arm of the double-armed suture through the other side of the defect. Once the two arms of the suture are now adjacent to one another, ensure that the suture and the future knot will not be touching the surface of the eye and tie the

knot, keeping the tails short (cut on the knot). The ideal vertical mattress suture here will evert the eyelid margin. Two sutures are then passed in a partial-thickness fashion through the tarsus to stabilize the eyelid. A final stabilizing suture is passed in a buried, interrupted fashion to reapproximate the eyelashes. Finally, the skin is approximated using interrupted or running 6–0 plain gut sutures (▶ Fig. 4.4).

Lateral Canthotomy/Cantholysis

Lateral canthotomy and cantholysis commence with a cut along the lateral canthus about 1 cm in length. A toothed forceps is used to grasp the lateral lid margin and retract this anteriorly. Scissors are used to strum and cut the desired arm of the lateral canthal tendon. For example, in a lower lid defect, this would be the inferior arm. Successful cantholysis can be confirmed when the lateral eyelid pulls away from the globe with ease. This allows the eyelid to be moved medially and can allow for direct closure (▶ Fig. 4.5). Once the primary defect site is closed via direct closure, the lateral canthus can be reformed with a buried, interrupted 6–0 plain gut suture at the desired location of the new canthal angle. An additional interrupted

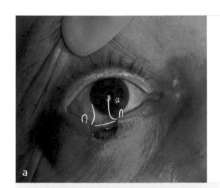
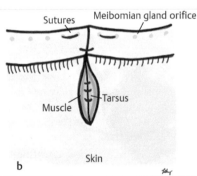
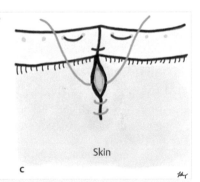

Fig. 4.4 Eyelid margin closure. **(a)** In a full-thickness defect that can be closed directly, the eyelid margins are first aligned and approximated with an interrupted, buried vertical mattress suture in the plane of the tarsus, taking care to avoid any suture exposure to the eye. This can be repeated in the plane of the eyelashes or a simple, buried interrupted suture can also be used at this location. **(b)** Two partial-thickness, interrupted sutures through the tarsus stabilize the eyelid margin. (Figure courtesy of Tiffany Cheng.) **(c)** The skin is then closed, using running or interrupted sutures. (Figure courtesy of Tiffany Cheng.)

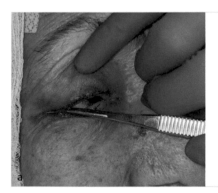
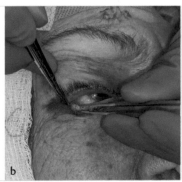

Fig. 4.5 Lateral canthotomy and cantholysis. **(a)** A lateral canthotomy commences with using scissors to incise the lateral canthus toward the lateral orbital rim. **(b)** Toothed forceps are then used to grasp the lateral eyelid margin and closed scissors used to palpate for the tendon. In the lower lid, the scissors should be pointed at the tip of the nose. The scissors are then used to cut through the tendon until the eyelid is lax enough to be pulled with ease away from the globe.

suture placed laterally at the level of the eyelashes reinforces this corner and the skin of the lateral canthal area can be approximated with the 6–0 plain gut suture as well.

Moderate Defect

Moderate defects (33–50% of the horizontal eyelid margin) can be addressed with the addition of a Tenzel semicircular flap to the direct closure. This consists of advancing tissue from the temple to form a new eyelid margin (▶ Fig. 4.6).

Commence by marking the Tenzel flap: in the lower lid; the curve will be superior, looking like a hill. The larger your "hill" is, the more tissue will be available to mobilize. Perform a superiorly angled, lateral canthotomy and lower cantholysis as described earlier in section "Small Defect." Incise and dissect the myocutaneous flap, staying in a superficial plane to avoid a branch of the facial nerve, which passes between the tragus of the ear and the tail of the brow. Once the margins of the defect can be opposed without tension, anchor the flap to the lateral orbital rim periosteum with a buried partial-thickness suture, such as a 5–0 polyglactin suture. Repair the eyelid margin as described in section "Direct Closure." The lateral portion of the eyelid will be now made of this flap and, thus, will be without eyelashes. This may require one or two interrupted, buried 6–0 polyglactin sutures to recreate a smooth eyelid margin.

Large Defect

Large defects (> 50% of the horizontal eyelid margin) can be addressed with a Hughes flap in the lower lid. Alternative options include a tarsoconjunctival graft with skin flap or a laterally based tarsoconjunctival flap with full-thickness skin graft or skin flap.

A Hughes procedure is used to reconstruct the tarsoconjunctival layer of a full-thickness defect of the lower eyelid that is too wide for reconstruction via a Tenzel flap. The Hughes flap carries its own blood supply and requires attachment to the upper lid for 4 weeks postoperatively. As the visual axis is completely covered for about a month, it should be avoided in patients who are monocular and using only that eye to see or in children younger than 10 years, who are at risk of developing amblyopia.

Commence by holding each edge of the defect toward each other with gentle traction and measuring the horizontal size of the defect. This will be the horizontal length of the Hughes flap. Place a 4–0 silk suture through the upper lid as a traction suture and evert the lid over a Desmarres retractor. On the posterior surface of the eyelid, mark 3 mm from the eyelid margin to indicate the inferior extent of the Hughes flap. Then mark the horizontal size of the flap using the measurement made initially. Use a no. 15 blade to carefully incise the conjunctiva and tarsus along the markings. Follow with a blunt-tipped Westcott scissors to dissect the tarsoconjunctival flap from the orbicularis oculi muscle. This should be extended superiorly into the conjunctiva to the point that the flap easily covers the defect. When suturing the flap in place, the superior border of the tarsus within the flap should be level with the superior border of the tarsus that is present medial and lateral to the defect. Use a 6–0 polyglactin suture to fixate the flap in this position with partial-thickness, interrupted sutures (▶ Fig. 4.7). This will need to remain in place for 3 to 4 weeks before undergoing the second stage of the Hughes flap procedure. The second stage requires local anesthesia into both the upper lid and the superior portion of the flap. Use Westcott scissors to divide the flap, erring on the side of leaving the flap edge too high, as this can always be trimmed more. If the margin appears wide or irregular, one or two interrupted, buried 6–0 polyglactin sutures can smooth out the eyelid margin. The remaining tarsoconjunctival flap in the upper lid should be either excised or recessed back into the upper lid fornix with buried interrupted

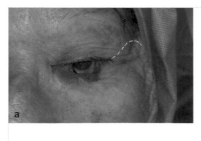
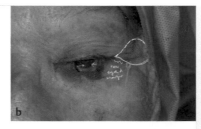
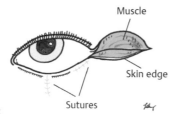
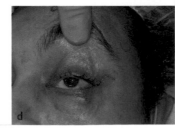

Muscle

Skin edge

Sutures

Fig. 4.6 The Tenzel semicircular flap. **(a)** The flap is marked in a semicircle on the opposite side of the defect. **(b)** The flap is dissected and rotated medially. **(c)** A suture is placed at the desired canthus to decrease tension on the eyelid margin defect and the eyelid margin defect is closed. (Figure courtesy of Tiffany Cheng.) **(d)** The end result is a newly formed eyelid margin laterally, which will not have eyelashes.

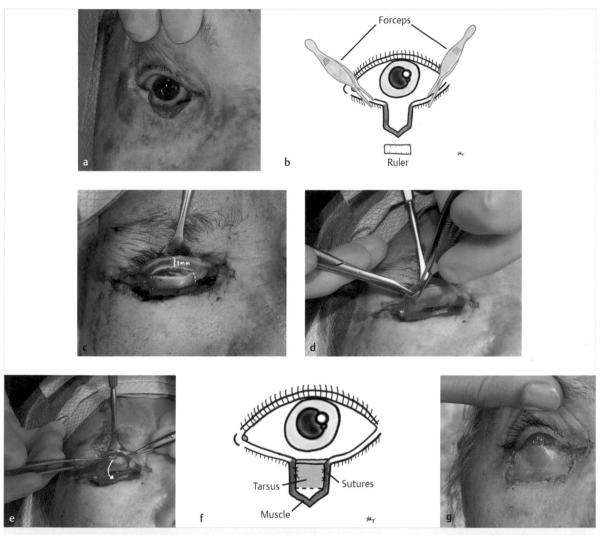

Fig. 4.7 The Hughes tarsoconjunctival flap. **(a)** In a large, lower lid defect, a Hughes tarsoconjunctival flap can be used to create a posterior lamella. **(b)** Use forceps to pull the edges of the defect together with gentle traction and measure the horizontal width of the defect. This will be the horizontal width of the flap. (Figure courtesy of Tiffany Cheng.) **(c)** On the tarsal conjunctival, mark 3 mm from the eyelid margin and incise with a no. 15 blade. This will be the inferior aspect of the flap. Then mark the medial and lateral aspects using the measurement from part **b**. **(d)** Use a Westcott scissors to extend the flap until it can cover the defect. **(e)** Rotate the flap inferiorly. **(f)** Fixate the flap with partial-thickness sutures so that the flap's superior border of the tarsus is flush with the superior border of the existing tarsus. (Figure courtesy of Tiffany Cheng.) **(g)** In this case, a full-thickness skin graft was used as the anterior lamellar substitute. In about 4 weeks, the eyelids can be separated in a second stage.

6–0 polyglactin sutures. The latter prevents retraction of the upper lid postoperatively.

At this point, the skin layer will need to be replaced. This can be done via a flap or graft. A myocutaneous flap can be rotated from the lateral area as done by a Mustarde flap (which is like a very large Tenzel flap). An inferior-based flap should be used cautiously as this has a risk of causing a cicatricial ectropion. Another alternative is a full-thickness skin graft. Press a nonadherent dressing into the defect and cut the impression out to create a template for the graft. Keep in mind that the template tends to be larger than necessary, so recheck the template's size

once it has been cut out. Then use the template to mark the skin at the donor site. Donor sites such as the upper eyelid can be closed with a 6–0 plain gut suture and sites like the pre- or postauricular skin can be closed with deep, buried 5–0 polyglactin sutures and the skin with a 5–0 chromic suture.

If the Hughes flap is not appropriate, other reconstructive options include a laterally based tarsoconjunctival flap from the upper lid or a tarsoconjunctival graft from the ipsilateral upper lid or the contralateral upper lid. Typically, two grafts should not be layered on top of one another due to the risk of poor vascular supply, so if a tarsoconjunctival graft is used, consider using a skin flap. Likewise, if using a skin graft, consider a tarsoconjunctival flap.

4.2.3 Key Points

The lower eyelid is unique in that skin closure along skin relaxing lines (where wrinkles typically form) should be avoided in most situations. This prevents vertical tension, which can cause an ectropion. Full-thickness defects can be addressed via direct closure ± lateral canthotomy and cantholysis, Tenzel flap, and Hughes tarsoconjunctival flap with skin flap or graft.

4.3 Upper Lid Unit

The upper lid can be approached similarly to the lower lid with a few small changes, mostly pertinent in defects categorized as large (> 50% of horizontal eyelid margin). Start by examining the defect for depth of involvement: skin only versus both skin and tarsus. Take note of the location medial to or involving the punctum, as this will require additional reconstruction in the form of a stent (see section "Medial Canthal Subunit").

4.3.1 Skin-Only Defects

Just like in the lower lid, skin-only defects be closed via healing by granulation, primary closure, primary closure with undermining, myocutaneous flaps, and full-thickness skin grafts. The only difference is that upper lid defects are less likely to result in ectropion, so closure can be done along skin relaxing lines (falling into or parallel to the preexisting rhytids; see section "Location").

4.3.2 Full-Thickness Defects (Skin and Tarsal Defects)

As in the upper lid, the horizontal width of the full-thickness defect determines the type of closure with some differences related to the vertical height of the tarsus in the upper versus lower lid (see section "Depth"). Additionally, full-thickness defects of the lateral portion of the eyelid may involve the lacrimal gland. The lacrimal gland is made of two lobes, the palpebral and orbital. The palpebral is more superficial, can be seen on eversion of the eyelid, and contains the ducts, which allow passage of tears from the gland to the surface of the eye. Damage to the palpebral lobe can result in severe dry eye issues, so manipulation should be avoided if possible.

Small Defect

A small defect (consisting of < 33% of the horizontal eyelid margin) can be reconstructed with direct closure with or without lateral canthotomy and cantholysis. This is described in section "Depth."

Moderate Defect

Moderate defects (33–50% of the horizontal eyelid margin) can be addressed with direct closure with Tenzel semicircular flap. This is described in section "Depth" with the only difference being that the lateral canthotomy should by inferiorly angled (instead of superiorly) and the Tenzel flap marked as a "U" shape (instead of as a hill).

Large Defect

Large defects (> 50% of the horizontal eyelid margin) can be addressed with a Cutler–Beard flap in the upper lid. Alternative options are similar to the lower lid and include a tarsoconjunctival graft with skin flap or a laterally based tarsoconjunctival flap with full-thickness skin graft or skin flap.

A Cutler–Beard procedure is used to reconstruct a full-thickness defect of the upper eyelid, which is too wide for a Tenzel flap. This carries its own blood supply and requires attachment to the upper lid for 6 to 8 weeks postoperatively. Therefore, it should be avoided in patients who are monocular and using only that eye to see or in children younger than 10 years, who are at risk of developing amblyopia. It is also more challenging technically with higher likelihood of revision surgery than a Hughes procedure.

Commence by holding each edge of the defect toward each other gently and measuring the horizontal size of the defect. Place a 4–0 silk suture through the lower lid as a traction suture and evert the lid over a cotton-tipped applicator. The original procedure describes the next step as marking 2 mm inferior to the inferior border of the tarsus to represent the superior aspect of the Cutler–Beard flap. Next, mark the horizontal size measured initially medially and laterally on the conjunctival surface and use a no. 15 blade to carefully incise along the newly marked superior border of the flap, extending inferiorly along the medial and lateral aspects using Westcott scissors. This extension inferiorly should be sufficient to allow the flap to easily cover the defect. Some surgeons have amended the procedure to split the anterior and posterior lamella and suture in a firmer material, like ear cartilage, to provide more stability to the postoperative upper lid. Use a 6–0 polyglactin suture in a partial-thickness interrupted fashion to fixate the flap into the defect (▸ Fig. 4.8). This will need to remain in place for 6 to 8 weeks before undergoing the second stage of the Cutler–Beard flap procedure. The second stage requires local anesthesia into both the upper lid and the superior portion of the flap, followed by Westcott scissors to divide the flap. If the margin appears wide or irregular, one or two interrupted,

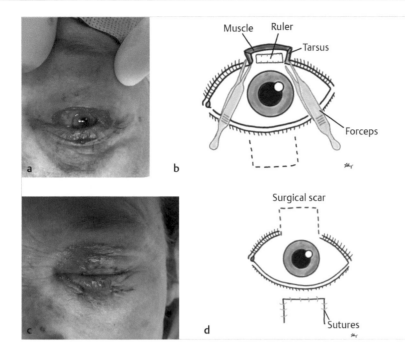

a

b

c

d

Muscle Ruler
Tarsus
Forceps
Surgical scar
Sutures

Fig. 4.8 The Cutler–Beard flap. **(a)** In a large, upper lid defect, a Cutler–Beard flap can be used for reconstruction. **(b)** Use forceps to pull the edges of the defect together with gentle traction and measure the horizontal width of the defect. This will be the horizontal width of the flap. Use this to mark the flap's horizontal width on the lower lid. Then, mark the superior aspect of the flap 2 mm from the eyelid margin. (Figure courtesy of Tiffany Cheng.) **(c)** Use a no. 15 blade to incise along the skin markings and mobilize the flap underneath the lower eyelid margin bridge. Fixate with sutures into the upper lid defect. Some surgeons utilize autologous ear cartilage between the conjunctiva and the skin to provide stability to the future upper lid. **(d)** The eyelids are separated in a second stage after about 6 to 8 weeks. (Figure courtesy of Tiffany Cheng.)

buried 6–0 polyglactin sutures can smooth out the eyelid margin.

Other reconstructive options are similar to the lower lid (see section "Depth").

4.3.3 Key Points

The upper eyelid is unique in that reconstructive options are limited by the shorter height of the lower lid. Full-thickness defects can be addressed via direct closure ± lateral canthotomy and cantholysis, Tenzel flap, and Cutler–Beard full-thickness flap.

4.4 Lateral Canthal Subunit

The lateral canthal area is more straightforward, requiring skin flaps or grafts without a tarsal replacement. One of the few important principles here is that the lateral canthal tendon is typically 2 mm higher than the medial canthal tendon and inserts on the inside of the lateral orbit rim. When recreating the lateral canthus, a lateral tarsal strip can be used.[2] If a lateral canthotomy/cantholysis is performed to allow more laxity, the canthus can be reformed by approximating the eyelid skin in the canthal angle with a buried, interrupted 6–0 plain gut suture through the lateral canthus along the gray line and also along the lash line. If the lid is under too much tension horizontally due to lack of sufficient posterior lamella, extra tissue can be obtained by utilizing the periosteum in the lateral orbital area. A periosteal flap can be created and rotated medially to act as a tarsal substitute laterally for the upper or lower eyelid (► Fig. 4.9).[3]

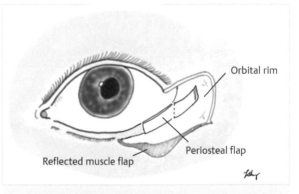

Orbital rim
Periosteal flap
Reflected muscle flap

Fig. 4.9 A periosteal flap can be created from the lateral orbital rim to create a lateroposterior lamella. (Figure courtesy of Tiffany Cheng.)

4.4.1 Key Points

The lateral canthal tendon inserts 2 mm superior to the medial canthal tendon and into the inside of the lateral orbital rim. Care should be taken during reconstruction over the zygoma to prevent damage to the frontal branch of the facial nerve as it passes over the zygomatic arch.

4.5 Medial Canthal Subunit

The medial canthal area includes the tear drainage system, as well as the medial canthal tendon.

The canaliculi, as mentioned earlier, require immediate stenting and reconstruction to prevent permanent epiphora. The simplest way to address this is to use a monocanicular, self-retaining stent, such as a Mini Monoka

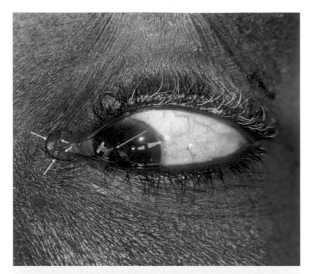

Fig. 4.10 This skin-only defect of the medial canthus was deep enough to involve the canaliculus. This was discovered on probing the lower lid punctum and irrigating saline, which promptly pooled into the defect, instead of entering the nasopharynx. A monocanalicular, self-retaining stent is featured here, already partially inserted into the punctum and canaliculus. The portion of the stent that allows for self-retention (*green arrow*) needs to be buried into the canaliculus so that the end of the stent lies flush with the eyelid margin. Once this is inserted completely, the skin can be closed in the direction of the *yellow arrows*.

(FCI Ophthalmics, Pembroke, Massachusetts, United States; ▶ Fig. 4.10). This avoids retrieval of the stent in the inferior meatus as required by prior stents. Once the stent has been placed through the punctum and the canaliculus, the eyelid margin can be repaired around this using buried, interrupted 6–0 polyglactin suture. It is important that the suture and its tails do not rub against the surface of the eye, as this can cause pain and can damage the vision permanently.

The medial canthal tendon provides structure for the eyelid and, if lax or misplaced, will cause an undesired aesthetic outcome and epiphora. Reconstruction of the medial canthal tendon is technically challenging and requires sutures to the periosteum of the deep medial orbital wall, near the posterior lacrimal crest. This is posterior to the lacrimal sac, so care should be taken to avoid damage to the nasolacrimal system. If the periosteum is not present, alternatives for medial canthal tendon reconstruction include anchors, plating, and transnasal wiring.

4.5.1 Key Points

Medial canthal defects should be evaluated for a damaged tear drainage system or medial canthal tendon.

Canalicular damage requires immediate reconstruction to avoid epiphora, typically with the insertion of a stent. If the medial canthal tendon is not properly reattached, this can result in telecanthus, unusual angling of the medial canthus, and epiphora.

4.6 Conclusion

Eyelid reconstruction is complicated but can be facilitated via an approach broken down into four main tenets. First, care must be taken at all times to protect the eye, both intraoperatively and postoperatively. Second, whereas skin-only defects can be addressed with skin-only reconstructive options, full-thickness defects require reconstruction of both the anterior and posterior lamellae. Third, damage to the upper tear drainage system, the canaliculi, requires immediate reconstruction to prevent permanent, postoperative epiphora. Finally, reconstruction of the defect requires categorization of location, depth, and horizontal size. In these complex cases, collaboration with an ophthalmic plastic surgeon (oculoplastics) can improve outcomes.

When addressing the upper and lower lid full-thickness defects, this is based on the horizontal length of the defect in comparison to the total horizontal length. These differ between the upper and lower lids, due to the short tarsal height of the lower lid.

Reconstruction of the lateral canthal defects requires understanding of the higher location of the lateral canthal tendon in relation to the medial canthal tendon and also its insertion onto the periosteum of the inner lateral orbital wall. Care during reconstruction over the zygoma prevents damage to the frontal branch of the facial nerve as it passes over the zygomatic arch.

Finally, reconstruction of the medial canthal defects is arguably the most complicated. Defects should be explored to rule out involvement of the tear drainage system or the medial canthal tendon. Canalicular damage should be repaired within days as treatments are limited once scarring occurs. Medial canthal tendon reinsertion is technically challenging and involves sutures, anchors, and/or transnasal anchoring into the medial orbital wall, posterior to the lacrimal sac.

References

[1] Black EH, Nesi FA, Calvano CJ, Gladstone GJ, Levine MR. Smith and Nesi's Ophthalmic Plastic and Reconstructive Surgery. New York, NY: Springer; 2011:551–569

[2] Anderson RL, Gordy DD. The tarsal strip procedure. Arch Ophthalmol. 1979; 97(11):2192–2196

[3] Weinstein GS, Anderson RL, Tse DT, Kersten RC. The use of a periosteal strip for eyelid reconstruction. Arch Ophthalmol. 1985; 103(3):357–359

5 Reconstruction of the Cheek

Jenna Wald and C. William Hanke

Summary

Reconstruction of surgical defects on the cheek is a common occurrence in micrographic dermatologic surgery. The cheek frequently has an excess of laxity allowing for most defects to be closed primarily in a curvilinear fashion. Due to tumor neglect because of hair coverage on the lateral/preauricular cheeks, field cancerization, and the diverse nature of the topography and skin quality of the cheek, some defects require more advanced repairs. This chapter provides a systematic approach to cheek reconstruction based on the subunit involved.

Keywords: cheek, cheek reconstruction, cheek anatomy, superficial musculoaponeurotic system, relaxed skin tension lines, V-to-Y flap, rotation flap, transposition flap

5.1 Introduction

The cheek is the largest cosmetic unit of the face. It is comprised of four aesthetic subunits, each with unique topography and skin characteristics. Each subunit, therefore, has unique cosmetic concerns and challenges during reconstruction. The abundance of tissue allows many repairs to be completed with primary closures arranged in relaxed skin tension lines (RSTLs). However, more complicated repairs are often necessary. The cheek has a smooth contour, which makes incisions difficult to camouflage. Reconstruction can affect facial symmetry and potentially alter functionality when tension distorts free margins. A number of factors should be considered when planning cheek reconstruction, including: RSTLs, adjacent structures with free margins, skin characteristics, and mobility of facial skin. The cheek can be divided into up to seven cosmetic subunits, but for the purpose of this chapter, it will be discussed as four subunits: the medial cheek, buccal cheek, zygomatic cheek, and lateral cheek (▶ Fig. 5.1). This chapter will explore the characteristics of each subunit and considerations for repair.

5.2 Anatomy

The cheek is the largest unit of the face with multiple flat, concave, and convex surfaces. The borders include the nasofacial sulcus, nasolabial fold, mandible, preauricular sulcus, zygomatic arch, and infraorbital rim. Depending on the subunit and size of the defect, the repair may be as simple as a primary closure or as complex as a regional or multicomponent repair. The cheek has several features that facilitate reconstruction including the following: (1) a rich and redundant vascular network, (2) several fixed anatomic points for tacking sutures, and (3) the

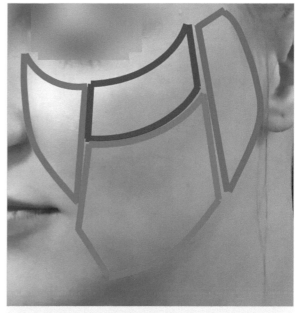

Fig. 5.1 The cheek can be divided into four cosmetic subunits: the medial cheek (*outlined in blue*), buccal cheek (*outlined in green*), zygomatic cheek (*outlined in red*), and lateral cheek (*outlined in orange*).

superficial musculoaponeurotic system (SMAS) for plication sutures. No matter the type of repair, understanding of innervation and anatomy is paramount. The goal of reconstruction should be to restore function, cosmesis, and facial symmetry.

5.2.1 Soft Tissue

Each subunit of the cheek is characterized by unique features. The superior periocular tissue of the medial and zygomatic cheek is characterized by thin, lightly pigmented skin. Due to the movement of the orbicularis oculi muscle, the periocular region is marked by both dynamic and static rhytids.[1] Inferiorly, the skin becomes thicker and more heavily pigmented as it covers the protruding malar eminence and zygomatic arch. The lateral subunit has less subcutaneous fat than adjacent subunits. The skin of the lateral subunit has variable hair abundance and quality.

Movement of tissue in both the zygomatic and lateral subunits is limited by its fixation to the SMAS and zygomatic-retaining ligament.[1] The zygomatic-retaining ligament is a point of fixation from the soft tissue to the zygomatic arch. Along with the orbicularis and the upper masseteric and mandibular ligaments, the zygomatic ligament resists cutaneous distension and creates cutaneous grooves as individuals age.[1] The cutaneous grooves deepen with age and provide an area to conceal surgical incisions. Division of these ligaments may increase tissue mobility.

Under the subcutaneous fat of the lateral and buccal subunits, the parotid gland courses perpendicular to the masseter muscle. It is located below the SMAS and above the fascia of the masseter.[2] The parotid duct (Stensen's ducts) lies in the buccal subunit. It is relatively deep and unlikely to be affected during reconstruction; however, if it is damaged, surgical repair is necessary.

5.2.2 Innervation

Motor innervation of the cheek is via cranial nerve VII (the facial nerve). The facial nerve exits the skull via the stylomastoid foramen and then enters the parotid gland where it is protected as it divides into five branches. The parotid gland therefore serves as a warning that caution should be exercised to prevent trauma or transection of the facial nerve branches. These branches exit the gland covered only by the SMAS and skin before they enter the deep surface of the muscles.[3,4]

In the lateral subunit of the cheek, the facial nerve is protected by the parotid gland, thereby reducing risk of damage. In the medial subunit of the cheek, damage to motor nerves is mitigated by anastomosing facial nerve branches. Additionally, the nerves are below the muscle in this subunit, decreasing the risk of trauma.[2,4]

The two branches of the facial nerve at highest risk of damage are the marginal mandibular and temporal branches. The marginal mandibular branch is covered only by skin, subcutaneous fat, and the platysma muscle as it crosses the mandible in the buccal subunit and is at high risk of trauma.[2] The marginal mandibular branch innervates the depressors of the lower lip. Damage therefore can lead to asymmetry of the mouth. The temporal branch of the facial nerve is at risk in the zygomatic subunit as the nerve crosses the zygomatic arch and enters the temple. During its path to the temporalis muscle, the temporal branch is covered only by the fascia, skin, and subcutaneous fat.[3] Damage to the temporal branch can result in paralysis of the ipsilateral frontalis muscle.

Sensory innervation of the cheek is through cranial nerve V (the trigeminal nerve). The maxillary branch (V2) innervates the medial and zygomatic subunits via the infraorbital, zygomaticofacial, and zygomaticotemporal branches. The inferomedial cheek is additionally innervated by the mental nerve. The mandibular branch innervates the lateral and buccal subunits via the buccal and auriculotemporal branches.[1,4]

5.2.3 Vascular Supply/Lymphatics

Two main arteries contribute to the vascularization of the cheek: the facial artery and the superficial temporal artery. Both arise from the external carotid artery. The facial artery traverses the cheek medially and then continues superiorly as the angular artery.[2] The facial artery and its branches supply much of the inferior face, including the parotideomasseteric region, the buccal, infraorbital, and paranasal cheek.[4] The superficial temporal artery arises within the parotid gland and runs anterior to the tragus where it branches into the transverse facial artery. The infraorbital artery, which exits the skull via the infraorbital foramen, connects with the facial artery. It is a minor contributor that arises from the internal carotid artery.[4] Almost all repairs of the cheek will be random and rely on the perfusion of the dermal plexus rather than a main artery.[2] Because of the rich plexus of anastomoses, transection of vessels rarely compromises vascular supply.[2,4]

Venous drainage of the cheek largely mirrors the associated arterial circulation. Their paths ultimately drain in a variable pattern to the external and internal jugular veins.

It is important to note that lymphatic drainage of the cheek involves several lymphatic chains, which may overlap. This requires a more thorough clinical examination to evaluate for metastasis. The periorbital and temporal regions drain into the intra- or periparotid nodes. Meanwhile, the medial cheek and adjacent regions drain into the submandibular nodes. The majority of the nodes, however, will eventually connect with the jugular chain.[4]

5.3 Clinical Considerations

Surgical defects on the cheek can often be closed primarily with the long axis in an RSTL or at the junction of cosmetic units.[5] Surgical incisions placed in the curvilinear RSTLs can result in fine-line scars. When planning reconstruction, it is important to consider the facial changes that will occur as the patient ages. Surgical planning should include evaluation of the patient in a seated position with their mouth (1) at rest, (2) smiling, and (3) open. Surgical repairs in young patients without rhytids, bony resorption, or atrophic fat pads should be designed to be camouflaged by the wrinkles and aging changes that will occur later in life. Additionally, primary closures in young or overweight patients may need to be longer than the traditional 3:1 ratio to prevent unsightly standing cones. Adjacent tissue is often adequate to close a surgical defect on the cheek. However, factors such as large surgical defect size, young age, chronic actinic damage, multiple surgical procedures or scarring, and proximity to adjacent free or fixed structures may limit available tissue, necessitating more complex reconstructions requiring nonadjacent tissue reservoirs.

When primary closure cannot be achieved, all efforts should be made to keep the subsequent repair within a single subunit in order to provide the best tissue match. Each cheek subunit has different characteristics such as skin thickness, color and quality, and presence or absence of hair. For example, the medial cheek skin is often thick because of increased numbers of sebaceous glands. The lateral cheek of men and some women may be hair bearing and it is important to consider the cosmetic problems that may result from transferring hair-bearing skin to non–hair-bearing portions of the cheek. Due to these features, skin grafts or healing by second intention often lead to poor cosmetic outcomes and are generally considered unacceptable.[6]

When defects are present near the junction of cosmetic units, the closure can be completely or partially hidden in the adjacent anatomic junction. For repairs extending beyond the cheek that involve multiple facial units, it is usually ideal to repair each subunit independently. This will result in multicomponent repairs. Multicomponent repairs of adjacent subunits are one of the few situations when second intention healing or a graft may be appropriate.

Although the cheek as a whole has considerations for repair, each subunit also has characteristics that will affect repair choices. Simple repairs are nearly always better. When necessary, more complex repairs are determined by the unique features of the subunit.

5.4 Algorithm for Cheek Reconstruction

Multiple approaches have been suggested for reconstruction of the cheek.[1,5,7,8,9] Although a strict algorithm is difficult to apply, predictable patterns may be applied to reconstruction.[1,5] Common themes in the algorithms include preference of primary closure when possible, followed by analysis of location and defect size. The various algorithms divide the cheek into three to five subunits.

Dobratz and Hilger begin their algorithm by a subunit in which the defect is located; as with this chapter, they consider four subunits for reconstruction (lateral, zygomatic, medial, and buccal).[1] Next, they consider the size of the defect. For all subunits, the closure of choice for small defects is primary. They point out that the lateral subunit, which has limited mobility, lacks of redundancy, and is in close proximity to the ear, may require a transposition flap even for small defects. For medium defects of the lateral subunit (2–3 cm), they recommend consideration of cheek advancement or rotation flaps. For large defects, they recommend the use of cervicofacial flaps and discuss the utilization of axial based flaps. The zygomatic unit is also limited in mobility and they recommend the use of transposition flaps for medium defects; this is to prevent ocular distortion. For closures of small defects of the medial cheek, the authors suggest the use of V-Y advancement flaps for maintenance of the melolabial fold. For medium and large defects of the medial cheek, they endorse advancement flaps, with emphasis on preventing distortion of the ocular unit as well as

placing surgical incisions at anatomic boundaries. When addressing the medium defects of the buccal subunit, they suggest transposition flaps, but acknowledge the scars are usually not ideal. For large buccal defects, they again recommend cervicofacial flaps. This algorithm, like others, focuses on location and size; it additionally addresses the possibility of free margin distortion. It does not, however, address skin quality such as hair and seems to encourage the use of larger repairs for medium to large defects that may be otherwise reconstructed with less morbid repairs.

Başağaoğlu et al divide the cheek into three subunits (suborbital, preauricular, and buccomandibular).[7] They begin by suggesting defects less than 2 cm on concave locations may be closed by secondary intention but do acknowledge the potential contraction and prolonged healing course. For surgical defects less than 2 cm not on concave surfaces, they suggest primary closure. The authors endorse the use of skin grafts, only for patients who are unable to tolerate larger procedures. Contrary to the prior algorithm, Başağaoğlu et al report that local flaps provide a good cosmetic result. They suggest the rabbit ear flap for intermediate defects of the zygomatic and buccal regions,[10] and the finger transposition flap for the medial cheek.[11] They endorse combination flaps. For intermediate to large defects, cervicofacial free flaps are useful. Although this approach takes size and other characteristics into account, it only minimally changes the approach by subunit.

Rapstine et al's approach was based on a review of 400 cases based primarily on size and then location.[5] They also divide the cheek into three zones, which mirror the three subunits of Başağaoğlu et al. Their preferred method for all defect locations and sizes is primary closure. If they are unable to close primarily, defects are differentiated by size less than or greater than 2 cm, and proximity to free margins. Defects of the medial and buccal unit approaching the nose or mouth less than 2 cm are closed via the crescentic advancement. Defects greater than 2 cm are closed with the cervicofacial advancement or full-thickness skin graft. The final leg of the algorithm suggests a bilobed or V-Y advancement flap for defects abutting the chin. The algorithm presented is simple. They report limited use of flaps due to an inability to provide color-matched skin. We feel this algorithm underutilizes local smaller flaps as repair options. Additionally, it encourages the use of grafts, which we have found to be typically unsuitable for cheek reconstruction.

Chandawarkar and Cervino divided the cheek into five zones (which correlate with the medial upper and lower, lateral upper and lower, and central cheek) for their approach based on a review of 160 patients.[8] Medial upper cheek defects were reconstructed with V-Y advancement flaps. The remaining subunits were repaired with transposition flaps with the pedicle determined by hair and defect size. They prefer laterally based flaps, but acknowledge the lateral inferior zone often requires a medial base due to its proximity to the ear. Although the approach does address repair directionality by zone, it is limited by utilizing two repairs and does not include discussion of other techniques.

Meaike et al divide the cheek into three zones (suborbital, preauricular, and buccomandibular).[9] Their approach is primarily determined by defect size. They endorse vertical primary closure as the preferred closure method. As with many others, they believe a longer linear scar is better than that of a transposition flap. If primary closure is not possible, transposition flaps are indicated. For defects greater than 3 to 4 cm, a cervicofacial flap is recommended. Free tissue transfer is discussed as an option for select situations.

We describe an algorithm that encompasses the various approaches and regions described by the aforementioned approaches. Our approach begins with stratification by location, followed by size, and finally skin characteristics. Our approach with order of preference is outlined in ▶ Fig. 5.2. Detailed discussion of the closure type and consideration by region can be found in ▶ Table 5.1. The following sections apply and discuss this approach, along with special considerations for each subunit.

5.5 Medial Subunit

The medial cheek is an area of significant cosmetic concern because it is a part of the central face that includes the nose, glabellar complex, and lips. The skin quality of

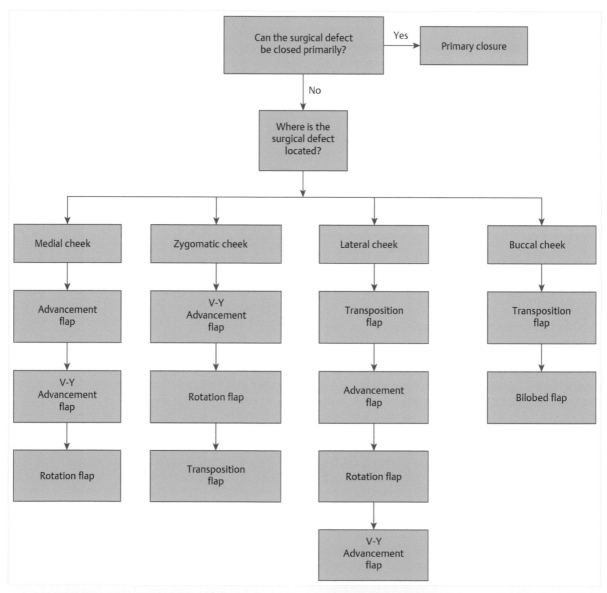

Fig. 5.2 Approach to reconstruction of the cheek.

Table 5.1 Repair options of the cheek

Repair type	Advantages	Disadvantages	Considerations	When to use
Skin graft	• Can be done in patients who cannot tolerate larger reconstructions	• Higher failure rate due to cheek movement	• May be used in combination with other repairs for large defects	• In combination with other repairs for large defects • Patients who cannot tolerate repair via other methods
Second intention	• Minimizes reconstructive surgery	• Prolonged wound care • Increased chance of distortion of free margins • Poor cosmesis	• Rarely used due to poor cosmesis and surrounding reservoirs of tissue available • May leave alopecic patch	• Use is unlikely but may be possible in small, superficial defects on the concave surface of the lateral subunit
Primary closure	• Simple repair • No change in hair or skin gradient • Scar easily hidden in RSTL • Camouflaged by rhytids of the buccal or periocular zygomatic/lateral subunit • Easy to monitor for recurrence	• Medial and zygomatic: may lead to ocular distortion • Use on large defects of buccal unit may cause eclabium	• May require M-plasty to prevent free margin distortion • Medial and zygomatic defects involving the convex surface frequently require apical angles < 30 degrees leading to scar elongation	• First-line repair when possible for all defects of all subunits
Advancement flap	• Good survival • Incisions can be hidden at unit junctions • Can maintain skin and hair gradients • Burow's triangle may be hidden in postauricular region	• Requires extensive undermining • Lateral tension may create free margin distortion	• Requires tissue laxity • May require thinning for superomedial subunit • Tacking sutures are frequently required to prevent free margin distortion when used in medial or zygomatic subunits • Fascial sutures are used to decrease tension on wound edges	• Medium to large defects of medial and lateral subunits
V-Y advancement flap	• Good survival • Random vascular base allows for utilization in all subunits • Incisions can be placed in RSTL and hidden in unit boundaries • Permits filling of deep defects • Significant movement achieved with minimal undermining	• Triangular shape may be notable • Risk of pincushion effect	• Tacking sutures should be used in medial and zygomatic subunit to prevent ocular distortion	• Used in place of larger more morbid flaps • Small to medium defects of the zygomatic cheek • Medium to large defects of medial and buccal cheek
Rotation flap	• Good survival • Incisions may be hidden at subunit junctions • Allows for recruitment of large amounts of tissue • Recruits tissue from multiple directions due to pivotal component	• Increased risk of hematoma • Requires large amount of undermining • Increased surgical time	• Tacking sutures may be used to prevent free margin distortion • Fascial sutures may be used to decrease tension on free edge	• Large defects of medial, zygomatic, and lateral cheek • Patients should be able to undergo large procedure

(Continued)

Table 5.1 (*Continued*) Repair options of the cheek

Repair type	Advantages	Disadvantages	Considerations	When to use
Transposition flap	• Good survival • Low complication • Redirection of tension vector • Recruit tissue from varying directions	• May transport/disrupt hair patterns • Create irregular multicomponent scars not easily hidden	• Tension should be directed to prevent free margin distortion • Movement is limited on lateral cheek	• Medium defects of the zygomatic cheek unable to be closed by other means • Medium to large defects of the lateral and buccal cheek
Bilobed flap	• Recruits tissue nonadjacent to the defect	• Requires significant undermining • May transport/disrupt hair patterns • Create irregular multicomponent scars not easily hidden	• Allows for closure of large defects of the buccal cheek	• Large defects of the buccal cheek unable to be closed by other means

Abbreviation: RSTL, resting skin tension line.

the medial cheek is variable. Superiorly, the skin is thin and fragile as it approaches the medial canthus. Inferiorly, it is thicker and more sebaceous. The malar eminence and fat pad add convexity to the medial subunit. As patients age, the fat pad undergoes atrophy and increased mobility of the skin often develops.[1]

The medial subunit is defined by the medial orbital rim, nasofacial sulcus, and nasolabial fold. These junctions can be useful to camouflage surgical incisions. However, caution should be exercised to prevent tension on free margins, which can cause distortion of the nasal ala, eclabium, or ectropion. It is also important to retain the definition of these junctions because blunting can cause facial asymmetry.

Depending on the size of the surgical defect, the patient's age and weight, and texture of the skin, many medial cheek defects can be repaired primarily. When this is not possible, additional tissue may be taken from the lateral and inferior tissue reservoirs by utilizing advancement flaps or V-Y advancement flaps.[6] Prior teaching advocated the use of larger repairs to hide suture lines in the anatomic unit junctions. However, current trends suggest smaller and simpler repairs utilizing local tissue. It has been our experience that even large defects of the medial cheek can be closed with local advancement flaps, avoiding larger flaps that require extensive tissue recruitment from the lateral cheek. For the medial cheek, flaps such as the rhombic, bilobed, or O-Z may be utilized to close the defect, but often produce unsightly scars.

5.5.1 Advancement Flap

The large surgical defect of the inferomedial cheek shown in ▶ Fig. 5.3a was repaired with an advancement flap. Standing cones superior and inferior to the defect were removed (▶ Fig. 5.3a). Adequate undermining of the cheek was performed (▶ Fig. 5.3b). Hemostasis was carefully achieved with electrocoagulation. A tacking suture was placed from the SMAS to the dorsal nasal periosteum to prevent distortion of the dorsal nose and maintain the position of the nasofacial sulcus. Additional tacking sutures were then placed from the SMAS to the pyriform aperture to prevent lateral traction on the nasal ala (▶ Fig. 5.3c). The deep layer was closed using 5–0 polyglactin 910 sutures and epidermal closure was achieved with 5–0 nylon sutures.

A primary closure of the large defect in ▶ Fig. 5.3a was not possible due to the proximity to the nose. Adequate adjacent tissue was present to repair the defect with an advancement flap. The advancement flap was selected because it required less undermining and constituted a smaller procedure. If unsuccessful, due to inadequate tissue movement or nasal distortion, the repair could be converted to a rotation flap with recruitment of tissue from the lateral cheek (▶ Fig. 5.3a). The additional arc along the orbital rim allows for additional tissue movement, creating a rotation flap.

In patients with skin laxity, medium to large surgical defects of the medial cheek can be repaired with relative simplicity. As with other cheek defects, incisions should be created in RSTL or along unit junctions (the nasofacial sulcus) when possible. When lateral tension is present, a tacking suture to the pyriform aperture can prevent distortion of the nasal ala and prevent spreading of the scar. Additionally, tacking sutures to the nasal periosteum can help maintain the nasofacial sulcus and prevent nasal distortion.

Key points for medial cheek repairs using advancement flaps are the following:
• Medium to large defects on the medial cheek can be closed with advancement flaps.

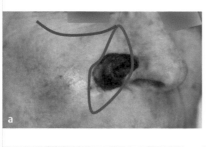
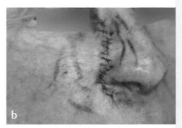
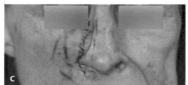
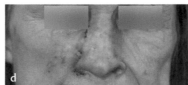

Fig. 5.3 **(a)** A large surgical defect is present on the inferomedial cheek approaching the nasal ala. The *blue outline* indicates the standing cones that were removed. If the surgical defect cannot be closed with the advancement flap (*outlined in blue*), an incision can be made along the orbital junction to create a rotation flap (*shown in orange*). **(b)** Suture closure of the surgical wound was achieved with an advancement flap. The *purple markings* indicate the extent of undermining that was performed. **(c)** Fascial sutures were placed in the superficial musculoaponeurotic system (SMAS) to prevent lateral displacement of the nasal dorsum. Tacking sutures were placed in the pyriform aperture to prevent lateral displacement of the nasal ala. **(d)** At the time of suture removal, no evidence of nasal distortion was present.

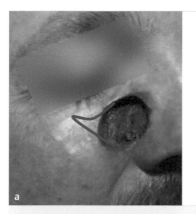
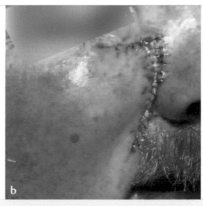
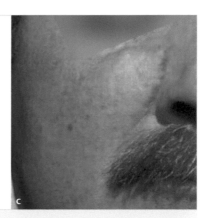

Fig. 5.4 **(a)** A large surgical defect on the medial cheek approaches the medial canthus. The surgical defect was repaired with a rotation flap. The inferiorly based rotation flap repair is *outlined in blue*. **(b)** The closure was achieved with the removal of a small standing cone laterally. Tacking sutures to the nasal bone periosteum were placed to prevent ectropion. Surgical incisions were placed in anatomic boundary lines. **(c)** Follow-up at 4 weeks demonstrated a well-healed erythematous surgical scar. At 6 months of follow-up, erythema resolved completely.

- Fascial sutures to the SMAS can prevent lateral nasal displacement and maintain the natural position of the nasofacial sulcus.
- Tacking sutures to the nasal periosteum and pyriform aperture are important to prevent nasal distortion.

5.5.2 Rotation Flap

The horizontally oriented defect in ▶ Fig. 5.4a was repaired with an inferiorly based rotation flap. The rotational arc was created along the nasofacial sulcus and nasolabial fold (▶ Fig. 5.4a). A small Burow's triangle was removed from the lateral wound edge, which allowed the incision to be hidden at the junction of the orbital rim (▶ Fig. 5.4b). The flap was undermined and hemostasis achieved. Tacking sutures from the SMAS to the orbital rim were placed to

prevent ectropion. The deep layer was closed using 5–0 polyglactin 910 sutures and epidermal closure was achieved with 5–0 nylon sutures.

Surgical defects on the medial cheek, which have a horizontal orientation, can often be repaired with a primary closure or advancement flap. However, as with the defect in ▶ Fig. 5.4a, larger defects on the medial cheek may require movement of additional tissue from the lateral and/or inferior cheek. This can be achieved with a rotation flap. Due to the large size and limited mobility of the surrounding tissue, the defect in ▶ Fig. 5.4a was repaired with an inferiorly based rotation flap. Alternately, a laterally based rotation flap would have required significant undermining and more potential morbidity. Although prior teachings frequently advocated larger flaps in order to keep the surgical lines in the anatomic junctions, it is our experience that smaller flaps outside of the junction lines often provide excellent results with less morbidity.

Rotation flaps combine advancement with a pivotal element, which allows for tissue movement from more than one direction. Rotation flaps are often useful in overweight or younger patients who typically have less skin laxity. The direction of rotation may be determined by the orientation of the defect. Repair of a vertically oriented defect, which requires movement of tissue from the lateral cheek, will extend the arc along the orbital rim/to the zygomatic cheek. A back cut may be made if necessary. When possible, this incision should be placed in lateral canthal rhytids. To prevent nasal distortion, tacking sutures to the pyriform aperture may be required. Horizontally oriented defects, on the other hand, will likely require movement of the tissue from the inferior cheek, and the arc of rotation will most likely follow the nasofacial sulcus and nasolabial fold. When moving tissue from the inferior cheek, it is important that vertical tension be limited in order to prevent ectropion. Tacking sutures to the orbital rim periosteum or the medial canthal tendon may decrease this risk of ectropion. For larger defects, placation sutures may be placed in the fascia to minimize tension on the flap.

Key points for medial cheek repairs using rotation flaps are the following:

- Medial cheek defects of almost all sizes can be repaired using rotation flaps.
- Vertically oriented defects can usually be repaired using laterally recruited tissue. In these instances, tacking sutures to the pyriform aperture can be utilized to prevent nasal distortion.
- Horizontally oriented defects can often be repaired using inferiorly recruited tissue. For these repairs, tacking sutures to the medial canthus or orbital rim may be required to prevent ectropion.
- When designing a rotation flap on the medial cheek, most surgical lines can be hidden in anatomic junctions.

5.5.3 V-Y Advancement Flap

The large surgical defect outlined in ▸ Fig. 5.5 was repaired with a V-Y advancement flap. The medial border of the flap was created along the nasofacial sulcus to camouflage the incision. The lateral incision was placed in the RSTL. Placement of the surgical incisions allowed for closure of the secondary defect (i.e., "kite-tail") to be placed in an RSTL (▸ Fig. 5.5). The flap was undermined in all directions with a central pedicle remaining until adequate movement was achieved. After hemostasis, the deep layers were closed with 5–0 polyglactin 910 sutures and the top layer was closed with 5–0 nylon sutures. The two key stitches to secure the flap were (1) tacking sutures to the nasal periosteum and (2) closure of the secondary defect.

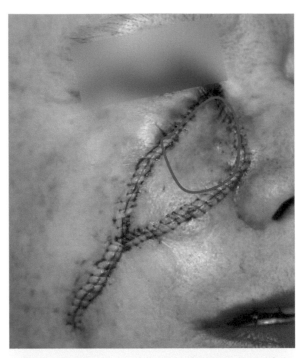

Fig. 5.5 A V-Y advancement flap was used to close a large defect on the superomedial cheek. The *blue outline* indicates a large surgical defect of the medial cheek that approaches the nasofacial sulcus and medial canthus. The majority of the incisions were placed at the anatomic unit junctions or along the relaxed skin tension line (RSTL). Tacking sutures were placed superiorly to the nasal bone periosteum to prevent ectropion. Additionally, plication sutures were placed medially to prevent nasal distortion.

Medium to large defects of the medial cheek are less likely to be repaired with a primary closure. For these defects, the repair choices include V-Y advancement flap or a large rotation flap. The V-Y advancement flap is a less complex repair than a rotation flap and has less morbidity. For this reason, it was selected for repair of the defect indicated in ▸ Fig. 5.5.

The V-Y advancement flap is characterized by a triangular island of tissue perfused by perforating vessels. The flap is released from surrounding tissue by dissection in the deep subcutaneous plane. The relative abundance of fat in the medial cheek allows for a well-vascularized flap. Proper depth of release allows for adequate movement without disruption of the musculature and motor innervation. Often, the surgical incisions for the V-Y advancement flap can be placed in the RSTLs or hidden in the nasofacial sulcus or nasolabial fold. When anatomic boundary lines are nearby, additional skin may be sacrificed so that surgical incisions can be placed at the junctions. When approaching the orbit, tacking sutures can be placed in the orbital rim, medial canthal tendon, or nasal periosteum to prevent ectropion. The V-Y advancement flap may sometimes develop a "trapdoor" deformity. This can be improved with intralesional triamcinolone or surgical debulking.

Key points for medial cheek repairs using V-Y advancement flaps are the following:

- The V-Y advancement flap can be used to repair large defects of the medial cheek that would otherwise require a large rotation flap.
- The surgical lines can often be hidden in anatomic unit junctions or in RSTL.
- Extensive undermining is required to create adequate movement without compromising the vascular supply.
- Secondary procedures may be required to correct "trapdoor" deformity.

5.6 Zygomatic Subunit

The zygomatic cheek is a convex surface with relatively thick skin. The skin in the majority of patients will lack hair. The lateral aspect of the zygomatic cheek will often develop rhytids as patients age. The zygomatic cheek can be a difficult unit to repair due to the absence of laxity due to retaining ligaments and proximity to the eye.[1] These factors can be especially notable in younger patients and overweight patients.

The zygomatic cheek extends lateral to the medial cheek along the zygoma. Similar to the medial cheek, the proximity of the zygomatic subunit to the orbit creates a high risk of ectropion; tacking periosteal sutures are useful to prevent ectropion and decrease tension on flaps. At the superior aspect of the zygomatic subunit, the temporal branch of the facial nerve is relatively superficial. Caution should be exercised to prevent injury to the nerve.

As with the medial cheek, primary closure is the repair of choice. When a surgical defect cannot be repaired primarily, a rotation or V-Y flap should be considered. Occasionally, a rhombic flap may be necessary for larger defects; however, the proximity to the eye requires attention to secondary vectors. Although the zygomatic cheek is not part of the central face, it can be visible from an anterior view. Repairs should be extended laterally, rather than medially, when possible to avoid moving incisions into the central face.

5.6.1 Primary Closure

The surgical defect of ▶ Fig. 5.6a was closed primarily. The repair was placed along the RSTL to minimize tension and achieve a fine-line scar. The inferior triangle of tissue was removed (▶ Fig. 5.6a—*blue outline*). No additional tissue was removed to extend the defect above the orbital rim. After limited undermining of the inferior portion, hemostasis was achieved with electrocoagulation. No undermining was performed above the orbital rim, in order to prevent lymphatic disruption. The deep layer was closed using 5–0 polyglactin 910 sutures and epidermal closure was achieved with 5–0 nylon sutures.

The majority of small to medium defects of the zygomatic cheek can be closed primarily; this is the repair of choice when possible. The surgical defect shown in ▶ Fig. 5.3a was amenable to a primary closure and a more complex repair was not necessary. When a primary closure extends beyond the orbital rim, the superior cone can be removed with an S-plasty or M-plasty to decrease proximity to the canthus. The S-plasty curves the repair along the junction of the orbital rim, removing the standing cone medially or laterally. M-plasty can be used to shorten the closure length. As demonstrated in ▶ Fig. 5.6c, removal of standing cones is not always necessary. If enough tissue laxity is not present to close a surgical defect, a small V-Y advancement can be performed. Alternatively, a rotation flap from the inferior cheek can be used to keep the incisions hidden at junctions of the orbital rim and nasofacial sulcus (▶ Fig. 5.6a—*orange outline*).

All primary closures on the zygomatic cheek should be placed in the RSTL. Repairs in the zygomatic cheek often approach or extend beyond the orbital rim. The thin eyelid skin above the orbital rim requires delicate handling. The thin skin of the lower eyelid can easily be affected by

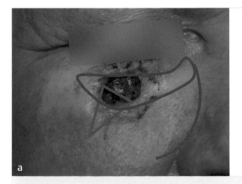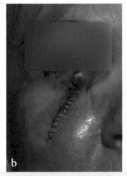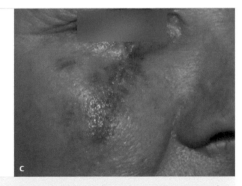

Fig. 5.6 (a) A surgical defect of the medial zygomatic cheek approaches the eyelid margin. The *blue outline* indicates the tissue to be removed to prevent an inferior standing cone. The *orange outline* indicates the surgical incisions for an additional closure option, that of an inferiorly based rotation flap with suture lines hidden at anatomic unit junctions. (b) A primary closure of a zygomatic cheek defect has been completed. The superior aspect was not undermined in order to prevent lymphatic disruption. Only limited undermining was performed in the inferior portion. (c) At the time of suture removal, there was no evidence of ectropion. Additionally, no standing cone was present at the superior margin.

nearby repairs. Additionally, repairs in this region are at risk of ectropion. It is important that tension be directed horizontally to prevent ectropion. By not removing a standing cone at the superior aspect of the surgical defect, the risk of ectropion and disruption of lymphatic drainage is significantly decreased. ▶ Fig. 5.6c demonstrates that excess skin will most likely settle due to the thin skin and lack of supporting subcutaneous structures.

Key points for zygomatic cheek repairs using primary closures are the following:

- Small to medium surgical defects of the zygomatic cheek can often be closed in a primary fashion.
- The incisions should be made along the RSTL or at cosmetic unit junctions to reduce tension on the wound and prevent scar spread.
- When surgical defects extend above the orbital rim, primary closures may not require the removal of the superior standing cone.
- The tension vectors for primary closures should be directed horizontally to prevent ectropion.
- Due to the convex nature of the zygomatic arch, primary closures may require greater than the typical 3:1 length-to-width ratio in order to prevent standing cone deformities.

5.6.2 V-Y Advancement Flap

The surgical defect of the medial zygomatic subunit in ▶ Fig. 5.7a was repaired with a V-Y advancement flap. The flap *outlined in blue* in ▶ Fig. 5.7a was designed to be slightly smaller than the defect to prevent "trapdoor" deformity. The flap was undermined in all directions with a central pedicle being preserved. No undermining was performed at the superior aspect of the surgical defect. The superior, or leading edge of the flap, was placed along the orbital rim. Placement of the surgical incisions was designed to create the tail, or secondary defect, in an RSTL.

The leading edge of the flap was tacked to the orbital rim to maintain the natural contour. After hemostasis, the deep layers were closed with 5–0 polyglactin 910 sutures and the epidermal layer closed with 5–0 nylon sutures.

Use of a triangular-shaped flap is not the preferred repair for the zygomatic subunit. However, when defects are too large to close primarily, the V-Y advancement flap can be a good option as it creates scars that can be hidden in the RSTL. In addition, there is less morbidity with a V-Y flap, compared to a large rotation flap. Bilobed or rhombic flaps are generally considered secondary repair options because of their inability to camouflage incision lines in anatomic boundary lines.

The V-Y advancement flap is a triangular island of tissue that is perfused by perforating vessels. The flap is released from the surrounding tissue by dissection in the deep subcutaneous plane. The relative abundance of fat in the zygomatic cheek allows for a well-vascularized flap. When undermining the flap to achieve adequate movement, release of the anterior edge may be required. This is due to the fixed nature of the tissue of the zygomatic cheek. When possible, surgical incisions of the V-Y advancement flap should be placed in RSTLs or hidden at the junction of anatomic units. When approaching the orbital unit, tacking sutures to the periosteum of the orbital rim or lateral canthus may be required to prevent ectropion. When oversized, the V-Y advancement flap is known to occasionally protrude resulting in a "trapdoor" deformity. This can be improved with intralesional triamcinolone or surgical debulking.

Key points for zygomatic cheek repairs using V-Y advancement flaps are the following:

- The V-Y advancement flap is not often the repair of choice for the zygomatic cheek, given the bulky pedicle and convex structure. However, it can be used for medium to large surgical defects with less morbidity than other flaps.

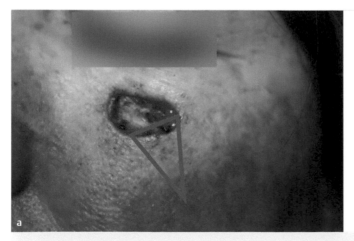 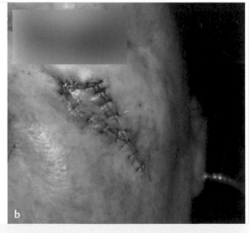

Fig. 5.7 (a) A surgical defect is present on the zygomatic cheek. Due to limited tissue movement, the defect was unable to be closed primarily. Rather than performing a large rotation flap, the defect was repaired with a V-Y advancement flap. The island pedicle, *outlined in blue*, was advanced superomedially after vertical undermining. **(b)** The V-Y advancement flap demonstrated was achieved without undermining at the superior edge of the defect. After closure, a slight lower lid swelling occurred, but with no evidence of ectropion. The V-Y flap was used to successfully close the defect with less morbidity than other repair options.

- The use of a V-Y advancement flap has less morbidity than large rotation flaps and is less likely to transfer unwanted hair or mismatched skin than a transposition flap.
- The placement of tacking sutures to the orbital rim decreases tension on the superior wound edge, and prevents ectropion.

5.7 Lateral Subunit

The skin of the lateral cheek is thinner and less sebaceous than that of the medial cheek. This subunit is also more uniform in characteristics than other subunits.[1] The skin is commonly less mobile than other cheek subunits due to the zygomatic-retaining ligament and the SMAS, which can create a need for more complex repairs. The SMAS contributes to the limited mobility, but the SMAS plication can be useful in minimizing tension on flaps. Rhytids may extend onto the lateral cheek from the periocular or perioral regions. The lateral canthal rhytids can occasionally be used to hide surgical incisions. The presence of both hair-bearing and non-hear-bearing skin makes it important to maintain normal anatomy.

In general, surgical repairs on the lateral cheek are not seen from an anterior view. When more complex repairs are performed in this region, the incisions are lateral to the field of view. Due to proximity to the ear, a fixed structure, skin movement is limited to the anterior and inferior reservoirs. Similar to the zygomatic cheek, it is important that repairs on the lateral cheek do not distort the ocular unit. Repairs approaching free margins may require use of an M-plasty to shorten the surgical line. When performing surgical procedures in the lateral subunit, caution should be exercised to prevent trauma to the temporal artery and the parotid gland.

Many surgical defects on the lateral cheek can be repaired primarily. For larger surgical defects or those with limited skin mobility, a more complex repair may be necessary. V-Y advancement flaps are often of limited utility in this region due to limited tissue mobility. A rhombic transposition flap is therefore the next choice, but caution must be exercised to prevent distortion of hair gradients. If hair patterns are a concern or the defect is too large, an advancement or rotation flap can be considered. When a defect is too large for repair with tissue from the cheek, large transposition or bilobed flaps may be used to move the skin up from the neck. These large flaps, however, have increased morbidity and risk of complications. Although it is generally not a reconstructive option, healing through second intention may be considered if a defect is small, superficial, and located on a concave surface such as the preauricular sulcus.[6]

5.7.1 Advancement Flap with Burow's Triangle

The surgical defect of the lateral cheek in ▶ Fig. 5.8a was repaired with an advancement flap with removal of a Burow's triangle in the postauricular region. The surgical defect was converted into an anteriorly oriented triangle (*outlined in blue*). The flap was released along the preauricular sulcus to advance tissue from the inferior reservoir. Adequate undermining of the flap was performed anteriorly, and inferiorly beyond the surgical incision. This allowed for adequate tissue movement. Hemostasis was then achieved. 4–0 polyglactin 910 fascial plication sutures were placed. After determining the degree of movement, a Burow's triangle was removed from the postauricular skin. Wound closure was then achieved with 5–0 polyglactin 910 sutures for the deep layer and 5–0 nylon sutures for the epidermal layer.

The surgical defect in ▶ Fig. 5.8a was not amenable to primary closure due to the large size and proximity to the

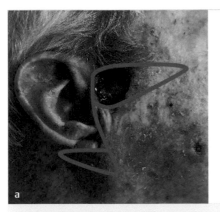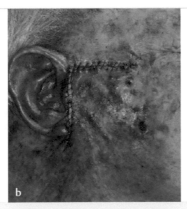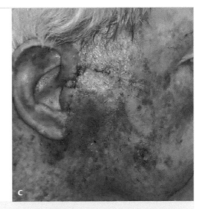

Fig. 5.8 (a) A surgical defect of the lateral cheek approaches the tragus. Primary closure was not possible due to proximity to the ear and lack of adjacent tissue mobility. Therefore, closure was achieved with an advancement flap with movement of tissue from the inferior reservoir. The *blue outlines* indicate (1) the tissue removed to prevent a standing cone medial to defect, (2) the edge of tissue advancement at the ear–cheek junction, and (3) the Burow's triangle hidden in the postauricular region. **(b)** The surgical defect was successfully repaired with an advancement flap. Fascial sutures were placed to minimize tension on the wound edges. **(c)** At the time of suture removal, there is no evidence of distortion of adjacent free margins or flap tip necrosis.

ear. The patient had limited skin laxity due to actinic damage. A rhombic flap was considered but was felt to be a poor choice because of the proximity to the ear and limited tissue reservoirs. In order to move tissue from the inferior cheek, an advancement flap was selected. Large preauricular defects that are unable to be closed primarily or with a rhombic flap can usually be repaired with an advancement flap. Flaps on the lateral cheek often create movement in the cephalic direction. However, there are times when anterior tissue will be moved, creating a rotation flap.

In order to prevent a standing cone, the original defect must be converted to a triangular shape. If necessary, it can be converted to an M-plasty to prevent eyelid distortion. The vertical portion of the repair will be hidden in the preauricular sulcus. Undermining of the flap must be performed beyond the inferior aspect of the flap to release more inferior tissue. Caution must be exercised in this region to prevent damage to the temporal artery and the parotid gland. The appeal of the advancement flap includes camouflaging the lateral incision in the preauricular sulcus and the Burow's triangle behind the ear. Additionally, by advancing tissue from the same cosmetic subunit, the directionality of the hair can be maintained. These benefits are not possible with a transposition or bilobed flap. Fascial sutures to the SMAS and tacking sutures to the lateral temple and zygomatic arch can help decrease vertical tension on the flap.

Key points for lateral cheek repairs using advancement flaps are the following:

- Defects of almost any size on the lateral cheek can be repaired with advancement flaps.
- Occasionally flaps will move tissue both medially and inferiorly, which creates an element of rotation.
- Advancement flaps on the lateral cheek are advantageous because they maintain hair gradients.
- Burow's triangles can be hidden in the postauricular area.
- Fascial sutures are critical to decrease tension on the wound edges.

5.8 Buccal Subunit

The buccal subunit of the cheek has similar thickness and mobility to the inferomedial cheek. Most women have no hair on the cheek; however, men will have variable hair patterns and demarcation lines. The quality of the skin and degree of fat pad atrophy will impact the repair selected in this subunit. Older patients commonly have increased laxity and increased rhytids. It is crucial that in this region the closures fall exactly in the RSTLs.

Repairs may move tissue from the preauricular area or from the neck inferiorly. The proximity to the nasolabial fold provides a reservoir of tissue. However, use of medial cheek tissue should be done judiciously to prevent oral distortion. Planning of surgical incisions in the buccal subunit must avoid distortion of the mouth and nose.

Evaluation of the patient with the mouth open and during a smile, in addition to resting, can help assess tension vectors and RSTLs.

Small to medium defects of the buccal subunit will be closed primarily. When this cannot be achieved, transposition or rotation flaps may be used. Flaps on the buccal cheek should be inferolateral based to minimize retraction on the periorbital and perioral area. Large defects may require movement of tissue from the neck. Flaps extending over the mandible transition from concave to convex structures. In order to accommodate this transition, extra length is required to prevent tension and tip necrosis. Extensive undermining may be required to achieve closure without tension. In all situations, the surgeon must be aware of the location of the marginal mandibular branch of the facial nerve.

5.8.1 Primary Closure

The small surgical defect of ▶ Fig. 5.9a was closed primarily. Planning of the direction of the apices of the ellipse should include evaluation of the patient with the mouth at rest (▶ Fig. 5.9a), open (▶ Fig. 5.9b), and while smiling (▶ Fig. 5.9c). This allows for precise placement of the surgical scar in the RSTL and to coincide with current and future rhytids (▶ Fig. 5.9d–f). Once the planned repair was evaluated with the aforementioned facial expressions, the inferior and superior standing cones, *outlined in purple*, were excised. Undermining was performed at all wound edges and hemostasis was achieved. The deep layer was closed with 5–0 Polyglactin 910 sutures and the top layer closed with 5–0 nylon sutures.

Small to medium defects of the buccal cheek can often be repaired primarily. This is the closure of choice when possible. For surgical defects that cannot be closed primarily due to large size, limited tissue mobility, or causation of eclabium, a transposition flap or rotation flap is considered. Reconstruction by transposition of tissue requires careful execution to prevent movement of poorly matched skin or tension vectors in unfavorable directions.

Repair of the buccal cheek with a primary closure commonly results in a curvilinear scar. Planning should include evaluation of the defect with the patient at rest, smiling, and with the mouth open. These positions will indicate the vectors of greatest tension and accentuate rhytids. It is important that the surgical incisions be placed exactly in these lines to prevent scar spreading or misalignment. In patients with full cheeks, the ellipse may require a length-to-width ratio greater than the traditional 3:1 to prevent standing cones. The buccal cheek is an area of great mobility and increased risk of hypertrophic scarring. Because of this, more undermining and support may be required than in other areas of the cheek. When surgical defects are next to the nasolabial fold, repairs may be camouflaged in the crease.

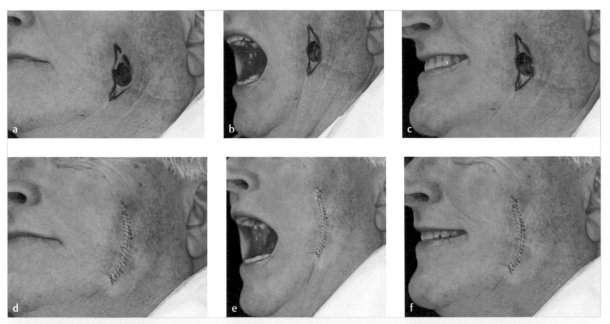

Fig. 5.9 **(a)** A small surgical defect is present on the cheek. A primary closure is *outlined in purple* with the patient's face at rest. The *blue outline* indicates an alternative primary closure that would have been selected had the various facial expressions not been evaluated. **(b)** When planning a primary closure anywhere on the cheek, it is important to evaluate the resting skin tension line (RSTL) with the patient's mouth open. This expression accentuates RSTLs and indicates the direction of least tension. This exercise helps with planning to determine whether elongation of the incision greater than the typical 3:1 elliptical ratio is necessary. **(c)** The next step in planning is to evaluate the closure with the patient smiling. The primary repair *outlined in purple* demonstrates that a proper closure will account for present and future rhytids. **(d)** The surgical repair was placed in the RSTL and coincides with rhytids. **(e)** Upon opening the mouth, the repair is oriented in the RSTL and tension on the closure is minimized. **(f)** When the patient is smiling, the repair is hidden precisely along the RSTL. The closure is perfectly aligned with both the perioral and periocular rhytids.

Key points for buccal cheek repairs using primary closure are the following:

- A primary closure is often the repair of choice.
- Primary closure can be used for small to medium wounds on the buccal cheek. Occasionally, even large wounds can be closed primarily if the patient has adequate tissue laxity.
- It is important that the patient be evaluated at rest, with the mouth open, and when smiling in order to align incisions precisely within the RSTL and rhytids.

5.8.2 Transposition Flap

The surgical defect of the superior buccal cheek in ▶ Fig. 5.10a was repaired with a transposition flap. The purple outline indicates placement of the initial surgical incisions. The surgical defect and flap were undermined and hemostasis was achieved. The secondary defect closure and flap placement were then approximated with nylon sutures. A standing cone was removed superiorly from the original surgical defect. The cone was removed superiorly to maintain a wide flap pedicle. The subcutaneous layer was closed with 5–0 Polyglactin 910 sutures and the epidermal layer closed with 5–0 nylon sutures.

The defect in ▶ Fig. 5.10a was too large to be closed primarily. Minimal skin laxity was present posterior, superior, or anterior to the defect. A rhombic flap was able to move tissue from the mandibular and neck area inferior to the defect. A bilobed flap from the neck was another option. A large bilobed flap from the neck, however, would have increased morbidity and risk of complications.

All repairs of the buccal cheek should be executed with caution to prevent damage to the marginal mandibular nerve. Large repairs on the buccal cheek may require movement of tissue from regions not immediately adjacent to the defect such as the neck. Due to the central location, camouflaging surgical incisions in anatomic boundary lines is not possible on the buccal cheek. For this reason, the broken lines of rhombic and bilobed flaps are often advantageous. When possible, surgical incisions in the RSTL can make the scars less notable.

Key points for buccal cheek repairs using transposition flaps are the following:

- Medium to large defects of the buccal cheek can be repaired with transposition flaps that require movement of nonadjacent (usually inferior or lateral) skin.

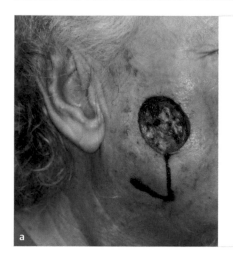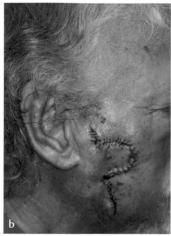

Fig. 5.10 (a) A large surgical defect is present on the superior buccal cheek. The defect was too large for primary closure. Alternative repairs included rotation flap and transposition flap. The transposition flap was selected due to an adequate inferior tissue reservoir and decreased morbidity. The *purple lines* indicate design of the transposition flap. **(b)** The surgical defect was successfully repaired with a transposition flap. Caution was exercised to prevent damage to the marginal mandibular nerve. A standing cone was removed at the superolateral aspect of the flap. The removal was oriented superiorly to maintain a wide flap pedicle.

- Additionally, tension vectors can be redirected.
- When creating a transposition flap, caution should be exercised to prevent transfer of nonmatching skin.
- Transposition flaps are useful because they do not sacrifice large amounts of normal tissue.

References

[1] Dobratz EJ, Hilger PA. Cheek defects. Facial Plast Surg Clin North Am. 2009; 17(3):455–467

[2] Summers BK, Siegle RJ. Facial cutaneous reconstructive surgery: facial flaps. J Am Acad Dermatol. 1993; 29(6):917–941, quiz 942–944

[3] Bernstein L, Nelson RH. Surgical anatomy of the extraparotid distribution of the facial nerve. Arch Otolaryngol. 1984; 110(3):177–183

[4] Marur T, Tuna Y, Demirci P. Facial anatomy. Clin Derm. 2014; 32:14–23

[5] Rapstine ED, Knaus WJ, II, Thornton JF. Simplifying cheek reconstruction: a review of over 400 cases. Plast Reconstr Surg. 2012; 129(6):1291–1299

[6] Pepper JP, Baker SR. Local flaps: cheek and lip reconstruction. JAMA Facial Plast Surg. 2013; 15(5):374–382

[7] Başağaoğlu B, Bhadkamkar M, Hollier P, Reece E. Approach to reconstruction of cheek defects. Semin Plast Surg. 2018; 32(2):84–89

[8] Chandawarkar RY, Cervino AL. Subunits of the cheek: an algorithm for the reconstruction of partial-thickness defects. Br J Plast Surg. 2003; 56(2):135–139

[9] Meaike JD, Dickey RM, Killion E, Bartlett EL, Brown RH. Facial skin cancer reconstruction. Semin Plast Surg. 2016; 30(3):108–121

[10] Kilinc H, Erbatur S, Aytekin AH. A novel flap for the reconstruction of midcheek defects: "rabbit ear flap.". J Craniofac Surg. 2013; 24(5): e452–e455

[11] Rebowe RE, Albertini JG. Complex medial cheek and lateral nasal ala defect. Dermatol Surg. 2016; 42(1):115–118

6 Reconstruction of the Upper and Lower Lip Unit

Gian Vinelli, Ramone F. Williams, David H. Ciocon, and Anne Truitt

Summary

Indisputably the aesthetic centerpiece of the lower face, the lips are both elegant in form and indispensable in function. From facial expression to phonation, sensation, and mastication, the lips are master orchestrators.

Keywords: lip cosmetic subunits, upper and lower lip reconstruction, lip subunits, lip flap repair, lip graft repair

6.1 Anatomic Considerations

The lip is composed of multiple aesthetic subunits: the philtrum, cutaneous upper lip, vermilion, cutaneous lower lip, and chin (▶ Fig. 6.1). Defects to these subunits necessitating repair may result from trauma, infection, inflammation, congenital malformations, and tumors.

For reconstructive purposes, the lip is divided into three layers: skin, mucosa, and muscle. The skin is composed of the cutaneous skin and the vermilion, which is separated by the vermilion border. The vermilion is the dry lip that becomes the mucosal wet lip that abuts the teeth. The red line marks the junction between the wet mucosal lip and the dry vermilion lip. Under the mucosal lip are a layer of minor salivary glands and then the muscle. Under the vermilion lip and the cutaneous lower lip are sebaceous glands and then muscle[1] (▶ Fig. 6.2).

The vermilion is the most striking aspect of the lips; it is displayed prominently in social interaction. Its red hue derives from the thin epithelium, lack of keratinization, and abundant underlying vasculature. The dry vermilion consists of a modified mucous membrane lacking pilosebaceous units, eccrine glands, and salivary glands. The vermilion and cutaneous portions of the lip converge to produce a line of variable prominence known as the white roll.[2]

The upper cutaneous lip spans the vertical distance from the nasal sill to the upper vermilion border. It is divided into three cosmetic subunits: one medial and two lateral. The medial philtral subunit encompasses the convex philtral crests and the central philtral groove, which connects the columella to the Cupid's bow. The lateral subunits extend symmetrically to the nasolabial folds. The apical triangle is a small but important cosmetic section of the cutaneous upper lip that extends from the ala laterally to the upper nasolabial fold with the inferior horizontal border being even with the nasal sill. The cutaneous lower lip is a single subunit bordered superiorly by the lower vermilion border, inferiorly by the mental crease, and laterally by the labiomental creases.[3]

The musculature of the lip can be grouped into the constrictors and dilators. The orbicularis oris is the primary muscle of the lip and functions as a constrictor. It is comprised of four distinct quadrants of muscle that interlace to give the appearance of circularity. Each quadrant contains two distinct sets of fibers best appreciated on the sagittal section: the pars marginalis, located more anteriorly, and the pars peripheralis, located more posteriorly. Thus, there are eight muscle parts, each with dermal insertions, near the corners of the mouth. It is thought

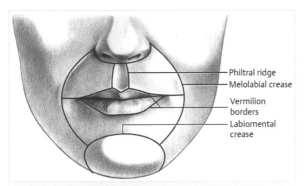

Fig. 6.1 Lip subunits. (Reprinted from Lips and Chin. In: Larrabee Jr W, Sherris D, Teixeira J, ed. Principles of Facial Reconstruction: A Subunit Approach to Cutaneous Repair. 3rd Edition. New York: Thieme; 2021.)

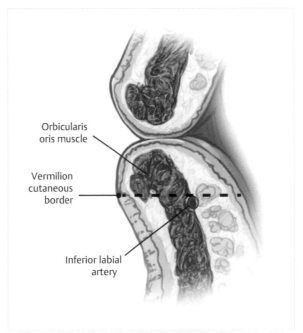

Fig. 6.2 Cross section of the lower lip. (Reprinted from Anatomy. In: Hanasono M, Butler C, ed. Handbook of Reconstructive Flaps. 1st Edition. New York: Thieme; 2020.)

the fibers of the orbicularis oris decussate in the medium plane creating the cosmetically distinct philtrum. The muscular segments of the orbicularis oris work synergistically to ensure oral competence while also providing support for the dilator muscles. The dilators of the mouth are located radially around the peripheral margin of the orbicularis oris and are grouped into the following categories: (1) the upper lip elevators (levator labii superioris alaeque nasi, levator labii superioris, zygomaticus major, zygomaticus minor, and levator anguli oris); (2) elevators of the corners of the mouth (levator anguli oris, buccinator, and risorius); and (3) lower lip depressors (the depressor anguli oris, depressor labii inferioris, and the mentalis).[3,4,5] The modiolus structure is the convergence of the orbicularis oris, lip elevator muscles, and lip depressor muscles, and it is located approximately 1 cm lateral to the oral commissures. As this neuromuscular bundle is a key unit to perioral expression and speech enunciation, preservation of the modiolus, while sometimes difficult with large defects and subsequent flap repairs, will aid in overall lip function if maintained[6,7] (▶ Fig. 6.3).

The superior and inferior labial arteries, branches of the facial artery, serve as the primary blood supply for the lips. The facial artery runs below the premasseteric notch and then courses upward toward the corner of the mouth. There it branches into serial tributaries including the superior and inferior labial arteries. The inferior labial artery perfuses the minor salivary glands and musculature of the lower lip. In most cases, the inferior labial artery runs along the lower vermilion border. Some anatomic studies suggest it may course along the labiomental crease. In these cases, the artery is termed the horizontal labiomental artery.[8] The superior labial artery branches from the trunk of the facial artery approximately 12 mm or one fingerbreadth away from the corner of the mouth.[9] The artery then courses along the upper vermilion border and produces a vertically ascending tributary termed the nasal septal branch.[10] The depth of the superior labial artery has been studied by anatomists in cadaveric studies. The superior labial arteries on either side anastomose in the middle of the lip. Most often, the superior labial artery is submucosal—coursing between the oral mucosa and the orbicularis oris. Although some reports have observed the superior labial artery to run intramuscularly, a subcutaneous course is quite rare being observed in only 2% of cases.[11]

The infraorbital and mental nerves, branches of the trigeminal nerve, provide sensory innervation to the upper and lower lips, respectively. Nerve blocks can be vital to the comfort of a patient during reconstruction. Understanding the location of the infraorbital and mental nerves will aid in producing a nerve block to provide effective anesthesia

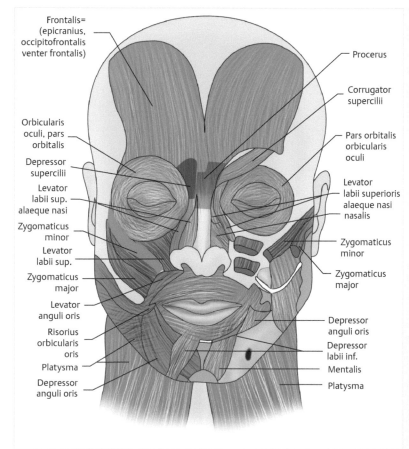

Fig. 6.3 Muscle diagram. (Reprinted from Browlift and Reshaping. In: Agrawal K, Singh K, Garg A, ed. Textbook of Plastic, Reconstructive, and Aesthetic Surgery: Volume VI Aesthetic Surgery. 1st Edition. Delhi, India: Thieme; 2021.)

with less anesthetic as well as less confusing lip distortion due to anesthesia volume during lip reconstruction. The infraorbital nerve exits the maxillary bone at the infraorbital foramen at approximately 1 cm below the orbital rim within the midpupillary line. About 1 to 2 mL of anesthetic should be injected deep just superficial to the maxillary bone periosteum. Another method of infraorbital nerve anesthesia is to inject intraorally between the first and second premolars moving cephalad toward the maxillary bone. The mental nerve exits the mandible bone in the midpupillary line and is best anesthetized through the intraoral route. Using a 0.5-inch needle, injection is between the first and second lower premolars extending caudally toward the bone to about the mid-chin level.[7] A small injection of anesthetic with epinephrine at the site of repair will aid in hemostasis without causing significant distortion, but adequate anesthesia through a nerve block will deliver significant comfort to patients with less anesthetic while also providing less distortion of the area.

Motor innervation is provided by branches of the facial nerve (cranial nerve VII). The buccal branch innervates the orbicularis oris and lip elevator muscles, whereas the marginal mandibular branch innervates the orbicularis oris and lip depressor muscles. Injury to the buccal branch is uncommon during lip reconstruction; however, injury to the marginal mandibular branch can occur given its more superficial location over the anterior jaw and extending close to the oral commissure. If the marginal mandibular branch is injured, the depressor anguli oris and depressor labii inferioris muscles no longer provide counter movement to the lip elevators, producing an asymmetric smile.[12]

Lymphatic drainage of the lip occurs primarily through the submandibular and submental nodes. For more aggressive cancers of the lips, lymph nodes should be clinically assessed prior to any surgical procedure. As there is cross-communication between the lymphatic systems, which could allow drainage to the contralateral side, examination of bilateral nodal regions should be performed.

6.2 Approach to Reconstruction of the Lip Unit

Reconstruction of a lip defect requires consideration of how best to restore function, cosmesis, adequate oral aperture, and sensation. Aesthetic goals of reconstruction include maintaining lip height, vermilion border, cosmetic subunits when possible, and color-matched skin. Functional goals of reconstruction include restoration of oral competence, sensation, expression, and dynamic activity as well as maximization of the oral aperture (for eating, brushing teeth, and removal of dentures as needed). Minimizing scarring is not only vital for the aesthetic outcome but also functional by decreasing the risk for microstomia.

Traditional teaching in lip reconstruction is based upon the location, tissue involved, and size of the defect. We present an anatomic approach to the reconstruction of the lip unit. Although there are different classification schemes of lip defects and reconstruction options, the algorithmic approach to this chapter will involve location, then branch into anatomic subunits, and then by size of the defect (▶ Fig. 6.4, ▶ Fig. 6.5).

Thus, the first step of the algorithmic tree is assessment of the location of the defect: upper or lower lip, medial or lateral. This is an important initial determination as a defect of the lateral upper or lower lip may have a different repair in comparison to the central upper lip even if the defect is the same size. As such, subunit analysis should be performed—this is particularly important for upper lip reconstruction. Refer to the illustration of the cosmetic subunits of the lip in ▶ Fig. 6.1. Next, the anatomic tissue involved should be assessed (i.e., cutaneous skin with or without vermilion lip), and then finally the size of the defect in proportion to the size of the overall lip. These initial assessments of the defect are necessary for an algorithmic anatomic approach to lip reconstruction.

Finally, there are two general rules for lip reconstruction that should be followed: (1) careful reassembly of the trilaminar structure (skin, muscle, mucosa) in order to restore function and form and (2) prior to any lip closure as anesthetic can distort and blur the vermilion border, it should be outlined with a skin marker or suture to ensure meticulous realignment as a "step-off" will be a permanent, easily noticeable cosmetic detraction.

6.3 Upper Lip

6.3.1 Philtral Subunit

Cutaneous Lip with or without Vermilion Lip Involvement

Less than 50% Involvement

After determining the location and tissue involvement of the defect, the next assessment should be the size of the defect. If the medial upper lip defect is smaller than 50% of the philtrum and not full thickness, then options for closure include primary closure, full-thickness skin graft (FTSG), and wedge resection (although wedge resections can also be used for full thickness).

Primary Closure

A primary closure includes adequate undermining above the muscle and good skin eversion while placing subcutaneous dissolvable sutures to ensure better cosmesis. Prominent skin eversion of the upper lip will help reduce the appearance of the surgical line over time. A bit "tongue in cheek," but several excellent Mohs surgeons have lectured that "there is no such thing as too much

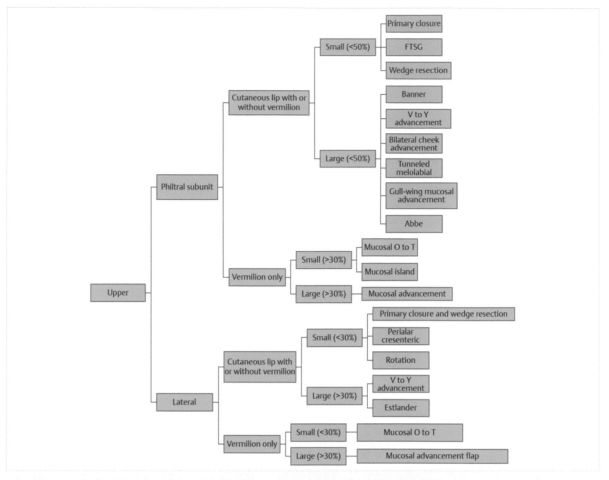

Fig. 6.4 Upper lip algorithmic tree showing location, branch into anatomic subunits, and size of the defect.

eversion on the cutaneous lip." The long axis of linear closures should be oriented along perioral relaxed skin tension lines, which run perpendicular to the horizontal axis of the lip. In the philtral subunit, the philtral crests are excellent for the camouflage of scars (▶ Fig. 6.6). If removal of the primary closure of the inferior Burow triangle involves extension through the vermilion border, again meticulous realignment of this border is imperative. Restoration of Cupid's bow can be more complicated with primary closures that cross the philtral vermilion border; particular attention to the formation of the dip and rise of Cupid's bow is required (▶ Fig. 6.7). Another option is to perform a W-plasty at the inferior border to reduce the length of the standing cone and perhaps not necessitate crossing the vermilion border; however, again, precise reapproximation of the border is required if crossed.

Sometimes a larger defect may need a "mini-wedge" with removal of some of the distal fibers of the orbicularis oris muscle to reduce the risk of a lip pucker deformity. Careful reapproximation of the muscle layer with durable and absorbable suture is required for function and cosmesis.[13]

Full-Thickness Skin Graft

An FTSG is also an excellent option for repair of a philtral defect. The donor site is often the preauricular cheek or the nasolabial fold as there is good texture and color match of the cutaneous lip skin. Despite the incision line being at an angle at the nasolabial fold, ensure horizontal tension vectors for the subcutaneous suturing of this line to avoid eclabium.

To improve cosmesis and reduce the risk of the "postage stamp" look, it is often recommended to remove the entire cutaneous philtrum as opposed to simply grafting the smaller defect portion. A graft that covers the entire cosmetic subunit of the philtrum can be more easily concealed at the natural borders of the nasal sill, philtral crests, and vermilion border. Standard technique of suturing from the graft to the surrounding skin ("ship to shore") is recommended. Simple interrupted tacking sutures are placed centrally to help create the concavity of the philtrum as well as prevent lifting of the graft from serous exudate (▶ Fig. 6.8).

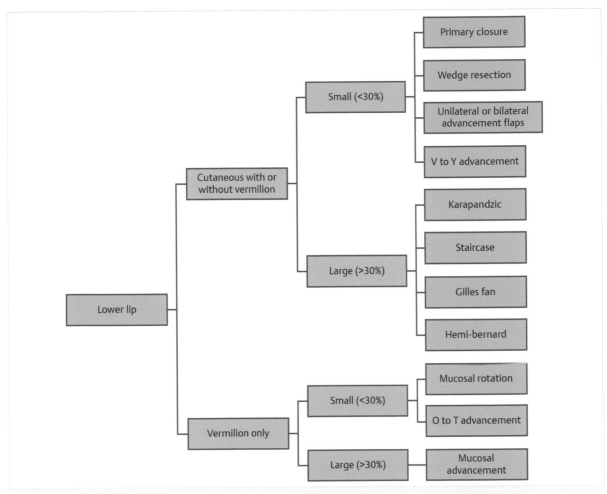

Fig. 6.5 Lower lip algorithmic tree showing location, branch into anatomic subunits, and size of the defect.

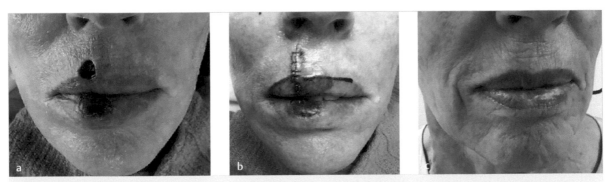

Fig. 6.6 (a) Mohs defect at the philtral crest. (b) Repair of the defect with vermilion border outlined and reforming of Cupid's bow angle. (c) Eight months postoperative.

Wedge Resection

As mentioned earlier, for full-thickness defects less than 50% of the philtrum, a wedge resection can be performed taking care to preserve the deeper orbicularis oris muscle bands if possible. A triangular, or wedge-shaped, excision is made extending to the nasal sill. The labial artery is ligated or electrocauterized and then the closure is completed in a multilayer fashion. Realigning from inside out (mucosa, muscle, and then skin) with a buried absorbable

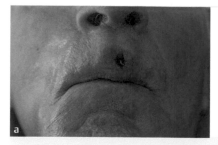
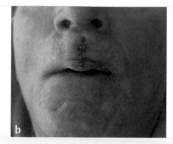
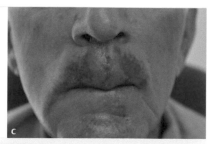

Fig. 6.7 A medial philtral defect closed by primary closure. **(a)** A Mohs defect less than 50% of the philtrum. **(b)** Closure performed by primary closure with good reapproximation of the vermilion border. **(c)** Repair at 1 week showing good reformation of Cupid's bow.

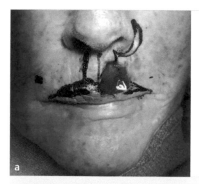
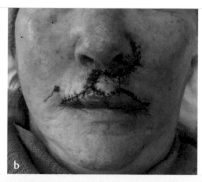
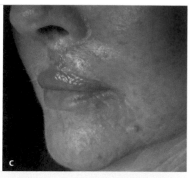

Fig. 6.8 **(a)** A philtral defect in combination with vermilion lip and left cutaneous lip defect. Repair with combination mucosal advancement, perialar advancement flap, and full-thickness skin graft (FTSG) at the philtrum. **(b)** Repair complete. **(c)** Ten weeks postoperative.

suture is preferred for ease of technique and better cosmesis. Care should be taken to still perform moderate undermining at the level of the subcutaneous tissue to ensure good skin eversion with buried suture placement. As mentioned previously, realignment of the vermilion border can be more challenging at the philtral upper lip, especially in younger patients with a more prominent Cupid's bow.

Defects Greater than 50% of the Philtrum

For defects that involve more than 50% of the philtrum, repair options include banner transposition flaps, V-Y advancement flap, bilateral advancement flaps, tunneled-pedicle flap, and for full-thickness defects the Abbe flap.

Banner Transposition Flap (Nasolabial Flap)

The banner transposition flap from the cheek–nasofacial sulcus is an excellent option for women (or men who have no desire for a mustache). Incision lines for this flap hide well along the nasofacial sulcus and the vermilion border. Care should be excised to perform generous (but not too thin) undermining of the flap laterally on the superior and inferior cheek as to allow transfer of the flap to the cutaneous lip with no tension. The key suture is deep and placed at the base of the nasofacial sulcus

pulling the cheek medially toward the nose to close the secondary defect, thus allowing the flap to gently drape over the cutaneous lip. The horizontal width of the flap at the nasofacial sulcus should match the vertical height of the cutaneous lip defect. If it is felt that the height of the defect is bigger the width of the flap, an FTSG (or Burow's graft from the tip of the flap) can also be added to the closure. First, ensure the transposed flap is lined up against the vermilion border and then place the graft closer to the nasal sill; this will reduce the risk of eclabium and also help camouflage the surgical lines under the nasal sill. The inferior Burow triangle can easily curve around the lateral oral commissure taking care to not cross the vermilion border[14] (▶ Fig. 6.9).

V-Y Advancement Flap

A V-Y advancement flap (island pedicle flap) is also an excellent option for a larger medial upper lip defect. This flap uses similar hair-bearing skin so as to cause little disruption for male facial hair. Consider enlarging the defect to the level of the vermilion border as to allow better concealing of the inferior base of the flap along this natural border of the cosmetic unit. Traditional flap design involves a 3:1 ratio of flap to defect size and curving the tail of the flap inferior and medial if possible to mimic the natural curve of the marionette line. Generous undermining of

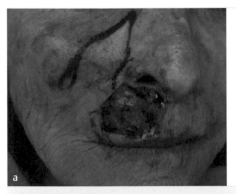
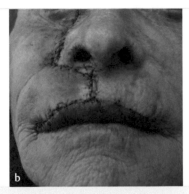
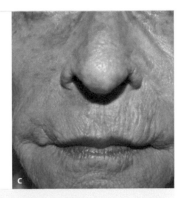

Fig. 6.9 Mohs cutaneous upper lip defect closed with a nasolabial transposition flap. **(a)** The defect with the design for closure. **(b)** The final defect with creation of a new vermilion border and reapproximation of the existing border. Note Burow's triangle at the nasal sill. **(c)** The patient at 6 months postoperative.

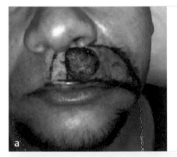
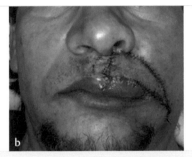
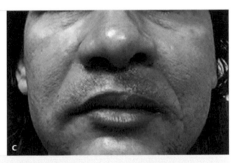

Fig. 6.10 (a) Defect with V-Y advancement flap design, (b) V-Y advancement flap in place, and (c) V-Y advancement flap at 2 months postoperative. (Photograph courtesy of Dr. David H. Ciocon.)

the flap and surrounding skin while maintaining a healthy-sized central muscular pedicle is recommended to ensure less tension and good vascularity of the flap. Once again, prominent skin eversion where the flap meets the surrounding skin (excluding the vermilion border) will help conceal the surgical lines over time[5] (▶ Fig. 6.10).

Bilateral Cheek Advancement

A bilateral cheek advancement is an exceptional closure technique for defects of the medial upper lip as it follows the horizontal natural cosmetic boundaries and thus obscures the scar lines. With appropriate undermining, this flap will share the tension bilaterally, thus reducing any unilateral pull. As the flap is created from tissue surrounding the defect, the color, texture, thickness, and hair density are more precise matches. Moreover, the heavy vascular supply provided by the labial arteries allows for quick wound healing and excellent cosmesis. Similarly, when properly designed, there is significantly less risk of hypoesthesia and sphincter dysfunction compared to other reconstructive techniques.

Extensive undermining of the bilateral flaps is necessary for tension-free approximation. The undermining plane should be superior to the orbicularis oris muscle

to ensure continued sphincter function. Undermining through the musculature and into the mucosa can lead to delayed infection, hematoma, and flap necrosis. It is important to ensure sufficient tissue laxity is recruited with each flap or there is potential for increased height of the vermilion and cutaneous lip as well as distal flap tip necrosis from excess tension.

Burow's triangles are often needed at the distal edges of the flaps, though these are particularly well suited for the central upper lip as the lines can be angled around the ala superiorly and the oral commissure inferiorly. Squaring off the defect and positioning the crossbar of the "H" (remember, the "H" is turned 90 degrees in this design) vertically at a philtrum column will aid in hiding the scar line. Careful attention to the positioning of the white roll and vermilion lip is pivotal in ensuring proper cosmesis with a smooth vermilion border.

An alternative to creating a surgical line along the vermilion border with this closure, it is possible depending upon size of the defect and oral aperture of the patient to excise any inferior redundant tissue similar to a wedge excision. The bilateral flaps are created superiorly with Burow's triangles curving around the bilateral ala as with a traditional bilateral advancement; however, once the superior edge of the flaps are brought together beneath

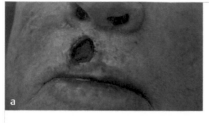
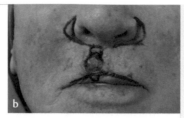
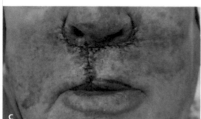
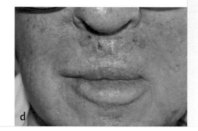

Fig. 6.11 Bilateral cheek advancement for repair of Mohs defect on patient with scar tissue from previous cleft lip repairs. **(a)** Mohs defect centered on the philtral crest. **(b)** Flap design extending the defect to the nasal sill. **(c)** Closure with concealing of surgical lines around the bilateral ala. **(d)** Postoperative view at 2 weeks.

the nasal sill, the remainder of the inferior redundant tissue is excised and the trilaminar layers are brought together as a wedge excision. Care is advised to ensure this modification does not result in microstomia (▶ Fig. 6.11).

Tunneled Melolabial Flap

The tunneled melolabial flap takes advantage of the generous full-sized cheeks that can often be found in older patients. A melolabial flap is raised with de-epithelialization of the proximal flap, whereas the distal flap retains the epidermis in the same size as the defect. The flap is then tunneled through the subcutaneous tissue and pulled medially through the defect. The epidermis is then oriented as to the defect, and cuticular sutures are placed. The melolabial donor defect is then realigned as per the natural cosmetic boundary with layers of both subcutaneous and cuticular sutures. Advantages of this flap include maintaining the size of the lip structure and the apical triangle while hiding surgical lines within natural subunits[16] (▶ Fig. 6.12).

Gull-Wing Mucosal Advancement Flap

The gull-wing mucosal advancement flap is an excellent reconstruction option for a partial-thickness oblong defect that involves the vermilion lip and the cutaneous upper lip where the horizontal length is greater than the vertical height. The gull-wing is aptly named as it spans the central philtrum as the arched wings of a seagull recreating the natural Cupid's bow. Care needs to be taken to ensure bilateral equal triangle removal (vermilionectomy) as to create a balanced upper lip; extending the excision of these triangles further toward the commissures will often aid in this endeavor. Undermining of the mucosa toward the gingival sulcus staying below the glands and above the muscle will allow the mucosa to gently rise to meet the new vermilion border. Soft absorbable cuticular sutures are recommended along the new vermilion border, and no subcutaneous

sutures are required. Generous bland moisturizing of the mucosal lip is often required for several weeks post repair as there is prominent scaling until the mucosa becomes the dry vermilion[17] (▶ Fig. 6.13).

A modification of this flap can be performed with double simultaneous cutaneous and vermilion lip defects. Using a similar technique to that of Dr. Mellett, a vermilionectomy is performed medially between the defects to allow lifting of the flap and creation of a new Cupid's bow. Removal of the bilateral Burow triangles is as mentioned earlier. The flap is then undermined and lifted to create a new vermilion lip and sutured into place (▶ Fig. 6.14).

Abbe Flap (Lip-Switch Flap)

The Abbe flap (also called the lip-switch or cross-lip flap) is a staged flap based upon the labial artery and can be used for both upper and lower lip defects. It is more commonly used for full-thickness central upper lip defects that do not involve the lateral commissures. The flap is designed to be half the size of the defect as to allow for a more balanced cosmetic look of the upper and lower lips after the flap has been transposed. The flap is designed to pivot and rotate into place with the pedicle being more lateral to allow for greater oral aperture and a more proximal based blood supply. As the flap is based on axial blood supply, a greater deal of thinning of the pedicle while preserving the artery can be performed to allow for more pivoting and less tension on the flap. A thorough discussion with the patient prior to the procedure is recommended as the patient needs to understand the pedicle will be in place for 3 weeks and will impede eating, speaking, and social comfort. Realigning of the vermilion border and white roll can also be more difficult with this type of flap.[18]

A few technical adjustments will aid in the creation of this flap: (1) small distal horizontal extension or tabs in the flap can be created to insert into the nasal sill

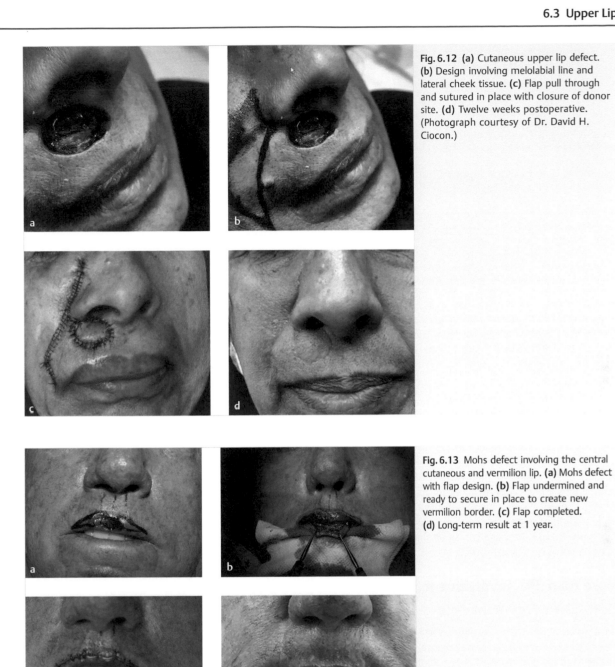

Fig. 6.12 (a) Cutaneous upper lip defect. (b) Design involving melolabial line and lateral cheek tissue. (c) Flap pull through and sutured in place with closure of donor site. (d) Twelve weeks postoperative. (Photograph courtesy of Dr. David H. Ciocon.)

Fig. 6.13 Mohs defect involving the central cutaneous and vermilion lip. (a) Mohs defect with flap design. (b) Flap undermined and ready to secure in place to create new vermilion border. (c) Flap completed. (d) Long-term result at 1 year.

bilaterally; (2) as the labial artery is at the level of the vermilion border but on the deep mucosal aspect, incisional release of the white roll is possible, thus allowing proper inset of the vermilion border and white roll at the receiving location on bilateral aspects of the pedicle[19]; and (3) similar to other full-thickness lip repairs, suturing of the Abbe flap should be done in a trilaminar fashion with good skin eversion of the cutaneous upper and lower lips.

6.3.2 Philtral Subunit: Vermilion Lip Only

Less than 30% Involvement

Primary Closure versus O-T Advancement Flap

For small defects confined to the vermilion lip, a primary closure can be performed or a small O-T advancement flap if there is concern for vermilion border distortion

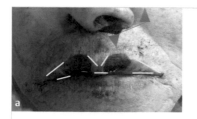
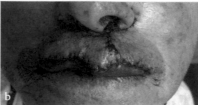
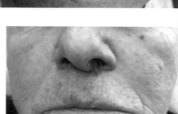

Fig. 6.14 Triple Mohs defects on the cutaneous and upper lip repaired with two separate flaps. **(a)** Mohs defects with a design of the mucosal advancement flap and perialar crescentic flap. **(b)** Closure in place. **(c)** Two days postoperatively demonstrating the normal edema of lip reconstruction. **(d)** Postoperative view at 2 months with edema resolution.

("lip pucker") by the redundant tissue. Undermining of the vermilion is required taking care to stay above the muscle. Use of only a soft cuticular suture (i.e., chromic suture) is recommended as subcutaneous sutures are not needed.

Mucosal Island Pedicle Flap

Mucosal island pedicle flaps are a good reconstruction option for defects confined to the vermilion lip as it helps maintain a natural vermilion border. The mucosal island is incised bilaterally toward the gingival sulcus and then elevated and moved to the vermilion border all while maintaining a central pedicle. Adequate undermining of the flap should be performed to ensure ease of movement while maintaining good vascular perfusion of the pedicle. This type of flap is best used on small shallow defects that do not involve significant muscle loss.

More than 30% Involvement

Mucosal Advancement Flap

This flap is similar to the gull-wing mucosal advancement flap, but it does not design a new vermilion border as the cutaneous lip is not involved. It simply brings the mucosa to the existing vermilion border. This is a commonly used technique for the repair of large defects involving the vermilion lip. The entirety of the vermilion can be repaired by advancement of the labial mucosa. This flap is accomplished by wide undermining of the labial mucosa posterior to the defect. The appropriate plane is below the level of the salivary glands but above the orbicularis oris musculature. The flap is then advanced to the most anterior edge of the defect. Undermining to the labiogingival groove is often not necessary for flap advancement. The unaffected lateral edges of the vermilion lip need to be removed as Burow's triangles prior to advancement as this will allow bilateral balance. The advancing layer of the mucosa is not well suited for deep sutures, and soft superficial sutures will suffice.

This flap is generally well tolerated with favorable cosmesis. However, there is a potential concern for contracture and inward rounding of the lip, which can lead to irritation from hairs projecting toward the lip on the new vermilion border. As with any surgical scar, there is risk of hypoesthesia, which can be minimized with limiting the area of undermining. Damage to salivary glands during the advancement can lead to postoperative dry lips, necessitating petrolatum. Moreover, it has been noted that a deeper red color is often seen in the newly generated vermilion.

6.3.3 Lateral Subunits

Cutaneous Lip with or without Vermilion Lip Involvement

Defects less than One-Third of the Upper Lip

Primary Closure and Wedge Resection

Common and excellent closure options for lateral upper cutaneous lip defects, which are a third or less of the length of the upper lip, are primary closures and wedge resection closures. A primary closure is often used for defects that are not full thickness. As mentioned earlier, the distal orbicularis oris muscle bands may need to be excised to ensure no downward "lip pucker" or lip distortion. Moderate undermining below the skin and above the muscle is recommended to reduce the tension of the two sides being brought together as well as promote good skin eversion. The lip is then closed in layers ensuring good alignment of the vermilion border.

A wedge resection is often performed for deeper or full-thickness defects. A transmural triangular wedge is removed to the gingival sulcus (or modified wedge without full extension to the gingival sulcus). The labial artery can be cauterized or ligated. Suturing of the layers is done posterior to anterior starting with the mucosa, then muscle, dermis, and ending with the cutaneous

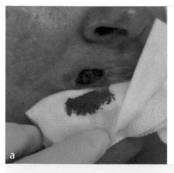
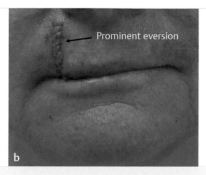
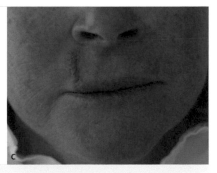

Fig. 6.15 Lateral upper lip defect repaired with primary closure. (a) Mohs defect. (b) Primary closure after moderate undermining and showing good skin eversion. (c) Postoperative view at 1 week showing good alignment of the vermilion border.

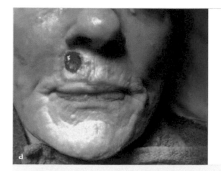
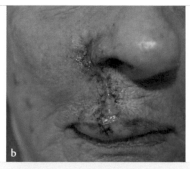
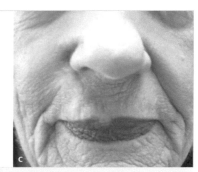

Fig. 6.16 Repair of Mohs defect at the upper lateral cutaneous lip. (a) Final Mohs defect. (b) Perialar crescentic flap repair showing good vermilion border alignment. (c) At the 7-week postoperative visit with skin eversion resolving to thin surgical line.

skin taking care for alignment of the vermilion[20] (▶ Fig. 6.15).

For smaller defects, it is recommended to stay within the subunit boundaries; if it is thought the superior Burow triangle needs to extend past the melolabial line crossing onto the medial cheek, then curve the dog-ear medially in line with the melolabial fold or possibly choose another closure option.

Perialar Crescentic Melolabial Advancement Flap

This flap is frequently used for smaller, partial-thickness defects of the superior area of the cutaneous upper lip, and it is so named for essentially the curving of the superior Burow triangle around the ala for better cosmesis. The elegance of this flap stems from the amount of tissue that can be recruited laterally as well as the hidden surgical line around the ala extending inferiorly to the vermilion lip in a relaxed skin tension line or possibly a philtral crest. When designing this flap, it is best to take an appropriate-sized Burow triangle so as not to push the ala medially in an attempt to make the flap stretch across the defect. It is also best to leave 1 to 2 mm between the ala and the medial incision line of Burow's triangle to eliminate cutaneous sutures being placed through the ala.

Undermining of the flap should be performed above the musculature to avoid damage to the facial nerve branches. The critical suture approximates the leading edge of the flap laterally to the medial edge of the defect just inferior to the nasal sill with a strong tacking suture to the periosteum to avoid alar pull and distortion. As with previous reconstructions, good skin eversion and vermilion alignment are cosmetic tenets[21] (▶ Fig. 6.16).

Rotation Flap

The rotation flap is a cosmetically appealing, fast, and easily performed flap; however, its use is primarily confined to smaller defects of the upper, lateral area of the cutaneous lip. The flap is designed by drawing an arc from the superolateral aspect of the defect along the melolabial line extending below the level of the oral commissure as needed for larger defects. To preserve the cosmetic look of the apical triangle as well as hide the surgical lines along the natural cosmetic boundaries, the arc should be extended superiorly along the melolabial line to the ala enlarging the defect as needed to preserve the cosmetic look of the upper lip. The flap is undermined above the muscle from the melolabial line laterally to the vermilion lip inferiorly. The flap is then rotated into place around the oral commissure. The standing cone inferiorly may cross the vermilion border as needed with careful realignment of the vermilion border. This type of flap should be restricted to patients with

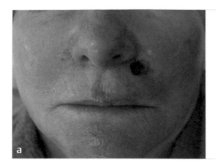
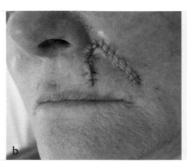

Fig. 6.17 (a) Mohs defect. (b) Rotational flap closure concealing surgical line within the nasolabial fold and extending to the top of the apical triangle.

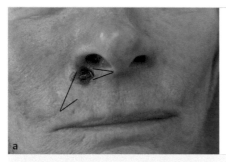
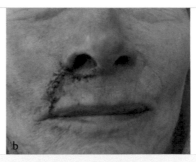
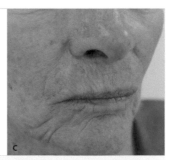

Fig. 6.18 Upper cutaneous lip repair with an inferiorly based hatchet flap. (a) Defect with design. (b) Post repair. (c) One-year postoperative image showing no eclabium and minimal scarring due to extensive undermining and good skin eversion during reconstruction.

small defects and a relatively large upper cutaneous lip as too much rotational torque on the flap to repair a large defect on a small cutaneous lip can cause a sneering distortion of the oral commissure[22,23] (▶ Fig. 6.17).

For smaller horizontal defects just below the nasal sill or within the apical triangle, a modified version of this flap involves doing a small back-cut extending medially and superiorly at the end of the melolabial incision to allow for more rotation of the flap. This back-cut can easily be hidden within the arc line of the melolabial fold with final closure. Extensive undermining of the cutaneous lip above the muscle will allow the flap to easily rotate into place with little risk of eclabium (▶ Fig. 6.18).

Defects Greater than One-Third of the Upper lip

V-Y Flap (Island Pedicle Flap)

The V-Y flap is versatile as it can be used for small defects as well as defects larger than one-third of the upper lip. In fact, the V-Y flap can be used for lateral subunits up to 3 cm in size. The design is as previously mentioned for philtral defects. Wide undermining of the flap while preserving a central pedicle to the overlying orbicularis oris muscle will ensure a well-vascularized flap with little tension. Test the tension of the flap by using a skin hook to guide the flap into place; further undermining may be required to release any restraints. Undermining of the surrounding skin should be performed to reduce possible pincushioning.[24]

Larger defects will require a larger flap, which may actually extend across the melolabial fold to the mandible, but gentle curving of the inferior, lateral portion of the flap mimicking the natural marionette line will produce a better overall cosmetic look. Undermining of a flap of this size may actually need severing of the pedicle to the orbicularis oris muscle while maintaining a peripheral pedicle gaining vascularity from the adipose tissue of the medial cheek.[25,26]

A drawback of this flap is that it may be difficult to conceal one of the three limbs of the island, compromising the aesthetics. This flap is better for a defect where one of the limbs can be concealed along a natural cosmetic boundary, such as the melolabial fold, vermilion border, or border of the ala.

Estlander Flap

A full-thickness lateral defect encompassing more than 30% of the upper lip can be a challenge to reconstruct. The lip-switch flaps are a good option for repair if the more common advancement flaps or wedge repairs are thought to be unsuitable. The Abbe flap is designed for repair of defects medial to the commissure, whereas the Estlander flap is a good option for defects that involve the commissure. The Estlander flap can be used to repair the upper lip, but it is more commonly used on the lower lip.[22] It is a one-stage variant of a cross-lip flap. It was first described in 1972 to help restore large defects of the lateral lip.[27] It is indicated for defects involving one-third to one-half of the lateral lip with involvement of the oral commissure. The flap is similar in execution as the Abbe flap except that it includes the oral commissure. The contralateral lip and commissure are transferred into the full-thickness defect and sutured into place. The donor site is then sutured. As with all full-thickness defects, significant care must be taken in the alignment of the vermilion border and layers for optimal cosmetic and functional results. Historically the flap was designed as a triangular wedge, but modifications to a more rounded appearance to hide the surgical lines within the melolabial fold have merit.[28]

The main advantage of the Estlander flap is that it is a single-stage procedure capable of repairing large full-thickness defects with similar tissue from the opposing lip.

However, the flap results in a blunted vermilion border at the commissure, lacking the normal tapered appearance. The discrepancy between the nonaffected commissure and the newly formed commissure is most visually apparent when the lips are open. The blunted commissure is often revised with further procedures to improve appearance, but returning the natural appearance of the commissure is difficult. Proper patient counseling prior to the procedure and during the repair is vital for improved patient satisfaction. There is also significant hypoesthesia associated with the flap, which can take more than a year to improve and may never fully return.

A commissuroplasty can be performed about 3 weeks after reconstruction in order to improve the cosmesis and function of the affected commissure. Ciocon and colleagues provide an elegant Z-plasty description at the oral commissure ensuring symmetric upper and lower lip lateral points.[29]

6.3.4 Vermilion Lip Only

Less than One-Third of the Upper Lip

Mucosal O-T Advancement Flap

This is a versatile flap that can be used for defects up to approximately 2 cm in diameter on the vermilion lip. Undermining is performed below the glands and above the muscle, which protects the orbicularis oris muscle and the neurovascular structures. Surgical lines can be hidden along the vermilion border and within the oral cavity. No dog-ears need to be removed as the difference can be worked out along the vermilion border. No deep sutures

are required. Soft cuticular sutures, such as chromic, are recommended for patient comfort and are removed 6 to 7 days postoperatively (▶ Fig. 6.19).

More than One-Third of the Upper Lip

Mucosal Advancement Flap

As discussed previously, the mucosal advancement flap creates a new vermilion lip by extending the mucosa from the internal mouth outward to the vermilion border. With larger defects, it is recommended to remove the remainder of the upper lip mucosa, creating a new lip in order to achieve a contoured, symmetric upper lip. The undermining is performed above the muscle and below glands as to decrease bleeding and risk to neuromuscular bundles. The amount of undermining required is based upon the anterior to posterior width of the lesion. Narrower longer lesions often require minimal undermining, whereas lesions of greater width extending into the mouth may necessitate more undermining to obtain less flap tension and greater flap movement. Too much tension on the flap can pull the lip into the mouth, creating a less desirable cosmetic look. Care to recreate the central Cupid's bow is paramount to a more natural upper lip (▶ Fig. 6.20).

6.4 Lower Lip Reconstruction

6.4.1 Cutaneous Lower Lip with or without Vermilion Involvement

Less than One-Third of the Lip Length

Primary Closure

Primary closure is the first technique that should be considered when designing a lower lip reconstruction. Defects of one-third (and possibly up to one-half) of the lower lip may be closed primarily without disrupting oral competence.[30,31] Primary closure will allow for an excellent cosmetic outcome while maintaining orbicularis muscle sphincter function. The goal is to have the final suture line well hidden within the natural skin tension lines surrounding the lip. Primary closures are best suited for defects not involving the commissure and within the same cosmetic subunit. It is important to note when designing linear closures that failure to properly debulk

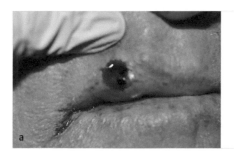
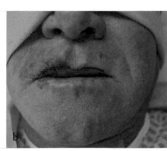

Fig. 6.19 (a) Mohs defect confined to vermilion lip only. (b) O-T advancement flap with T crossbar along the vermilion border.

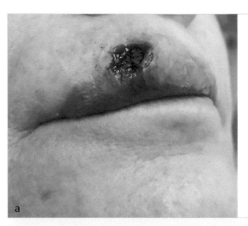
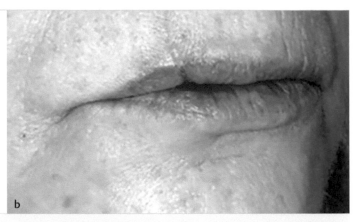

Fig. 6.20 (a) Mohs defect confined to the vermilion lip. (b) Postoperative view at 2 months after mucosal advancement flap with well-contoured Cupid's bow. (Photograph courtesy of Dr. David H. Ciocon.)

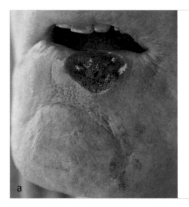
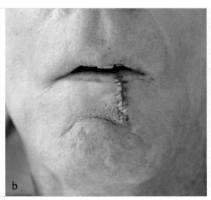

Fig. 6.21 (a) Mohs defect encompassing both the vermilion lip and the lower cutaneous lip. (b) Completed primary closure with "mini-wedge" removal of the distal orbicularis oris muscle. Note the vermilion border and the mental crease outlined prior to repair.

the orbicularis oris muscle ("mini-wedge") may lead to poor cosmesis with puckering deformities.[13] The primary closure has the benefit of restoring the orbicularis oris muscle and not altering the position of the modiolus with risk of sensation loss.[32] When possible, preserving mucosa is preferred as this will lead to quicker recovery times and decreased infection risk.[33]

For defects involving the lower cutaneous lip extending toward the chin, it is important to properly design the flap within cosmetic subunits. Outlining the anatomic boundaries of the vermilion border and mental crease prior to reconstruction will guide the design and execution of the repair. The apex of the repair of the lower lip should not extend beyond the mental crease as repairs that cross the mental crease can risk poor cosmesis. Curving the Burow triangle to follow the mental crease laterally is preferred to crossing this line. Finally, good approximation of the vermilion border and proper skin eversion is necessary for cosmesis (▶ Fig. 6.21).

Wedge Resection

Wedge resection is a versatile reconstruction for either the upper or lower lip and is often used for full-thickness defects, and can often produce a tension-free and aesthetically pleasing repair.[33] This repair can be used on both the lateral and central areas of the lower lip. Lateral defects are often V-shaped excisions, whereas for central defects, a W-plasty (inverse M-plasty) may be used to ensure the repair does not cross the mental crease. The two apices of the W-plasty are oriented away from the vermilion border and the angles should not exceed 30 degrees.[23,34] Excision of remaining tissue within the wound site extending toward the gingival sulcus is removed to produce a full-thickness V-shaped defect. Although undermining is often limited in this repair, it is still important to be aware of the mental nerve as it provides innervation for the lower lip and several different branching variations have been characterized.[35] It is prudent to make patients aware of the risk of lower lip hypoesthesia for defects in this area, especially deeper defects.

The repair is transmural and needs to be closed in layers. Careful reapproximation of the different layers is important for function and cosmesis. The labial artery can be ligated or cauterized, and then close each layer from inner to outer starting with mucosa, then muscle, subcutaneous tissue, and finally the cuticular layer. Meticulous alignment of the vermilion border and good eversion of the cutaneous lip are cosmetic requirements.

Unilateral or Bilateral Advancement Flaps

This is an excellent closure option for deeper partial-thickness defects or full-thickness defects. The unilateral flap approach will suffice for small defects. For defects in the central area and depending upon the size of the oral aperture, the bilateral advancement flaps may possibly be used for defects larger than one-third the size of the lip. The area is converted to a full-thickness rectangular defect to facilitate closure with the base of the rectangle at the level of the mental crease (▶ Fig. 6.22). The design is then carried inferiorly in an arciform line on the bilateral sides of the mental crease. Although a staircase method along the mental crease is also an option to allow advancement of the flaps,[36] following the curve of the mental crease and taking dog-ears as needed provides an easy and elegant form of flap advancement and acceptable cosmesis for smaller defects. The closure is in a transmural fashion, ensuring good approximation of the muscle and vermilion border.

Partial-thickness bilateral advancement flaps can also be performed for modest-depth defects. These flaps are designed to either side of the primary defect with the incision lines at the vermilion border and the mental crease.[22] As the flap is created from tissue surrounding the defect, the color, texture, thickness, and hair density are excellent matches. Moreover, the heavy vascular supply provided by the labial arteries allows for quick wound healing and excellent cosmesis. Similarly, when properly designed, there is significantly less risk of hypoesthesia and sphincter dysfunction compared to other reconstructive techniques. This repair has also been described in vermilion-only defects with good success.[37]

This bilateral advancement flap utilizes tissue from both sides of the defect. Extensive undermining of both the lateral aspects and the superior and inferior edges is necessary for tension-free approximation. The undermining plane should be superior to the orbicularis muscle to ensure continued sphincter function. Undermining through the musculature and into the mucosa can lead to delayed infection, hematoma, and necrosis. It is important to ensure sufficient tissue laxity is recruited with each flap or there is potential for increased height of the vermilion and cutaneous lip as well as distal flap tip necrosis from excess tension.

Burow's triangles are often needed at the distal edges of the flaps, though these are particularly well suited for central upper and lower lips. The distal angled surgical lines can be well hidden along the curvature of the

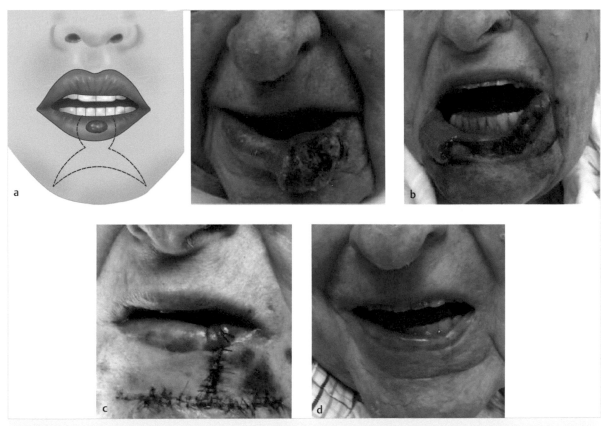

Fig. 6.22 (a) Design on cartoon showing Burow's triangles following mental crease. **(b)** Large squamous cell carcinoma (SCC) of the lateral lower lip. **(c)** Squaring off of defect after Mohs completed. **(c)** Closure. **(d)** Postoperative view at 2 months. (Photograph courtesy of Dr. David H. Ciocon.)

commissures and the labiomental crease in lower lip defects. This repair can also be combined with a mucosal advancement or smaller mucosal rotation if the vermilion is involved. This will ensure the subunits remain separate.[25]

In lower lip defects, the lateral surgical lines can be hidden in the labiomental crease. The central line of the "H"-shaped flap may be a source of poor cosmesis, especially if under high tension; appropriate undermining and good skin eversion at closure will help improve cosmesis. The subsequent scars will be well hidden within the natural cosmetic boundaries. Failure to properly design the flap abutting the vermilion will lead to an unfavorable result and may necessitate scar revisions. Z-plasties are particularly effective in these circumstances.

V-Y Advancement Flap (Island Pedicle Flap)

This is a versatile flap in that it can be used on either the upper or the lower cutaneous lip. Similar to the upper lip, the design entails an approximate 3:1 ratio of the flap to the defect size, and the key suture is at the point of the V (or island) with the forces extending horizontally. This suture is especially important for the lower lip as it will help support the flap and counteract the downward gravitational pull. Undermining of the flap while retaining a central muscular pedicle will allow good flap movement and vascularity. Undermining of the surrounding skin should also be performed to reduce pincushioning. Good cuticular eversion as mentioned previously will improve long-term cosmesis.

If the mucosa is involved with this defect, then a mucosal rotation or advancement flap should be performed in order to respect the subunits. The mucosal flap should be brought outward after undermining to meet the new vermilion border and secured into place with soft cuticular sutures. The repair can be a full advancement flap with vermilionectomy for larger defects or rotational flap depending upon size and location of the defect. As an

added benefit, the mucosal repair can also provide pull in the opposite direction to alleviate the downward pull of the V-Y flap (▶ Fig. 6.23). Bocchi et al reported excellent results with this flap in their cohort.[38]

More than One-Third of Lip Involvement or Involving the Commissure

Karapandzic Flap

The Karapandzic flap is a modified full-thickness circumoral rotation-advancement flap first described in 1857 by von Bruns.[39] The flap was designed as both a rotation and an advancement to move around the commissure. The modification by Karapandzic in 1974 improved upon the original version by maintaining the innervation. The flap is designed to ensure preservation of neurovascular structures and maintain sphincter function.[40] It is classically used in the reconstruction of full-thickness defects of the lower lips as upper lip defects that are not centrally located are generally not suitable for this repair given the distortion of the philtrum. This method is reliable for defects involving up to two-thirds of the lower lip. Other investigators have reported success with defects up to 80%.[41,42]

For lower lip defects, the flap is created by circumoral incisions parallel to the free margin of the lips along the mental and melolabial creases. The incisions should terminate near the lateral projection of the nasal ala. When designing the two circumoral flaps, it is important to maintain symmetry as much as feasible given the variation in symmetry in the melolabial creases. The next step as described by Karapandzic involves partial-thickness incisions made to the subcutis to facilitate the dissection and identification of the neurovascular pedicle. The peripheral muscle fibers are dissected and preserved and then only divided and repositioned as needed for flap advancement. Every care is made to avoid incision of the mucosa unless necessary. The flap is then advanced to the defect and sutured into place with special care taken to

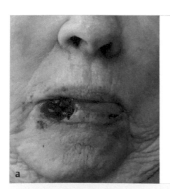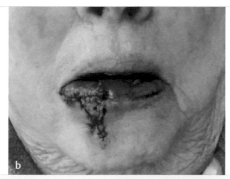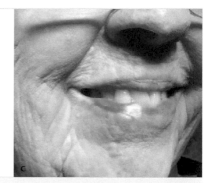

Fig. 6.23 V-Y advancement flap (island pedicle flap) and mucosal rotation flap. (a) Mohs defect after removal of squamous cell carcinoma (SCC). (b) V-Y advancement flap with mucosal rotation flap ensuring good realignment with the vermilion border. (c) Postoperative view at 10 weeks.

ensure each layer is sutured into place. Failure to properly align the flaps can result in a distorted and clownlike appearance.[43]

The Karapandzic flap is a one-stage procedure that can reliably reconstruct large defects of the lower lip. Hypoesthesia and loss of sphincter function, which plague other larger flaps, is less frequently seen. There is some blunting of the commissures, but unlike with the Estlander flap, commissuroplasty is rarely indicated.[44]

Staircase/Stepladder Plasty

The staircase or stepladder plasty was first described by Johanson and is utilized for defects of up to two-thirds of the lower lip.[45] This flap is a modified advancement flap that utilizes numerous small incisions in a staircaselike fashion. The defect is converted into full thickness with a rectangular shape with free margins. The short incisions or "steps" are directed horizontally and then vertically downward in an overall 45-degree angle away from the defect's squared-off edges. The individual steps are progressively smaller than the last leading away from the defect. The individual steps of the flap are incised full thickness at the same level as the converted defect. The flap is advanced horizontally and the mucosa, subcutis, and muscle are then sutured into place. In practice, two to four steps are needed for sufficient tissue laxity for tissue approximation. For larger central lesions, a bilateral staircase flap can be utilized, whereas a single set of steps is sufficient for lateral defects less than 2 cm. Though classically considered a repair for the lower lip, Dado and Angelats have shown that the technique can also be utilized in upper lip defects.[46]

There is a modified version of the Johanson technique designed by Kuttenberger and Hardt that does not involve full-thickness incisions in the lower lip.[47] The key difference in this modification lies in the fact that the flap is undermined above the orbicularis and depressor labii inferioris muscle, thereby leaving the musculature intact. This modification removes the risk of possible sphincter and depressor dysfunction that can potentially occur with the classic reconstruction.

Similar to a Z-plasty, the stepwise fashion of the flap elongates the wound, preventing contracture. Moreover, the flap does not result in a diminished aperture of the oral cavity as is a potential drawback of many of the repairs for large defects of the lips. When hidden in the mental crease, the cosmetic outcome is generally excellent.

Gilles Fan Flap

First described in 1957 by Gillies and Millard, this flap is a type of fan or rotational flap that can be used for both upper and lower lip defects,[22,47,48] but more commonly used in lower lip defects. Similar to the staircase flap, it can be modified for lateral or central defects with unilateral and bilateral tissue mobility. The flap utilizes the tissue reservoir of the cheek and lips to fill the defect. The defect is converted to full thickness and squared off with free margins. A radial full-thickness incision is then made on the contralateral lip toward the nasolabial and then directed toward the labiomental crease. The flap is then rotated into the defect and sutured into place. Similar to other full-thickness flaps, special care must be taken to ensure each layer of the donor flap is appropriately sutured into the recipient site, especially to maintain some degree of concurrent muscular function.

The main advantage to this flap is that it is a single-stage procedure that can repair large defects of the lip. There are potential drawbacks to this technique, most notably the decrease in the oral aperture and the formation of a rounded commissure. In bilateral based flaps, there is complete loss of oral commissure on both sides. Although the repair is single staged, often the patient must return for a scar revision to improve the appearance of the commissure. Finally, there is often hallowing of the cheeks noted as well as decreased function of the rotated orbicularis muscle and decreased sensation.

Hemi-Bernard Flap

This flap is a unilateral version of the Bernard–Burow bilateral flap and does not alter the continuity of the orbicularis oris muscle or the modiolus–commissure relationship. This flap is best for a lateral lower lip defect where microstomia may be of a concern with more commonly used repairs. It combines a unilateral advancement cheek flap with the advancement of the remaining contralateral lower lip while preserving the orbicularis oris muscle and the mental nerve. By preserving these two structures, function and sensation are spared.

The design involves incision along the vermilion border laterally curving around the oral commissure to the nasolabial line. The contralateral incision runs along the mental crease laterally following the natural curve. Redundant tissue is excised along the nasolabial fold and commissure and bilaterally along the arcs of the mental crease. The two flaps are slid together ensuring transmural reapproximation and good realignment of the vermilion border.[32]

6.5 Vermilion Involvement Only

6.5.1 Less than One-Third of the Lip Length

Mucosal Rotation Flap

Small rotation flaps are good for the lateral vermilion lip where the defect does not cross the vermilion border. It is best to widen the defect as needed to extend to the vermilion border, thus allowing the flap to follow the cosmetic subunit. The flap is incised extending toward the gingival sulcus and undermining is performed above the muscle and below the glands. The flap is then rotated (often around the oral commissure) and lifted outward to be in line with the vermilion border. A small advancement flap from the medial direction can aid with providing less tension on the rotational flap while allowing a small amount of thinning of the subcutaneous tissue medially for better lip contour and transition along the vermilion lip. After ensuring good approximation of the vermilion border, the flaps are sutured into place with only cuticular sutures (▶ Fig. 6.24).

O-T Advancement Flap

The mucosal rotation flap is of similar design to the O-T advancement flap on the upper vermilion lip. This flap is of exceptional good use for fuller lower lips and may possibly be used for defects slightly larger than one-third of the lower lip as there is adequate flap movement with good undermining of the vermilion lip and mucosa. Undermining is above the muscle and below the glands. Burow's triangles are not needed as the difference can be worked out along the vermilion border. Subcutaneous sutures are not needed as cuticular soft sutures will suffice[49] (▶ Fig. 6.25).

6.5.2 Greater than One-Third of the Lip Length

Mucosal Advancement Flap

Mucosal advancement is an excellent option for vermilion lesions greater than one-third of the lip length and may also be used if only 1 to 2 mm of the cutaneous lip is involved. The design is similar to the upper lip mucosal advancement and gull-wing flaps; however, it is considered simpler in that there is no Cupid's bow to recreate. A vermilionectomy of the bilateral Burow triangles is required to ensure a contoured lower lip. The flap is created by undermining inward toward the sulcus below the glands and above the muscle.[25] The amount of undermining is determined by the width of the defect as narrower defects may require only minimal undermining and not extending all the way to the sulcus. This flap creates an entirely new vermilion and vermilion border as the mucosa is brought outward and sutured into place. The key suture is placed in the middle of the lip connecting the mucosa to the cutaneous lip and subsequent sutures are placed on one side of the key suture and then the other, working back and forth until completed (▶ Fig. 6.26).

One drawback of this flap is that for men it may eliminate the small 2- to 3-mm area between the vermilion border and the start of the beard line. It may be disconcerting to have stiff beard hairs in such close proximity to the lip. Another disadvantage of this flap is the inward pull of the lower lip, thus reducing the cosmetic appearance of a full lip. Patients should also be advised that this flap will require the use of moisturizers for many months until the mucosa keratinizes.

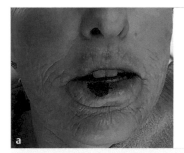
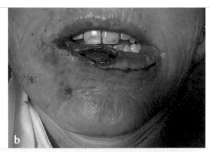
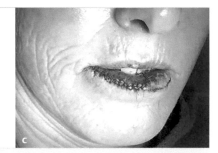

Fig. 6.24 Mucosal rotation flap after Mohs procedure. **(a)** Mohs defect involving only the vermilion lip. **(b)** Mucosal rotational flap with first suture at mid flap along vermilion border. **(c)** Repair complete.

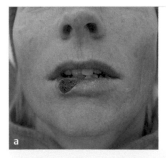
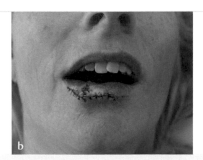
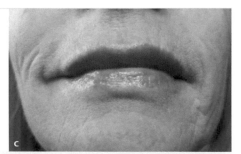

Fig. 6.25 (a) Mohs defect of the vermilion lip. **(b)** O-T advancement flap with good alignment of the vermilion border and no Burow's triangles needed. **(c)** Postoperative view at 6 months.

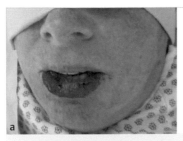 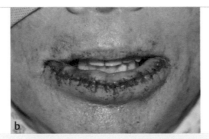 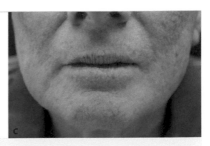

Fig. 6.26 (a) Mohs defect after removal of extensive squamous cell carcinoma (SCC). (b) Mucosal advancement flap with undermining to the sulcus and using chromic sutures. (c) Postoperative view at 12 months.

References

[1] Sanniec KJ, Carboy JA, Thornton JF. Simplifying lip reconstruction: an algorithmic approach. Semin Plast Surg. 2018; 32(2):69–74

[2] Jacono AA. A new classification of lip zones to customize injectable lip augmentation. Arch Facial Plast Surg. 2008; 10(1):25–29

[3] Pepper JP, Baker SR. Local flaps: cheek and lip reconstruction. JAMA Facial Plast Surg. 2013; 15(5):374–382

[4] Rogers CR, Mooney MP, Smith TD, et al. Comparative microanatomy of the orbicularis oris muscle between chimpanzees and humans: evolutionary divergence of lip function. J Anat. 2009; 214(1):36–44

[5] Krunic AL, Weitzul S, Taylor RS. Advanced reconstructive techniques for the lip and perioral area. Dermatol Clin. 2005; 23(1):43–53, v–vi

[6] Tong CCL, Vandegriend ZP, Lee YH, Lawson W. Anatomical basis for lip reconstruction: the role of the modiolus. Ann Plast Surg. 2019; 82 (5):565–569

[7] Bolognia JL, Jorizzo JL, Schaffer JV. Dermatology. 3rd ed. Amsterdam: Elsevier Saunders; 2012

[8] Lee SH, Lee HJ, Kim YS, Kim HJ, Hu KS. What is the difference between the inferior labial artery and the horizontal labiomental artery? Surg Radiol Anat. 2015; 37(8):947–953

[9] Lee SH, Lee M, Kim HJ. Anatomy-based image processing analysis of the running pattern of the perioral artery for minimally invasive surgery. Br J Oral Maxillofac Surg. 2014; 52(8):688–692

[10] Lee HJ, Won SY, O J, et al. The facial artery: a comprehensive anatomical review. Clin Anat. 2018; 31(1):99–108

[11] Samizadeh S, Pirayesh A, Bertossi D. Anatomical variations in the course of labial arteries: a literature review. Aesthet Surg J. 2019; 39 (11):1225–1235

[12] Tulley P, Webb A, Chana JS, et al. Paralysis of the marginal mandibular branch of the facial nerve: treatment options. Br J Plast Surg. 2000; 53(5):378–385

[13] Zitelli JA, Brodland DG. A regional approach to reconstruction of the upper lip. J Dermatol Surg Oncol. 1991; 17(2):143–148

[14] Luce EA. Upper lip reconstruction. Plast Reconstr Surg. 2017; 140(5): 999–1007

[15] Thornton JF, Harirah MH. Discussion: elegance in upper lip reconstruction. Plast Reconstr Surg. 2019; 143(2):585–588

[16] Yim E, Tinklepaugh AJ, Libby TJ, Ciocon DH. Reconstruction of a deep cutaneous lip defect involving the nasal sill. Dermatol Surg. 2020; 46 (1):123–125

[17] Paniker PU, Mellette JR. A simple technique for repair of Cupid's bow. Dermatol Surg. 2003; 29(6):636–640

[18] Baumann D, Robb G. Lip reconstruction. Semin Plast Surg. 2008; 22 (4):269–280

[19] Culliford A, IV, Zide B. Technical tips in reconstruction of the upper lip with the Abbé flap. Plast Reconstr Surg. 2008; 122(1):240–243

[20] Godek CP, Weinzweig J, Bartlett SP. Lip reconstruction following Mohs' surgery: the role for composite resection and primary closure. Plast Reconstr Surg. 2000; 106(4):798–804

[21] Wang SQ, Behroozan DS, Goldberg LH. Perialar crescentic advancement flap for upper cutaneous lip defects. Dermatol Surg. 2005; 31(11, Pt 1):1445–1447

[22] Krunic AL, Weitzul S, Taylor RS. Advanced reconstructive techniques for the lip and perioral area. Dermatol Clin. 2005; 23(1):43–53, v–vi

[23] Guanning NL, Desai SC. Lip reconstruction: primary full thickness closure and superficial partial thickness closure. Oper Tech Otolaryngol Head Neck Surg. 2020; 31:2–9

[24] Braun M, Jr, Cook J. The island pedicle flap. Dermatol Surg. 2005; 31 (8, Pt 2):995–1005

[25] Goldman GD, Dzubow LM, Yelverton CB. 2013

[26] Griffin GR, Weber S, Baker SR. Outcomes following V-Y advancement flap reconstruction of large upper lip defects. Arch Facial Plast Surg. 2012; 14(3):193–197

[27] Estlander JA. Methode d'autoplastie de la joue ou d'une levre par un lambeau emprunte a l'autre levre. Rev Mens Med Chir. 1877; 1:344

[28] Baker SR, Swanson NA. Local Flaps in Facial Reconstruction. St. Louis, MO: Mosby; 1995

[29] Songco JAP, Routt E, Vinelli G, Ciocon D. Reconstruction of a full-thickness defect of the left upper lip, cheek, and oral commissure. Dermatol Surg. 2021; 47(12):e220-e223

[30] Soliman S, Hatef DA, Hollier LH, Jr, Thornton JF. The rationale for direct linear closure of facial Mohs' defects. Plast Reconstr Surg. 2011; 127(1):142–149

[31] Pelly AD, Tan EP. Lower lip reconstruction. Br J Plast Surg. 1981; 34 (1):83–86

[32] Boukovalas S, Boson AL, Hays JP, Malone CH, Cole EL, Wagner RF, Jr. A systematic review of lower lip anatomy, mechanics of local flaps, and special considerations for lower lip reconstruction. J Drugs Dermatol. 2017; 16(12):1254–1261

[33] Barry RB, McKenzie J, Berg D, Langtry JA. Direct primary closure without undermining in the repair of vermilionectomy defects of the lower lip. Br J Dermatol. 2012; 167(5):1092–1097

[34] McCarn KE, Park SS. Lip reconstruction. Otolaryngol Clin North Am. 2007; 40(2):361–380

[35] Alsaad K, Lee TC, McCartan B. An anatomical study of the cutaneous branches of the mental nerve. Int J Oral Maxillofac Surg. 2003; 32(3): 325–333

[36] Ebrahimi A, Kalantar Motamedi MH, Ebrahimi A, Kazemi M, Shams A, Hashemzadeh H. Lip reconstruction after tumor ablation. World J Plast Surg. 2016; 5(1):15–25

[37] Ohtsuka H, Nakaoka H. Bilateral vermilion flaps for lower lip repair. Plast Reconstr Surg. 1990; 85(3):453–456

[38] Bocchi A, Baccarani A, Bianco G, Castagnetti F, Papadia F. Double V-Y advancement flap in the management of lower lip reconstruction. Ann Plast Surg. 2003; 51(2):205–209

[39] von Bruns V. Chirurgischer Atlas: Bildliche Darstellung der chirurgischen Krankheiten und der zu ihrer Heilung erforderlichen Instrumente, Bandagen und Operationen, II Abt, Kau- und Geschmaks-Organ. Tubingen: Luupp; 1857/1860

[40] Karapandzic M. Reconstruction of lip defects by local arterial flaps. Br J Plast Surg. 1974; 27(1):93–97

[41] Neligan PC. Cheek and lip reconstruction. In: Neligan PC, ed. Plastic surgery. Vol. 6. 3rd ed. London: Elsevier Saunders; 2013:254–277

[42] Neligan PC. Strategies in lip reconstruction. Clin Plast Surg. 2009; 36 (3):477–485

[43] Renner GJ. Reconstruction of the lips. In: Baker SR, ed. Local Flaps in Facial Reconstruction. 3rd ed. Philadelphia, PA: Saunders; 2014:481–529

[44] Anvar BA, Evans BCD, Evans GRD. Lip reconstruction. Plast Reconstr Surg. 2007; 120(4):57e–64e

[45] Johanson B, Aspelund E, Breine U, Holmström H. Surgical treatment of non-traumatic lower lip lesions with special reference to the step technique. A follow-up on 149 patients. Scand J Plast Reconstr Surg. 1974; 8(3):232–240

[46] Dado DV, Angelats J. Upper and lower lip reconstruction using the step technique. Ann Plast Surg. 1985; 15(3):204–211

[47] Kuttenberger JJ, Hardt N. Results of a modified staircase technique for reconstruction of the lower lip. J Craniomaxillofac Surg. 1997; 25(5): 239–244

[48] Gillies H, Millard DR. The Principles and art of Plastic Surgery. Vol. 2. Boston, MA: Little, Brown, & Co.; 1957

[49] Hirokawa D, Samie FH. Lip reconstruction with a mucosal A-to-T flap, revisited. Dermatol Surg. 2014; 40(6):696–698

7 Reconstruction of the Mental Unit

Thomas K. Barlow, Arjun Dayal, and Vineet Mishra

Summary

The chin is a foundational facial feature and one of the most prominent parts of facial anatomy. Although it serves as an osseous foundation for the face and a site of muscle attachment, it is thought that a large part of its function is aesthetic. For centuries, a strong chin has been associated with strength, power, confidence, and to this day remains as one of the most important structures when assessing facial aesthetics. An observer's gaze typically focuses on the eyes and the central face, especially in conversation. However, any conspicuous disfigurement of the chin can break this eye contact, creating uncomfortable downward glances. In the profile, a youthful attractive chin forms a smooth curve, providing balance to the prominence of the forehead and nose, and sharply defining the border to the submental area and neck. Given its prominent role in facial aesthetics, it is important to carefully reconstruct the chin after skin surgery.

Keywords: chin reconstruction, submental unit, central chin, lateral chin, O-T flap, double rotation flap

7.1 Anatomy

The shape of the chin is defined by the mental protuberance of the mandible. The form is refined by the muscle above the bone, a layer of subcutaneous tissue, and the skin, which is thicker here than in any other area of the face.[1] The skin of the chin has direct insertion of the mentalis muscle, which allows for complex movement and expression.[2] The chin's surface is primarily convex with a flat or concave area near the junction with the lower lip. Because of its convexity, wound healing with secondary intention in this location tends to cause unsightly contour irregularities with depressed or hypertrophic scars.[3,4]

The chin is defined superiorly and laterally by the labiomental crease and inferiorly by the submental-cervical crease (▶ Fig. 7.1).[5] These creases provide for reasonable concealment of scar lines. With facial aging, patients also develop melomental or "marionette" lines, which delineate the chin from the cheeks and can also serve as creases for scar concealment. However, there is significant variability in the location and presence of these creases on the lower face, making advance planning of reconstruction in this area challenging.[6]

The skin of the chin tends to be thick, oily, and dynamic—moving with both mastication and facial expression. Mouth opening stretches the skin of the chin, exacerbating tight scars and tissue deficits. Local reservoirs for skin laxity for the chin include the cheeks and the submental area. Excessive recruitment of soft tissue from the lower cutaneous lip may cause eclabium and oral incompetence, and therefore must be avoided.[2,7]

Facial expression in the chin involves the mentalis muscle, which originates from the depths of the mental protuberance and inserts into the overlying skin. It is useful to convey facial expressions of doubt and pout and is also involved in indirect elevation of the lower lip.[8] As the mentalis muscle attaches directly to the skin, it is prone to disruption with undermining and tissue rearrangement. Although loss of function of the mentalis is usually acceptable to patients, asymmetry of the muscle should be avoided. When undermining a portion of the mentalis, thought may be given to undermining it entirely to allow for symmetrical healing. Mentalis asymmetry or dyskinesis, should it occur, may be treated with neuromodulators.[9]

Just superficial to the mentalis lies the depressor labii inferioris (DLI), which originates from the mandible and inserts into the skin of the chin along with fibers from the orbicularis oris. As the name implies, the DLI depresses the lower lip and moves it laterally. Also arising from the mandible and running superficial to the DLI is the depressor anguli oris (DAO), which also inserts into the skin of the chin and the orbicularis oris and depresses the corner of the mouth during frowning.[10] The platysma envelops the anterior neck, drapes over the submental space, and inserts into the mandible. It does not reach the anterior portion of the chin, but does rise more superiorly at the lateral jawline, crossing over the mandible to insert into the muscles of the cheeks (▶ Fig. 7.2).[11]

The chin has a robust blood supply, suitable to support random flaps in many configurations. The primary supply comes from the mental artery, which is a terminal branch of the maxillary artery. Paired mental arteries exit the mental foramina on each side and run medially, forming an anastomosis with one another. Additional blood supply to the area is provided by branches of paired inferior labial and labiomental arteries (not pictured), which course medially along the chin and lower lip, and inferiorly from contributions of the submental artery (▶ Fig. 7.3).[12,13,14]

The motor innervation of the mentalis and the oral depressors is provided by the marginal mandibular branch of the facial nerve. This nerve exits the parotid gland and courses medially and inferiorly underneath the platysma muscle along the mandible, reliably crossing over the facial artery at the medial border of the masseter muscle, and running between the lip depressors and platysma muscle within 2 cm of the corner of the mouth.[5,15,16] It is especially prone to injury near the middle of the mandibular body where the overlying platysma-SMAS layer is often unpredictably thin (▶ Fig. 7.4).[17,18] Furthermore, this branch of the facial nerve often only has a single

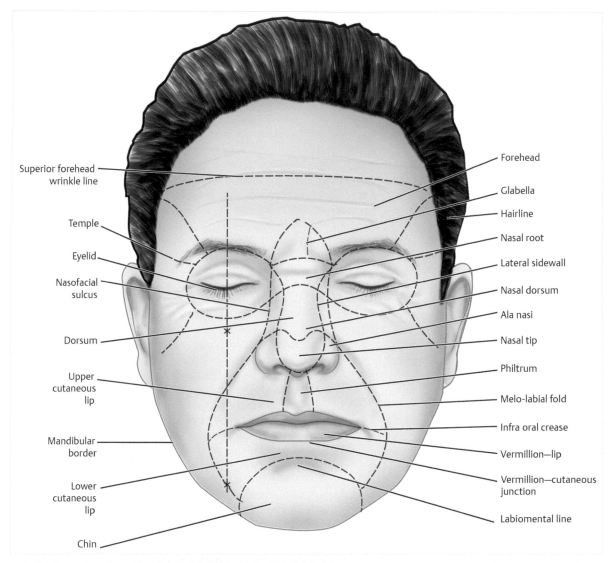

Superior forehead wrinkle line
Temple
Eyelid
Nasofacial sulcus
Dorsum
Upper cutaneous lip
Mandibular border
Lower cutaneous lip
Chin

Forehead
Glabella
Hairline
Nasal root
Lateral sidewall
Nasal dorsum
Ala nasi
Nasal tip
Philtrum
Melo-labial fold
Infra oral crease
Vermillion—lip
Vermillion—cutaneous junction
Labiomental line

Fig. 7.1 Cosmetic units and junctions of the face.

ramus after leaving the parotid gland, increasing the chance of complete denervation and permanent paralysis of the target muscles should it be accidentally transected.[10,15,16] Fortunately, within the mental unit, the marginal mandibular nerve lies deep to the lip depressors, which makes injury in this area rare.

The mental nerve, a branch of the mandibular division (V_3) of the trigeminal nerve, supplies sensory innervation in this area. The mental nerve exits the mandible along with the mental artery and vein through the mental foramen and immediately divides into three branches: one providing sensation to the chin and the others innervating the skin and mucous membranes of the lower lip as shown in ▶ Fig. 7.5. Because of the early branching beneath the DAO muscle, this nerve is usually injured only when deep tissue near the foramen are manipulated

and with procedures that expose the mandible.[10,19] However, injury to this nerve results in numbness along the ipsilateral half of the lower lip and chin. Patients may report they inadvertently bite their lower lip while chewing and find it difficult to keep food in their mouth after a mental nerve injury.[17]

An intraoral mental nerve block can be effectively used for larger surgical procedures in the mental unit. This is achieved by first applying a topical anesthetic such as 5% viscous lidocaine to the base of the first and second premolar teeth, adjacent to the mental foramina. Afterward, a 30-gauge needle is advanced approximately 1 cm through the mucosa toward the mental nerve, and between 1.5 and 3.0 mL of local anesthetic is instilled at the level of the mandibular periosteum (▶ Fig. 7.6).[20] Percutaneous approaches have also been described, but

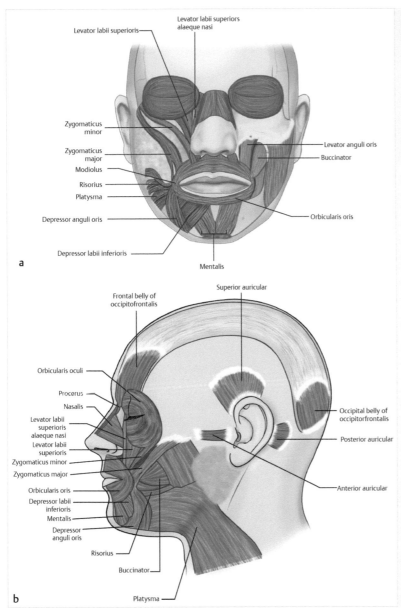

Fig. 7.2 (a, b) Musculature of the lower face.

a

Levator labii superioris

Levator labii superiors alaeque nasi

Zygomaticus minor

Zygomaticus major

Modiolus

Risorius

Platysma

Depressor anguli oris

Depressor labii inferioris

Mentalis

Levator anguli oris

Buccinator

Orbicularis oris

b

Frontal belly of occipitofrontalis

Superior auricular

Orbicularis oculi

Procerus

Nasalis

Levator labii superioris alaeque nasi

Levator labii superioris

Zygomaticus minor

Zygomaticus major

Orbicularis oris

Depressor labii inferioris

Mentalis

Depressor anguli oris

Risorius

Buccinator

Platysma

Occipital belly of occipitorfrontalis

Posterior auricular

Anterior auricular

these were found to be more painful than intraoral approaches in one study.[21]

7.2 Defects and Repairs

Due to the chin's convexity, movement, and skin quality, scars in this cosmetically sensitive location can be unforgiving. There is little inherent skin laxity in this subunit due to the adherence of the underlying soft tissue to the mandible. Excessive recruitment of the skin from the lower lip for repairs may lead to eclabium and oral incompetence, further adding to the challenge of mental unit reconstruction.[22] The relatively thick and oily nature of the mental subunit skin makes this area unfavorable for repair by skin grafting.[7] Healing by secondary intention, which yields favorable scars when used in concave areas, is rarely used on the chin given the predominantly convex nature of the mental unit.[4] Zitelli found that secondary intention healing in this area often leads to stellate, hypertrophic scars, whereas others report scarring with a depressed groove. Becker et al found that secondary intention healing of deeper defects in this area lead to scarring with contracture.[3]

Flaps with a digitate form will constrict as they contract, highlighting the outline with a pincushion effect. If such a scar overlies the dermal insertion of the mentalis, muscle contraction will exacerbate the deformity.

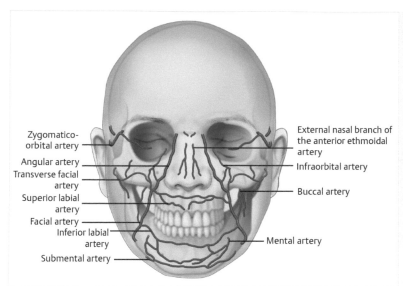

Fig. 7.3 Vascular supply to the mid and lower face.

Zygomatico-orbital artery
Angular artery
Transverse facial artery
Superior labial artery
Facial artery
Inferior labial artery
Submental artery

External nasal branch of the anterior ethmoidal artery
Infraorbital artery
Buccal artery
Mental artery

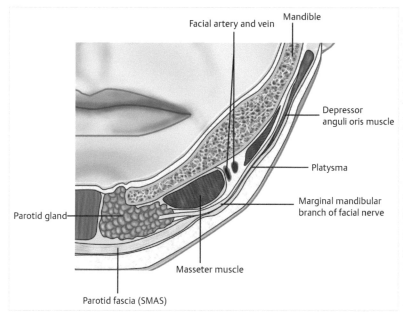

Facial artery and vein
Mandible

Depressor anguli oris muscle

Platysma

Marginal mandibular branch of facial nerve

Parotid gland

Masseter muscle

Parotid fascia (SMAS)

Fig. 7.4 Illustration depicting a transverse section of the right hemiface at the level of the mandible. Note the superficially located marginal mandibular branch of the facial nerve, covered only by a thin layer of superficial musculoaponeurotic system (SMAS)/platysma muscle, subcutaneous fat, and skin at this level.

Even the passive motion of the mental skin during talking or eating can highlight scars. For these reasons, repairs should be carefully designed with scars in mind, and designs should be reconsidered if they result in an ill-placed scar line. When using flaps on the chin, the surgeon may consider the use of Z-plasty or zigzag design at the leading and lateral edges. This strategy, along with adequate undermining, will limit the pincushion effect that can result from concentric constriction with scar contraction.

Linear repairs may be reasonably designed along the cosmetic unit junctions: the labiomental crease, the melomental or "marionette" lines, and transversely across the submental skin. Additionally, scars are usually well concealed when placed vertically along the midline, where the creation or recapitulation of a cleft does not create an unnatural feature. Even along these favorable lines, wounds should be carefully everted during repair since there is a significant tendency for scar depression and contraction on the chin.

We will now consider the defects of the central, lateral, and submental chin and discuss reconstruction strategies and pitfalls.

7.3 Central Chin

Although the Mohs surgeon has numerous closure techniques available, often a direct linear closure will

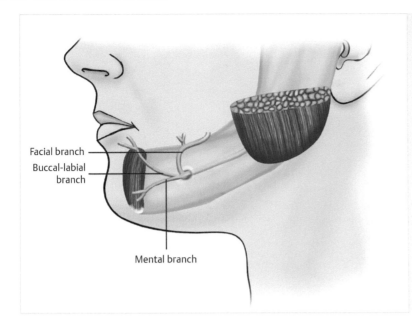

Fig. 7.5 The mental nerve as it emerges from the mental foramen. Note the early division of the nerve into buccal–labial, mental, and facial branches.

Facial branch
Buccal-labial branch
Mental branch

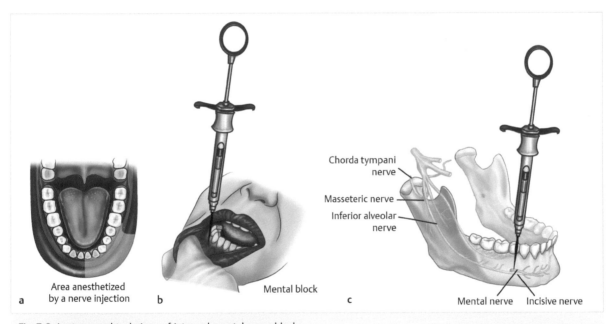

Chorda tympani nerve
Masseteric nerve
Inferior alveolar nerve
Mental nerve   Incisive nerve

Area anesthetized by a nerve injection
a

Mental block
b

c

Fig. 7.6 Anatomy and technique of intraoral mental nerve block.

achieve superior aesthetic results while minimizing the amount of tissue dissected and avoiding complications such as flap necrosis.[6,22] A retrospective review of chin reconstruction techniques employed after Mohs excision found that defects up to 2.2 cm could be successfully closed by linear closure.[22]

Small to medium defects near the midline of the chin may be repaired with a linear closure oriented vertically along the midline. Many patients have a natural midline cleft or depression on the chin and therefore a subtle scar along the midline may not be very conspicuous

(▶ Fig. 7.7). In patients without a preexisting cleft, the closure should be performed with moderate eversion in order to minimize depression of the final scar, which tends to occur in this area.[1] For defects that are just off the midline, the surgeon may consider modifying the wound so that it is symmetric across the midline prior to repair. The closures can also be oriented along the circumoral relaxed skin tension lines to reduce the visibility of the resulting linear scars.[23] An M-plasty may be used to avoid crossing into the lower lip and vermillion cosmetic units with vertical closures. Wide undermining

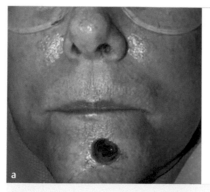
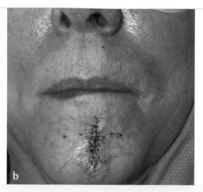
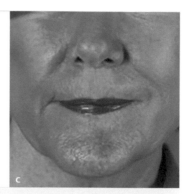

Fig. 7.7 (a–c) Reconstruction of a central chin Mohs defect with vertical linear closure. The defect was widely undermined and dog-ears were excised before vertical linear closure. The rightmost panel shows the 1-month postoperative results.

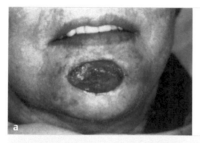
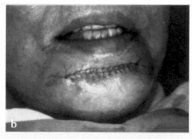
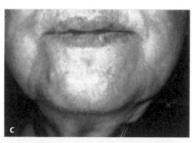

Fig. 7.8 (a–c) A defect on the central chin after Mohs excision. The defect was successfully closed with a horizontal linear closure. The rightmost panel shows the 4-month postoperative results.

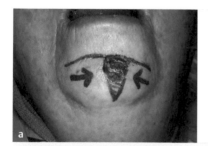
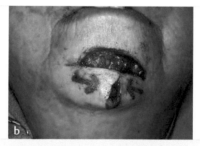
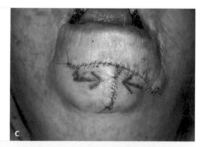

Fig. 7.9 (a–c) A 1.5 × 1.5 cm central chin defect is repaired with an O-T advancement flap. The direction of flap advancement is demonstrated by *arrows* and the anticipated triangular standing cutaneous deformity is drawn in panel A and subsequently excised and repaired in panels B and C.

in the subcutaneous plane may be required to allow for closure under minimal tension.

It may be tempting to close defects in the central chin with a horizontal linear closure along the labiomental crease (▶ Fig. 7.8), but the surgeon must carefully evaluate tension with the patient's mouth open and closed to avoid inadvertent creation of eclabium, oral incompetence, and difficulties with smiling, talking, and other mouth movements, especially when repairing larger defects.

For larger central chin defects that cannot be repaired by simple linear closures, the surgeon should consider using the O-T advancement and O-Z rotation flaps. The O-T advancement flap is ideal for small, midline defects that are adjacent to the labiomental crease (▶ Fig. 7.9). A horizontal linear incision is made along the labiomental crease and bilateral flaps are dissected in the subcutaneous plane. The flaps are then advanced medially into the defect, pivoted toward each other, and sutured together. An inferior vertical standing cutaneous deformity is created by tissue advancement and is excised, resulting in the vertical limb of the final T-shaped repair. The horizontal incision is closed by minimal inferior advancement of the lower lip skin. Rarely, small standing cutaneous

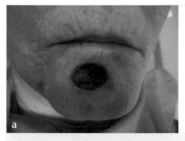
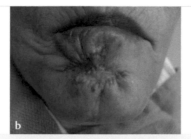
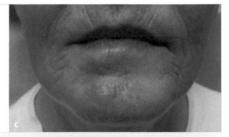

Fig. 7.10 (a–c) Off-center oval Mohs defect on the chin repaired with bilateral O-Z rotation flap. The rightmost panel shows the 8-week postoperative results.

deformities may arise along the horizontal incision. Excision of these deformities, if required, should be done along the melomental folds.

The O-Z bilateral rotation flap, which is typically used in areas of thick, inelastic skin (like the trunk), can also be used to repair small to medium-sized central chin defects. It is particularly helpful when the defect does not align well with the midline, but when there is still sufficient tissue adjacent to the defect that can be recruited. With adequate undermining, this type of flap is well suited to the chin because it results in a scar with broken, angular segments, avoiding long lines and digitate outcroppings that accentuate themselves as the scar contracts.

Jenkins and Lequeux-Nalovic published a case series of small to medium-sized circular chin defects (< 4 cm in diameter) that were repaired with the O-Z flaps with good cosmetic and functional outcome (▶ Fig. 7.10).[2] To execute this flap, curvilinear incisions are made on opposite sides of the defect so that the length of each flap is approximately four times the radius of the original defect. Each flap is created with an acute takeoff angle to minimize closure tension.[24] The skin flaps are elevated by dissection in the subcutaneous plane and the surrounding skin is undermined as shown in ▶ Fig. 7.11.[24,25] Note that the base of each flap was undermined to minimize pivotal restraint and improve mobilization. The flaps are then rotated toward each other into the primary defect and sutured in place. Next, the secondary defects are closed. Standing cone redundancies may form near each flap's pivot point, which can be excised or redistributed using the "rule of halves" suturing technique.[26,27]

For larger central chin defects, it may be necessary to recruit skin from the submental area and neck for closure (▶ Fig. 7.12).[28] This can be achieved using transposition flaps such as the bilobed flap, which transfer the area of maximum wound closure tension to a location considerably far away from the primary defect.

The first lobe is adjacent to the primary defect and is typically situated in the submental area. This lobe is oriented approximately 45 degrees from the axis of the primary defect to minimize the size of the standing cutaneous deformity that develops with rotation of the lobe about its pivotal point with a greater arc of rotation. The

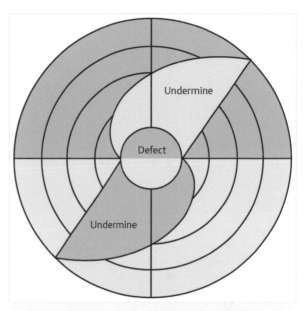

Fig. 7.11 Optimal flap design to minimize closure tension in the O-Z rotation flap.

first lobe is generally smaller than the primary defect, but the exact size depends on the laxity of skin adjacent to the defect as greater advancement of adjacent tissue is required when using an undersized lobe. The second lobe is designed on the neck and should be adjacent to the first lobe and oriented another 45 degrees from the axis of the first lobe, thereby being oriented 90 to 110 degrees from the primary defect's axis. Because of the greater amount of skin available for advancement in the submental area and neck, the second lobe is generally smaller than the first lobe.

Once planning is complete, the bilobed flap is elevated by dissection in the deep subcutaneous plane (remaining above platysma) and the surrounding tissue is widely undermined to facilitate flap movement.[7,29] Extreme care must be taken to avoid transection of the marginal mandibular branch of the facial nerve, which is only protected by a thin layer of the platysma muscle and has a variable course along the mandible, often crossing into the

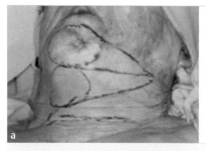
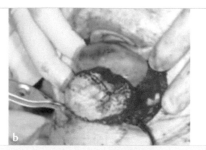
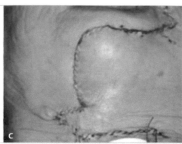

Fig. 7.12 (a–c) A large central chin defect repaired with a large bilobed flap.

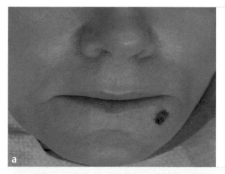
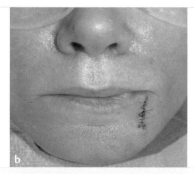
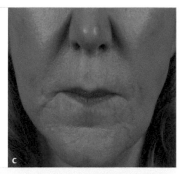

Fig. 7.13 (a–c) A 3-cm defect on the lateral chin closed with a vertical linear closure. Good cosmetic outcome seen at the 1-year follow-up.

submandibular region.[15] The first key suture closes the tertiary defect and mobilizes the first lobe toward the primary defect. The next suture secures the first lobe into the primary defect. If needed, the standing cutaneous deformity is now excised. Finally, the second lobe is transposed, trimmed, and secured.[30,31]

As on the nose, there is a risk of pincushioning with bilobed flaps on the neck and chin. This risk can be minimized by widely undermining, which should include symmetrical freeing of the mentalis insertion from the dermal surface. The mentalis will eventually reinsert into the newly configured overlying skin as healing occurs. V-Y advancement flaps and skin grafts have also been described for defects in this region; however, we feel that these techniques result in suboptimal postoperative appearance and contour.

7.3.1 Central Chin Key Points

- Linear repairs are useful along the mental crease and midline cleft.
- O-Z rotation flaps can be used when adequate tissue is present on two sides of the defect.
- Bilobed flaps may be used for large defects and utilize skin laxity present in the submental area and neck.
- V-Y flaps and skin grafts usually yield suboptimal cosmetic results.

7.4 Lateral Chin

Lateral chin defects are challenging to repair with excellent cosmetic outcomes due to the indistinct cosmetic subunit junctions and lack of naturally occurring creases. In patients with developed rhytids and redundant skin, linear closure to recapitulate the melomental fold is ideal. Younger patients without visible lines may be disfigured by the creation of an unnatural straight line at this convex juncture, so a repair resulting in broken lines, such as after a Z-plasty, is favored.

Surgical defects near the melomental fold can be repaired with a vertical linear closure with placement of the closure along the circumoral lines or along the melomental fold (▶ Fig. 7.13). Single advancement flaps may be appropriate when the resulting lines recapitulate natural skin creases (▶ Fig. 7.14).

An O-T bilateral advancement flap can also be used for lateral chin defects. This is similar to the O-T flap described earlier for central chin defects, except here there is greater advancement from the cheek than from the medial chin.[1] As described earlier for central chin defects, O-Z flaps and bilobed flaps can also be used for this area.

Larger defects of the lateral chin can be reconstructed using the redundant tissue of the medial cheek and melolabial fold using an inferiorly based melolabial transposition flap (▶ Fig. 7.15). A long flap with a base adjacent to the defect is planned parallel to the melolabial fold. The

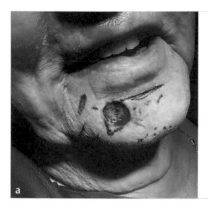

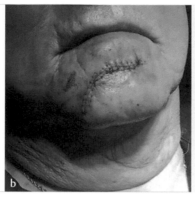

Fig. 7.14 (a, b) Single advancement flap repair of right lateral chin defect.

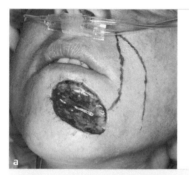

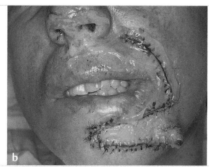

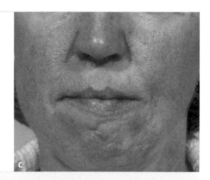

Fig. 7.15 (a–c) A 5 × 4 cm defect on the left chin repaired with an inferiorly based melolabial transpositional flap. The center panel also shows the resulting standing cone deformity that resulted after the flap was secured. This deformity was eventually excised 4 months later. The rightmost panel shows the postoperative results at 3.5 years of follow-up.

flap is elevated by dissecting in the subcutaneous plane above the underlying muscles.[32] Wide undermining is performed around the flap and recipient site to minimize closure tension and prevent pincushioning. The key stitch is placed at the base of the secondary defect allowing transposition of the flap into the primary defect. The flap is then secured with sutures. Height mismatch of the flap is managed by trimming the base of the recipient site rather than by thinning the flap to prevent vascular compromise.[30] Flaps that are too narrow may create a downward displacement at the lip and unfortunately leading to eclabium.

While technically a random pattern flap, the rich vessels of the subdermal plexus are oriented along the flap's long axis, allowing for the viability of a flap of such length with a narrow pedicle.[34] However, to avoid flap necrosis some authors recommend either excising the resulting standing cutaneous deformity in a second stage once the flap has healed or planning the excision away from the flap pedicle to avoid compromising vascularity of the flap.[30,33]

Finally, V-Y advancement flaps have also been described for lateral chin defects but often lead to inferior cosmetic results.[7,35]

7.4.1 Lateral Chin Key Points

- Linear repairs are useful in patients with well-formed rhytids. In younger patients without visible lines, the closure may be modified with Z-plasty or broken line repair to improve cosmesis.
- Consider O-T bilateral advancement flaps with greater tissue recruitment from the lateral chin and cheek or the bilateral O-Z rotational flaps for defects not amenable to linear closure.
- Larger defects may be repaired with the bilobed and melolabial transposition flaps.
- V-Y flaps usually yield suboptimal cosmetic results.

7.5 Submental Chin

The submental chin often has sufficient laxity even in young patients for linear closures for small to medium-sized defects. Linear repairs can be performed either in a side-to-side fashion along a sagittal plane or anteriorly to posteriorly along a coronal plane.[36] Larger defects may be repaired using a bilobed transposition flap or V-Y island pedicle advancement flap, which recruits excess skin from the anterior neck (Fig. 7.16).[37]

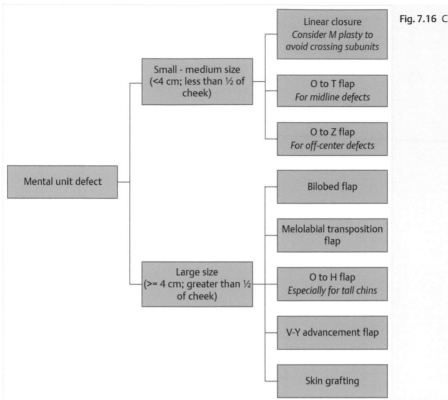

Fig. 7.16 Closure algorithm for the chin.

References

[1] Larrabee YC, Moyer JS. Reconstruction of Mohs defects of the lips and chin. Facial Plast Surg Clin North Am. 2017; 25(3):427–442

[2] Jenkins S, Lequeux-Nalovic KG. Reconstruction of chin defects using an O to Z bilateral rotation flap. J Cosmet Dermatol Sci Appl. 2012; 2(2): 41–44

[3] Becker GD, Adams LA, Levin BC. Outcome analysis of Mohs surgery of the lip and chin: comparing secondary intention healing and surgery. Laryngoscope. 1995; 105(11):1176–1183

[4] Zitelli JA. Wound healing by secondary intention. A cosmetic appraisal. J Am Acad Dermatol. 1983; 9(3):407–415

[5] Salasche S, Mandy P. Anatomy. In: Flaps and Grafts in Dermatologic Surgery. 2nd ed. Philadelphia, PA: Elsevier; 2007:1–15

[6] Wheeland RG. Reconstruction of the lower lip and chin using local and random-pattern flaps. J Dermatol Surg Oncol. 1991; 17(7):605–615

[7] Thornton JF, Carboy J. Chin reconstruction. In: Facial Reconstruction after Mohs Surgery. 1st ed. New York, NY: Thieme; 2018:151–153

[8] Carney JM. Implants. In: Surgery of the Skin: Procedural Dermatology. 3rd ed. Philadelphia, PA: Elsevier Inc.; 2015:409–206

[9] Sykes JM. Complications of Facial Implants. In: Eisele DW, Smith RV, eds. Complications in Head and Neck Surgery. 2nd ed. Philadelphia, PA: Mosby; 2009:671–676

[10] Afifi Ahmed M, Sanchez R, Djohan R. Anatomy of the head and neck. In: Aesthetic Surgery. Vol. 2. Plastic Surgery. 4th ed. London: Elsevier; 2017:24

[11] Drake RL, Vogl AW, Mitchell AWM. Head and neck. In: Gray's Anatomy for Students. 4th ed. Philadelphia, PA: Elsevier; 2020:823–1121.e4

[12] Tansatit T, Apinuntrum P, Phetudom T. A typical pattern of the labial arteries with implication for lip augmentation with injectable fillers. Aesthetic Plast Surg. 2014; 38(6):1083–1089

[13] Fang M, Rahman E, Kapoor KM. Managing complications of submental artery involvement after hyaluronic acid filler injection in chin region. Plast Reconstr Surg Glob Open. 2018; 6 (5):e1789

[14] Flowers FP, Goldsmith CB, Steadmon M. Surgical Anatomy of the Head and Neck. In: Dermatology. 4th ed. Philadelphia, PA: Elsevier; 2018:2425–2439.e2

[15] Batra AP, Mahajan A, Gupta K. Marginal mandibular branch of the facial nerve: an anatomical study. Indian J Plast Surg. 2010; 43(1): 60–64

[16] Liebman EP, Webster RC, Gaul JR, Griffin T. The marginal mandibular nerve in rhytidectomy and liposuction surgery. Arch Otolaryngol Head Neck Surg. 1988; 114(2):179–181

[17] Seckel BR. Facial danger zones: avoiding nerve injury in facial plastic surgery. Can J Plast Surg. 1994; 2(2):59–66

[18] Bard RL. Anatomy of the face for cosmetic purposes. In: Wortsman X, ed. Dermatologic Ultrasound with Clinical and Histologic Correlations. New York, NY: Springer; 2013:357–363

[19] Nguyen J, Duong H. Anatomy, Head and Neck, Mental Nerve. Treasure Island, FL: StatPearls Publishing; 2020

[20] Norton NS. Intraoral injections. In: Netter's Head and Neck Anatomy for Dentistry. 3rd ed. Philadelphia, PA: Elsevier; 2017: 567–588

[21] Syverud SA, Jenkins JM, Schwab RA, Lynch MT, Knoop K, Trott A. A comparative study of the percutaneous versus intraoral technique for mental nerve block. Acad Emerg Med. 1994; 1(6):509–513

[22] Soliman S, Hatef DA, Hollier LH, Jr, Thornton JF. The rationale for direct linear closure of facial Mohs' defects. Plast Reconstr Surg. 2011; 127(1):142–149

[23] Renner G. Reconstruction of the lips. In: Advanced Therapy in Facial Plastic and Reconstructive Surgery. Shelton, CT: PMPH-USA; 2010

[24] Buckingham ED, Quinn FB, Calhoun KH. Optimal design of O-to-Z flaps for closure of facial skin defects. Arch Facial Plast Surg. 2003; 5 (1):92–95

[25] Baker SR. Rotation flaps. In: Local Flaps in Facial Reconstruction. 3rd ed. Philadelphia, PA: Elsevier/Saunders; 2014:108–130

[26] Quatrano NA, Samie FH. Modification of Burow's advancement flap: avoiding the secondary triangle. JAMA Facial Plast Surg. 2014; 16(5): 364–366

[27] Goldman GD. Rotation flaps. In: Rohrer TE, Cook JL, Kaufman AJ, eds. Flaps and Grafts in Dermatologic Surgery. 2nd ed. Philadelphia, PA: Elsevier; 2018:71–81

[28] Mourad M, Arnaoutakis D, Sawhney R, Chan D, Ducic Y. Use of giant bilobed flap for advanced head and neck defects. Facial Plast Surg. 2016; 32(3):320–324

[29] Arnaoutakis D, Rihani J, Thornton J. Comparison of various techniques in the reconstruction of Mohs chin defects. Am J Cosmet Surg. 2015; 32 (4):258–263

[30] Bhatia AC. Transposition flaps. In: Rohrer TE, Cook JL, Kaufman AJ, eds. Flaps and Grafts in Dermatologic Surgery. 2nd ed. Philadelphia, PA: Elsevier; 2017:18

[31] Baker SR. Bilobe flaps. In: Local Flaps in Facial Reconstruction. 3rd ed. Philadelphia, PA: Elsevier/Saunders; 2014:187–209

[32] Singh S, Singh RK, Pandey M. Nasolabial flap reconstruction in oral cancer. World J Surg Oncol. 2012; 10(1):227

[33] Baker SR. Transposition flaps. In: Local Flaps in Facial Reconstruction. 3rd ed. Philadelphia, PA: Elsevier/Saunders; 2014:131–155

[34] Hynes B, Boyd JB. The nasolabial flap. Axial or random? Arch Otolaryngol Head Neck Surg. 1988; 114(12):1389–1391

[35] Thornton JF, Reece EM. Submental pedicled perforator flap: V-Y advancement for chin reconstruction. J Oral Maxillofac Surg. 2008; 66(12):2633–2637

[36] Bitner JB, Friedman O, Farrior RT, Cook TA. Direct submentoplasty for neck rejuvenation. Arch Facial Plast Surg. 2007; 9(3):194–200

[37] Benjegerdes KE, Jamerson J, Housewright CD. Repair of a large submental defect. Dermatol Surg. 2019; 45(1):141–143

8 Reconstruction of the Ear

David G. Brodland

Summary

The auricle is a primary anatomic and aesthetic structure of the head and neck and a common site for skin cancer. It is topographically complex and has the relatively simple function of transmitting sound to the middle and inner ear. The primary goal in reconstruction of the ear is to restore form and maintain function through patency of the external auditory canal. The vast majority of reconstruction for defects of the ear resulting from skin cancer removal are primarily for restoration of form. The aesthetics of ear reconstruction is somewhat simplified by the fact that the ears are not generally the focus of attention in social situations due to its lateral location on anterior view. Therefore, the primary aesthetic concern is projection of the ear from the head. Asymmetry of ear projection will be noticeable on the anterior view. It is interesting to consider that on lateral view, the specific form of the ear is less of an aesthetic issue due to the complexity of the contours and topography of the ear. Furthermore, from the lateral view, asymmetry is not as noticeable. Reconstruction of the ear requires in-depth assessment of the defect and the structural effect the defect and its reconstruction will have on it. Since the majority of the ear is a free margin, careful consideration of tension vectors induced by reconstruction is a constant requirement. This chapter provides fundamentals of reconstruction of defects ranging from simple to complex.

Keywords: ear reconstruction, helix, antihelix, conchal bowl, earlobe, postauricular sulcus, tragus, interpolation flap, advancement flap, transposition flap, cartilage graft, cartilage flap, full-thickness skin graft, split-thickness skin graft

8.1 Basic Concepts in Reconstruction of the Ear

The ear is a common site for skin cancer formation and represents a special challenge in reconstruction. The structure of the auricle is topographically complex and yet its function is relatively simple in transmitting sound to the middle and inner ear.

There are two primary goals in all reconstruction of head and neck structures, form and function. Maintaining and restoring form occupies the majority of reconstructive attention, while function is much less commonly an issue and limited to large defects directly affecting the external auditory canal (EAC).

The complex anatomic features make reconstruction of the auricle unique and challenging. And yet, the same complexity can result in aesthetic forgiveness. Minor alterations in normal anatomy are often not easily noticed by the casual observer. The essence of reconstruction can be summarized by three rules, in descending order of importance: Patency of the EAC, anterior profile, and lateral profile. Maintenance of EAC patency is fundamentally the prevention of scar-induced constriction of the canal and, in the case of near total or total loss of the canal structure, the repair and maintenance of the patency of this structure. It is a rare tumor that mandates the focus of reconstruction to be maintenance of the EAC patency.

The anterior profile supersedes the lateral profile in importance because the face-to-face appearance is most important. The anterior profile is characterized by a modest projection of the ear from the side of the head. This projection increases slightly from inferior to superior. Since slight variance in projection from one side to the other is normal, there is some leeway. But maintaining symmetry of projection is ideal.

The lateral profile is very important to reconstruct, but asymmetry is even more acceptable on the lateral profile since the profiles of the right and left ears are never seen simultaneously by the casual observer or the patient. Preserving the smooth exterior of the nautilus-shaped helix is the highest priority in aesthetic consideration, followed by the more complex and highly variable antihelical and conchal bowl structures of the ear.

The cartilaginous structure of the auricle, when preserved, serves as a sturdy framework upon which to restore the ear after tumor removal. If the cartilage can be safely preserved during tumor extirpation, it should be. In the event of significant loss of cartilage, its replacement and repair may need to be considered.

The exception to the otherwise well-supported structural foundation of the ear is the earlobe. In fact, the lobe is perhaps the subunit with the least structural support of all cutaneous features of the head and neck. With no cartilage, no fibrous or boney structure, it is perhaps the most vulnerable to distortion and disfigurement. This necessitates a very specialized approach to its reconstruction. Yet, mild asymmetries between left and right earlobes are manageable and, in fact, the loose, redundant tissue of the lobe is often utilized as a donor pool to resurface the helical ear.

Given the typical complexity of each ear and the manner in which each wound interacts with the appearance and structure of the ear, a dogmatic approach to its reconstruction is unrealistic. Yet, there are logical principles that are basic to a successful reconstructive approach that can be used to optimize results for each case (▶ Fig. 8.1, ▶ Fig. 8.2).

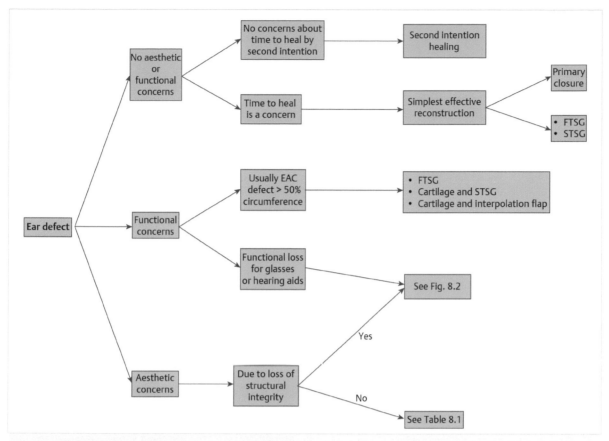

Fig. 8.1 Algorithm for ear reconstruction.

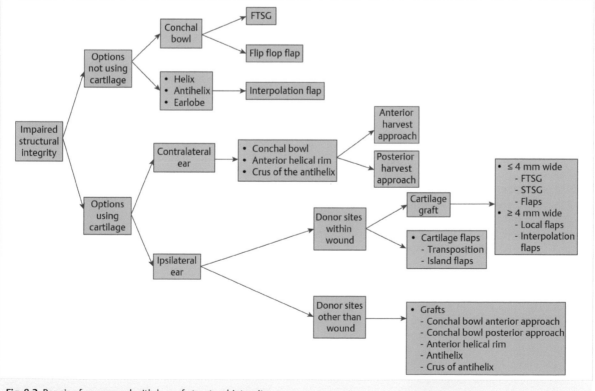

Fig. 8.2 Repair of ear wound with loss of structural integrity.

8.1.1 Superior Helix

Defects on the superior helix are some of the most challenging due to the relative lack of adjacent loose donor skin (▶ Table 8.1). Aesthetically, it is of moderate importance since on frontal view, most of the superior helix is not easily seen. Patients with short hair will be more concerned about scarring than those who wear their hair longer. On lateral view, a noticeable scar can be distracting if it interrupts the natural smooth helical curvature.

In this patient, we have a female who wears her hair short and has a high level of aesthetic expectation (▶ Fig. 8.3a, b). The first closure option to consider would be second intention since all cartilage structure is intact and it would be anticipated that the wound heal without distortion of the ear (▶ Fig. 8.1). However, the type of scar and, more importantly, the texture of the scarred skin may be unacceptable to a patient with a high aesthetic expectation.

Another reasonable consideration would be a helical advancement flap or bilateral advancement of the helix. As mentioned before, there are no easily accessible donor sites and this is true for the helical advancement flaps. Having said that, the anterior helix can occasionally be advanced. An incision would be made along the helical rim just superior to the level of the tragus and most likely a back-cut at the root of the anterior helix would be used rather than the traditional standing vertical cone, which would normally extend posteriorly around the helical rim for mid helical defects. The back-cut releases the tethering of the skin along with wide undermining around the helix and onto the posterior ear. A Burow's triangle would be taken extending from the defect onto the posterior ear perpendicular to the helical rim. The skin would be raised off of the helix and posterior ear and advanced superiorly and posteriorly. The anterior to posterior size of this defect would make closure with a unilateral helical advancement flap challenging. Therefore, the use of a bilateral helical advancement flap is a consideration as well. The anterior flap would be done as described earlier, while the posterior flap would be executed with an incision line extending along the helical rim as far as needed to recruit enough lax skin. As some patients have very loose skin on the mid to superior helix, a significant amount of tissue movement might be possible. If not, it is likely that the incision line will need to be made inferiorly to the level of the earlobe in order to recruit an adequate amount of tissue laxity. This would represent a very large flap and extensive tissue mobilization in order to effect a relatively small closure.

Interpolation flaps are possible and often useful for superior helical defects when their size and complexity merit a two-stage flap. In this case, the complexity of an interpolation flap outweighs the benefit. It was felt that a full-thickness skin graft (FTSG) harvested from the preauricular skin was optimal. There are numerous reasons for this including its relative simplicity, the

expected good cosmetic results, and the restoration and maintenance of the appearance not only from a structural standpoint but also texturally. The preauricular skin, located posterior to the hair-bearing sideburn region, routinely has an excellent match to helical skin in terms of thickness, in color and texture (▶ Fig. 8.3c). Other excellent donor sites for FTSGs on the helix include the postauricular sulcus and the conchal bowl. In this case, the more hidden donor site of the postauricular sulcus consisted of skin that was thought to be too thin to match the adjacent helical skin. The conchal bowl, on the other hand, had skin that was likely too thick to match perfectly.

FTSGs require an adequate vascular base. As can be seen, the perichondrium is intact in this defect, which has a very adequate blood supply to support the graft. When portions of the perichondrium are missing or blood supply is more questionable, then opting for one of the flaps previously discussed or a split-thickness skin graft (STSG) may be preferred. An STSG is an option when the vascularity of the wound base is more tenuous because of its inherent lower metabolic requirements.

The location of the ear represents a challenge to the patient during the inosculation period for the FTSG. This ingrowth of blood vessels from the underlying wound base into the graft requires that the graft not be moved or exposed to any shearing force. The first week is the most critical during which the graft is very susceptible to disruption of the ingrowing blood supply. Although the first week postoperatively is the most critical, the grafted skin is not able to endure normal bumps and bruises for about the first month. Therefore, a tie-over bolster dressing is often used and left in place for the first week. It is then removed and another dressing is applied and left in place for the entire second week. At the end of the second week, this bandage is removed and the patients are instructed to continue to be careful not to bump the area through the end of the first month postoperatively and to wear a light bandage over ointment, which can be changed daily. After a month, the patient is allowed to discontinue bandages but instructed to lubricate the graft as needed. As can be seen from the follow-up photograph, the cosmetic result is excellent (▶ Fig. 8.3d). The typical normalization of grafted skin is delayed compared to flap skin and typically takes 6 to 12 months to achieve an optimal cosmetic appearance.

Key Points

- Endeavor to understand the patient's aesthetic expectations.
- Choose the simplest closure when function and aesthetics are obtainable with multiple reconstruction options.
- FTSGs are simple and provide excellent function and aesthetics for helical defects not involving cartilage.

Table 8.1 Reconstruction options ranked (1, 2, 3) according to approximate frequency of use. Less frequently used (X) but appropriate reconstruction choice in certain circumstances

	Tragus	Superior Helix		Mid Helix		Ear Lobe		Antihelix	Posterior Ear	Conchal Bowl
		< 1.5 cm	> 1.5 cm	< 1.5 cm	> 1.5 cm	< 1 cm	> 1cm			
Primary	1	2	2						1	
FTSG	X	1	1	1	1	2	2	2	3	1
STSG		3						1	2	2
HAF		X	3	2	3	3	3			
Bilateral HAF			X		X					
Transposition flap	3	X	X						X	
Bilobe flap	X	X	X	3					X	
Wedge		X	X	X		1	1	X		X
Stellate wedge			X		X			X		X
V-Y flap	X	X				X				
Flip flop flap										3
Interpolation flap			X		2		X	3		X
Double tangent advancement flap	2		X							

1. Most common or primary consideration in typical defect.

2. Second most common consideration.

3. Third most common consideration for typical wound in this subunit.

X. Indicates a reconstructive option to consider it in certain circumstances rarely considered for most wounds in this subunit.

Abbreviations: FTSG, full thickness skin graft; HAF, helical advancement flap; STSG, split thickness skin graft.

- Pre- and postauricular skin as well as the conchal bowl are excellent donor sites for helical defects.
- Avoidance of shearing force injuries for 1 month is critical for ear defects closed with grafts.

8.1.2 Mid Helix

The mid helix is a critical portion of the helix with a high aesthetic value. Representing the midportion of the beautiful, smooth curvature of the helix, it is very conspicuous on lateral view and can easily be seen on anterior view as well. Topographically, the mid helix is probably the most "plain" subunit of the ear in that it is approximately 3 to 4 cm in length with minimal curvature and very delicate features as most notably represented by the helical rim. Because of the relative lack of topographical complexity, scars tend to be more noticeable than either above, below, anteriorly, or posteriorly on the auricular structure. There is significant variation from person to person in this area as well. Some have very lax, loose, and "fleshy" tissue, while others have a very rigid, inflexible constitution relatively void of subcutaneous tissue. Reconstruction obviously must take into account these individual characteristics (▶ Table 8.1).

In this case, the majority of the mid helical skin is absent, although the defect extends only minimally onto posterior ear (▶ Fig. 8.4a). It does extend into the antihelical groove, but there is minimal loss of the very delicate cartilage of the helical rim. This is a female who wears her hair short and has a high aesthetic expectation. Wound healing by second intention is unlikely to provide the patient satisfactory aesthetic result and would likely result in a noticeable loss of substance as well as a loss of the characteristic helical rim and groove.

An FTSG is a very good consideration with an adequate vascular wound base. However, it would be difficult to maintain the aesthetic features of the helical rim. The graft would likely heal with a deficiency of soft tissue further damaging the smooth helical curvature in this area. Finally, there is wound on three sides of this portion of the ear including the anterior helical groove, the posterior ear, and the helix itself. The likelihood of a perfectly healing graft is relatively low because of this and should be considered a somewhat risky wound closure option in a patient with high esthetic expectations.

Transposition flaps do not often play important roles in defects such as this, although they can be considered when there is adequate donor site on the posterior surface of the ear that can be accessed by, for example, a bilobed flap.

A two-staged retroauricular interpolation flap would be a very good consideration and could be expected to work very nicely in restoring this defect. Given that the cartilage is entirely intact and there will be no need for a cartilage graft, the benefit of the interpolation flap is lessened and a less complex closure should be sought. When cartilage grafting is needed to replace missing helical rim cartilage, the retroauricular interpolation flap is an outstanding choice and would be expected to not only heal well but also provide excellent blood supply for the cartilage graft. Since the anterior to posterior extent to the wound was so small, the interpolation flap option was not selected.

This defect is relatively close to an ample donor pool. The earlobe represents an excellent source for advancement of

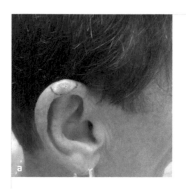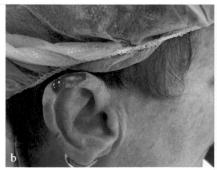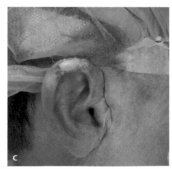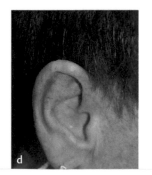

Fig. 8.3 (a) Basal cell carcinoma preoperatively involving the superior helix. **(b)** Defect after excision extends to the perichondrium. **(c)** Full-thickness skin graft harvested from the preauricular donor site, sutured into place with fast absorbing gut suture. A tie-over bolster dressing will be applied. **(d)** Six months postoperatively.

the tubular helical skin superiorly with minimal disruption of the lobe itself. And for this reason, an inferiorly based helical advancement flap was planned.

The initial incision is made along the helical groove inferiorly to the superior aspect of the earlobe (▶ Fig. 8.4b). Here, a crescentic Burow's triangle was incised onto the earlobe and over the inferior rim of the conchal bowl. The cartilaginous aspect of the auricle was identified and the skin was carefully dissected from the cartilage both anteriorly and around the posterior surface of the auricle. The flap is raised off of the posterior surface of the auricular cartilage to nearly the postauricular sulcus (▶ Fig. 8.4c) and a Burow's triangle is excised posteriorly from the defect perpendicular to the helical rim. All wound edges are undermined including over the superior-most portion of the defect separating the skin of the helical rim from the underlying cartilage. A small cartilaginous tubercle is identified under the skin just superior to the wound and

was contoured by slight shaving in order to optimize the continuity of the helical rim. For advancement flaps, the first critical suture to be placed is that which closes the donor site on the earlobe. This advances the flap naturally into the wound. The second key suture is used to close the Burow's triangle on the posterior surface of the ear. These two key sutures precisely position the flap so that it is easily positioned and refined by subsequent sutures. The final key suture is the placement of the anterior and superior-most corner of the advancing flap. In this case, the suture is placed in the helical groove (▶ Fig. 8.4d). It is important to emphasize wound eversion as the flap is sutured across the helix (▶ Fig. 8.4e). Without precise eversion, the junction of the flap with the native skin across the helix can develop a distracting notch, which can be persistent. It is best if this skin edge eversion is created by both the deep sutures and the top skin suture.

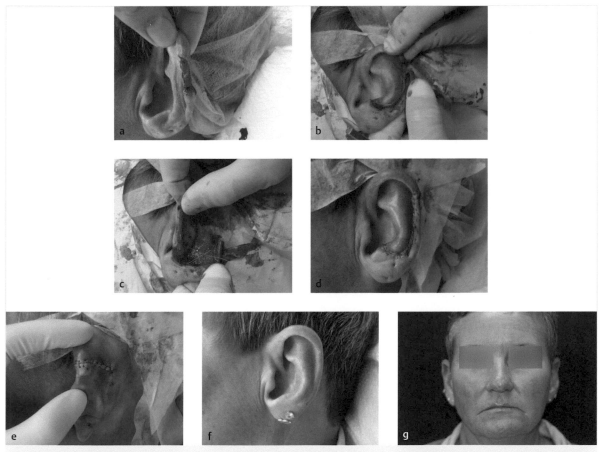

Fig. 8.4 (a) After Mohs excision of the defect extends anteriorly over the helical rim into the helical groove and posteriorly to the posterior surface of the helix. **(b)** The initial incision is made along the helical groove inferiorly to the superior earlobe where a crescent-shaped Burow's triangle is excised. **(c)** A flap is created by dissection along the posterior ear extending toward the postauricular sulcus. **(d)** Key dermal sutures are placed first in the crescentic Burow's triangle at the earlobe followed by a dermal suture closing the Burow's triangle on the posterior ear. And lastly, the superior and anterior leading edge of the flap in the helical groove to precisely advance and position the flap for epidermal suturing. **(e)** The suturing of the flap over the helix is maximally everted in order to prevent noticeable notching at the mid helix. **(f)** Lateral view at the 4-month follow-up. **(g)** The final results show preservation of symmetry.

The 4-month postoperative photograph shows excellent restoration of the contour of the helix and maintenance of the helical groove (▶ Fig. 8.4f, g). Although the earlobe was the donor site for the 1.9-cm defect, the change in size is subtle and not noticeable on frontal view.

Key Points

- The earlobe is an excellent donor pool for ear reconstructions, making helical advancement flaps excellent choices for mid and inferior helical defects (▶ Table 8.1).
- For advancement flaps, the first critical stitch closes the earlobe donor site.
- The second key suture closes the Burow's triangle on the posterior ear.
- Wound eversion is important for perpendicular incision lines crossing over the helix to avoid visible helical notching.

8.1.3 Earlobe/Inferior Helix

The earlobe is unique in that it is the only portion of the ear that does not contain cartilage. As such, it is entirely mobile and distensible. It is this feature that can be problematic when surgery is performed on it. Scar contraction can have a profound, undesirable effect on the shape, position, and texture of the earlobe. It is most prominently visible on lateral view and as long as its projection from the head is not conspicuous, the front-on view

can be aesthetically tolerated. Even minor asymmetries between the right and left earlobes can be minimally distracting since they cannot be easily viewed simultaneously. Having said that, the goals of reconstruction of the earlobe is to try to minimize asymmetry and normalize its position and projection from the adjacent jawline. As described earlier, the earlobe represents an area of laxity and source of donor skin. As such, smaller defects of the earlobe can be managed easily by taking advantage of its intrinsic flexibility and elasticity, as long as attention is paid to maintaining its natural curvature.

This defect of the earlobe is in a woman who wears her hair short and has a moderately high level of aesthetic expectation (▶ Fig. 8.5a). Approximately one half of the earlobe has been removed by full-thickness excision and the defect extends very slightly up on to the inferior helix. An incidental feature of her earlobe is that it is the "connected" variant in that it is connected to the cheek.

Second intention healing would be suboptimal in almost any patient. Even a patient with low aesthetic expectation would benefit from some form of closure. Simple primary closure, realigning the margin of the earlobe with the helix, would provide an improved aesthetic result not to mention easier postoperative wound care. Inferior advancement of the helix holds no advantage due to the relative lack of donor skin superiorly. An FTSG would do nothing to restore the contour of the earlobe/inferior helical junction and, in fact, would exacerbate notching of the earlobe. For large earlobe defects, a

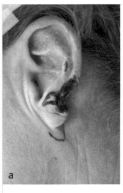
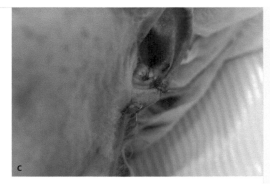
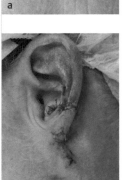
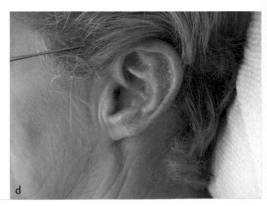

Fig. 8.5 (a) Post-Mohs defect involving both the inferior helix and the earlobe. Markings denote location of anticipated Burow's triangle as well as a V-Y advancement of infra-auricular skin to provide additional donor tissue for advancement of the remaining earlobe. **(b)** Direct advancement of the residual earlobe along with recruitment of infra-auricular skin to supplement the lobule. **(c)** Anterior view showing V-Y induced transfer of supplemental tissue from the infra-auricular skin onto the inferior earlobe. **(d)** Four-month postoperative view showing excellent reconstruction of the inferior helix and earlobe with reasonable reconstitution of the lobule.

two-stage interpolation flap can occasionally be very useful. This can be utilized not only for defects limited to the anterior or posterior surface of the earlobe but also for full-thickness earlobe defects in that the interpolation flap can be folded upon itself, recreating the absent lobule. In order to maintain the shape of the earlobe, cartilage grafts can be sandwiched between the folded interpolation flap providing some rigidity to the reconstructed earlobe and helping maintain a more natural shape. The source of cartilage is most conveniently the conchal bowl.

In this case, direct closure of the earlobe to the inferior helix was planned. This was accomplished through direct advancement of the lobe, which was stretched up to the superior portion of the defect. However, because of the broad nature of the defect, this would have effectively eliminated the lobule as the majority of the earlobe tissue would be recruited to fill the wound. In order to recreate the semblance of a lobule, a V-Y advancement of the cheek just inferior to the attachment of the earlobe was planned to recruit tissue onto the lobe.

First, a Burow's triangle was excised into the earlobe directly from the wound base. This triangle was intentionally made diminutive anticipating that the plasticity of the earlobe skin would accommodate the redundancy medially and superiorly. Next a V-shaped incision was made from the base of the attachment of the earlobe inferiorly toward the angle of the jaw. This V-shaped flap was incised deeply, intentionally including and incorporating the majority of the subcutaneous tissue. The flap was undercut with an incision from the inferior apex of the flap superiorly to the original earlobe–cheek junction. Here, as is usual, the earlobe was tethered by fibrous bands extending to and integrating with the superficial musculoaponeurotic system (SMAS). This fibrous tissue was transected, releasing the earlobe and mobilizing the entire V-Y flap. This enabled the V-Y flap to be folded upon itself adding substance to the now-depleted substance of the earlobe. The flap is then sutured upon itself and tucked up under the earlobe. The resulting defect on the cheek is closed primarily effectively completing the transfer of tissue from the cheek onto the inferior earlobe (▶ Fig. 8.5b, c).

The result at 4 months shows an inconspicuous scar with the semblance of an earlobe thanks to the V-Y plasty (▶ Fig. 8.5d). Without it, the result would have portrayed a less natural ear, void of a lobule, with the inferior rim of the conchal bowl effectively representing the ear–cheek connection. As with all closures on the helix, eversion sutures across the helical margin minimizes the notch shape that can on occasion be prominent.

Key Points

- The key to earlobe and inferior helix reconstructions is the maintenance or recreation of the lobular shape of the earlobe.

- Recruitment of infra-auricular skin in the form of V-Y flaps or interpolation flaps may assist in restoring the lobule in larger wounds.
- Cartilage grafts may be used to maintain the lobular shape if distorting scar contraction is likely.

8.2 Antihelix and Conchal Bowl

The antihelix/conchal bowl subunit of the auricle can present complex and fascinating reconstructive challenges. However, the vast majority of tumors that occur on these subunits are typically not highly destructive of its infrastructure. As such, wound management is often simply by second intention and alternatively as simple as resurfacing the wound with a skin graft. However, a good analogy of the relationship between the conchal bowl and antihelix to the helix is that it is the hub of the wheel to the tire. And as with the hub, the antihelix and conchal bowl provide the core structure to the auricle. A defect involving cartilage loss is typically quite extensive when it is enough to require reconstruction. But when extensive enough, it is important to reestablish its hublike structural integrity.

This case is of a relatively large defect involving the superior portion of the conchal bowl extending up onto the antihelix and the crus of the antihelix (▶ Fig. 8.6a). There is substantial cartilage exposure involving an area of approximately 3 × 2 cm. However, there is no structural compromise despite the size of the wound. This is an elderly gentleman with moderate esthetic expectations.

The first option that comes to mind is healing by second intention. This is an excellent option in most defects without structural compromise and involving primarily the antihelix and conchal bowl. Occlusive wound care with daily bandage changes will lead to granulation formation over the base of the wound and subsequently marginal re-epithelialization from the margins of the wound. The challenges for second intention healing in this wound include the size of the wound, which would result in a relative prolonged healing with an expected range of between 1 and 3 months depending on intercurrent complications and the patient's attentiveness to occlusive wound care. Another challenge is the relatively large area of what appears to be exposed cartilage devoid of perichondrium and its questionable blood supply. In wounds with exposed cartilage measuring more than 1 cm, a helpful technique to augment healing by second intention is the perforation of the cartilage with Keyes punches. A 3- or 4-mm punch through the cartilage creates a corridor to the posterior ear skin and exposes the underlying vascularized tissue. Through these perforations, granulation tissue will form serving to augment the healing. This also diminishes the risk of desiccation of the cartilage, which is more likely to occur when the wound healing process is over an extended period of time. This technique is also useful in providing vascular support for grafting over an area stripped of perichondrium.

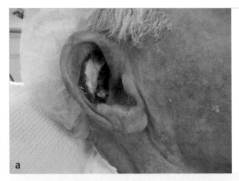 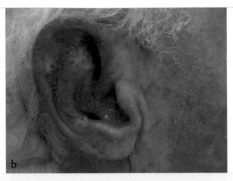 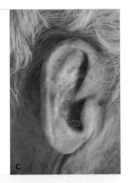

Fig. 8.6 **(a)** Defect after excision resulting in cartilage exposure of the antihelix and conchal bowl. **(b)** Sutured split-thickness skin graft harvested with a Weck blade from skin overlying the clavicle. A tie-over bolster dressing will be applied for 1 week. **(c)** Reconstructive results at 4 years postoperatively.

Another very common closure for this type of wound is an STSG. Even in the face of a diminished vascular supply in the wound base, the reduced metabolic requirements of an STSG make it more likely to survive under physiologically austere conditions and, if there is concern about adequate vascular support for an STSG, perforations through the cartilage with a Keyes punch would be useful for STSGs as mentioned earlier. One of the normal disadvantages of STSGs is the lack of adnexa and the very smooth and light-colored surface that is characteristic of these grafts. However, on the conchal bowl and antihelix, both the smooth texture and the light color approximate the natural appearance of this skin. Donor sites include, in addition to the traditional donor site of the thigh, the skin over the mastoid process, and the skin overlying the clavicle. In the case of the mastoid donor site, the hair is shaved and the graft is harvested using a Weck blade over the prominence of the mastoid. The superficial nature of the graft does not affect the underlying hair follicles and in fact the follicles contribute to very rapid re-epithelialization of the donor skin.

Another reasonable option would be an FTSG. The advantages are similar to those of STSGs; however, the FTSG has a higher metabolic requirement. Therefore, the paucity of blood supply in this wound is more of an issue for an FTSG. Once again if the FTSG is considered the very best option, then perforations of the cartilage, as mentioned earlier, is a reasonable technique to enhance vascular supply to the graft. Donor sites may include preauricular, postauricular, and supraclavicular areas and the choice of the donor site would depend on the size of graft needed, desirable thickness, and quality of donor skin.

Other considerations that might be entertained include the pull-through flap (flip-flop flap), retroauricular pedicle flap, or a preauricularly based interpolation flap. Although these options may be effective, they are substantially more complicated and costly without substantial benefit to the patient.

In this case, the patient was not interested in the prolonged period of healing by second intention and because

of the relatively good tissue match and low metabolic requirements, an STSG was used for reconstruction (▶ Fig. 8.6b). In this case, the STSG is harvested from the right clavicle using a Weck blade and a 12/100ths of an inch blade guard. This provides a very thin graft from an area that is simple for the patient to care for during second intention healing. The underlying bone provides an excellent firm surface that augments the harvesting of the graft. Once harvested, the graft is transferred to the defect and tacked into place. Thereafter, the graft is trimmed to fit the defect and sutured into place circumferentially. The use of a bolster is important in contoured areas such as these to assure that the graft remains undisturbed during the period of inosculation. The bolster can be nonstick gauze placed over a thin coat of ointment and bolstered in place with a fluffed gauze. The wetting of the gauze with saline makes it more malleable and moldable such that it can be packed into the complex contours of the conchal bowl and antihelix. Another excellent bolster material is Vaseline gauze. This can be readily packed into the contours of the ear and likewise affixed with sutures. Tie-over suture is placed to secure the bolster and the suture and bolster are removed in 1 week. Additional occlusive bandages are placed for a minimum of 1 additional week after initial bolster removal. After the second week, the graft is kept heavily lubricated with petroleum ointment for the balance of a month. Grafts are quite susceptible to minor trauma, necessitating protective coverage for 1 month.

▶ Fig. 8.6c shows the results of reconstruction 4 years later. Note the nearly imperceptible blending of the STSG without adnexa with the surrounding native skin. Unlike an FTSG, STSGs do not blunt or attenuate the complex contour of the antihelix, the crus of the antihelix, or the conchal bowl.

Key Points

- Healing by second intention is often the optimal approach to wounds not involving cartilage.

- Exposed cartilage void of perichondrium can be perforated with Keyes punch to promote granulation and revascularization from the transcartilage communication to the posterior ear.
- STSGs provide reasonable skin match to defects of the conchal bowl and antihelix.
- The traditional donor site for STSGs are from the upper thigh. However, the skin overlying the mastoid process and the clavicle are also excellent donor sites.

This antihelical defect measures over 2 cm in the vertical dimension and 2 cm in the horizontal direction (► Fig. 8.7a). What is difficult to appreciate is that the cartilage of the helix is entirely absent within the middle third of the helical groove defect despite the skin of the helix being intact. So the tasks at hand for this reconstruction include not only the resurfacing of the large area but also maintaining the form of the helix through repair of the cartilaginous structure.

Although second intention healing would occur, the consequence would be the folding and noticeable deformation of the smooth curvature of the helix. The skin would be fused to the anterior surface of the antihelix and the helical groove would be ablated. Skin grafts are also options (► Table 8.1). An STSG by itself would be an excellent repair of the portion of the defect limited to the antihelix. However, it would do little to prevent the deformation of the helical groove and curvature of the helix. Scar contraction is less inhibited by an STSG than an FTSG. An FTSG would be an option and may reduce the amount of contraction and the fusing of the anterior surface of the helix to the antihelix. However, there would be some contraction and it is likely that the structureless portion of the helix would not retain its normal curvature.

A retroauricular interpolation flap would be a reasonable option. It would very effectively resurface the antihelical defect and a cartilage graft could be placed where

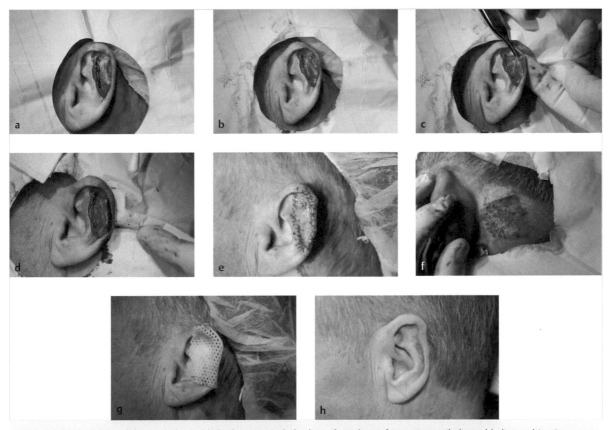

Fig. 8.7 (a) This defect of the antihelix and helical groove includes loss of cartilage of posterior antihelix and helix resulting in a structureless helical rim. The *purple marks* delineate the cartilage donor site, which will be placed within the cartilage-deficient helical rim. **(b)** Following harvest of cartilage graft and its placement into the recipient bed of the mid helix. The inferior-based cartilage flap has been incised and elevated. **(c)** Cartilage flap after dissection from the underlying skin and rotation posteriorly to fortify and maintain the shape of the ear at its perimeter. **(d)** Sutured cartilage flap and cartilage graft ready for split-thickness graft. **(e)** Split-thickness graft sutured into place. **(f)** Donor site of split-thickness skin graft harvested with a Weck blade over the mastoid process. **(g)** The graft is covered with ointment, nonstick gauze and then thermoplastic splint dressing. This dressing was manually molded after being made malleable when dipped in hot water. Upon cooling, the thermoplastic splint dressing is rigid and protects the flaps, grafts, and the shape of the ear for 1 week. **(h)** Five months postoperatively with reasonable preservation of the nautilus shape of the auricle.

the cartilage defect is and be expected to engraft thanks to the excellent vascular supply the interpolation flap and the skin of the helical groove would provide. The cartilage donor site could be the exposed cartilage of the defect in the conchal bowl.

A flip-flop flap or pull-through flap would also be a consideration and, in contrast to the retroauricular pedicle flap, would be a single-stage closure. A portal would need to be created to enable the passing-through of the flap. This would most likely be created at the anterior-most aspect of the defect and would involve full-thickness removal of a portion of the auricular cartilage large enough to pass the flap through and conduct the vascular pedicle for the flap. The patient was not interested in a two-stage procedure, which eliminates the retroauricular interpolation flap. The pull-through flap would be better suited for defects of the conchal bowl and this wound is not optimal for this flap.

The option that was chosen involves the use of a cartilage strut graft outlined in *purple* at the anterior-most aspect of the defect in ▸ Fig. 8.7a. The posterior rotation of the cartilage flap adjacent to the donor site of this cartilage graft was planned to provide additional support to the helix and helical groove. Finally, the defect and all of the cartilage components were covered with an STSG.

First, the cartilage strut is harvested and transferred to the recipient bed, the helical skin (▸ Fig. 8.7b). The cartilage graft is secured within that groove by 6–0 Vicryl loop sutures with the envelopment of the three sides of the graft by the helical skin. Next, the exposed cartilage of the antihelix located just posterior to the cartilage graft donor site is dissected from the underlying skin and raised upon an inferior base. The cartilage flap is rotated posteriorly, adjacent to the aforementioned cartilage graft (▸ Fig. 8.7c). This vascularized cartilage rotation flap is then sutured and affixed in its position at the posterior-most aspect of the defect in order to support and maintain the full size of the helix (▸ Fig. 8.7d).

Next, an STSG harvested from the ipsilateral mastoid process is sutured over the remaining wound, cartilage flap, and graft (▸ Fig. 8.7e, f). A very carefully constructed and precisely molded plastic cast (thermoplastic splint) is placed over the entire wound including the helix (▸ Fig. 8.7g). This has two purposes, as both a bolster for the graft and a cast for maintaining the shape of the helix during inosculation of the cartilage and skin graft. This cast is left in place for 1 week, after which the original nonstick gauze dressing is removed and then replaced with a new nonstick gauze over ointment and re-bandaged for a second week. The plastic cast can be reapplied for more prolonged protection of the delicate structure of the reconstructed helix. In fact, this cast can be utilized on a daily basis after the second week when the wound is simply covered by a light bandage.

Five months postoperatively, the helix is seen to be reasonably well maintained and aesthetically acceptable (▸ Fig. 8.7h).

Key Points

- The relationship of the conchal bowl to the helix is analogous to the hub of a wheel to the tire.
- Structural compromise of the conchal bowl or the antihelix (the "hub") necessitates repair to preserve the appearance of the helix (the "tire").
- Adjacent or exposed cartilage may be used as a donor site for cartilage grafts and cartilage flaps.
- Heat malleable plastic molds are useful as bolsters for grafts and to protect and maintain the shape of underlying cartilage grafts for extensively reconstructed ears.

8.3 Posterior Ear Defects

The vast majority of posterior ear defects are cosmetically inconsequential and therefore second intention wound healing is a very common wound management selection. As long as there is no structural compromise and the visible aspect of the helix is not involved, the primary reason to consider closure is for speed of healing and ease of wound care. In this case, both FTSG and STSG are relatively simple and effective for these cases (▸ Table 8.1). Should a posterior ear defect extend onto or over the helix onto the visible portion of the ear, more serious consideration for comprehensive reconstruction can be made.

This defect extends from the upper postauricular sulcus superiorly onto the temporal scalp and sideburn and onto the posterior ear with extension up and over the superior helix (▸ Fig. 8.8a, b). In this case, if the wound was allowed to heal by second intention, the exposed helical cartilage would be put at risk of distortion. Even if distortion did not occur, healing by second intention would leave the helix noticeably atrophic, lacking in any subcutaneous tissue. Considerations for closure might include a superiorly based transposition flap from the preauricular skin with transposition onto the helix. This technique nicely addresses anterior helical defects but would not be able to reconstruct the large posterior ear defect nor directly address the defect extending onto the temporal scalp. An FTSG could be used in combination with such transposition flaps to cover the remaining defect behind and above the ear.

Because of the defect involving the postauricular sulcus and scalp, a two-stage retroauricular flap would not be feasible.

A large STSG would resurface the skin; however, the thin nature of the graft would not address the aesthetic concerns well. Along those lines, a large FTSG would be a reasonable consideration and would provide a more

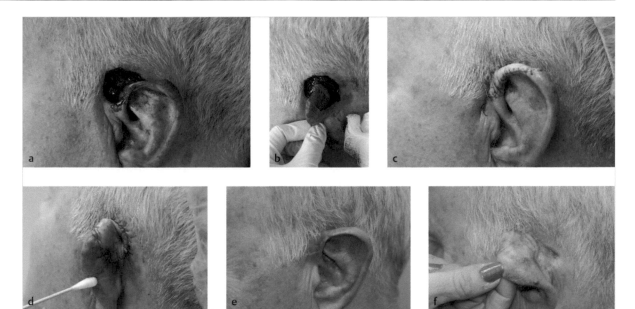

Fig. 8.8 **(a)** Large defect involving anterior helix, posterior ear, and extending onto the supra-auricular skin and scalp. **(b)** View of defect involving the posterior ear. **(c)** Following direct advancement of the scalp defect to the ear and full-thickness repair of the defect involving the anterior helix and posterior ear. **(d)** View of the posterior ear resurfaced with full-thickness skin graft harvested from the supraclavicular fossa. **(e)** Lateral view 3 months postoperatively showing excellent preservation of the appearance of the ear. **(f)** View of well-healed full-thickness skin graft reconstruction of the posterior ear.

aesthetically pleasing result on the visible portions of the helix and limit the scar contraction that would happen to a great degree in the case of an STSG or second intention.

The actual closure in this case utilized the principle of closing cosmetic subunits independently. As such, the skin of the temporal scalp and sideburn were advanced directly to the postauricular sulcus (▶ Fig. 8.8c) isolating the remaining wound to the posterior ear and helix. A template was made of this wound and an FTSG was harvested from the supraclavicular fossa and the donor site was closed primarily. The FTSG was aggressively thinned removing all subcutaneous tissue. It was then sutured into place (▶ Fig. 8.8d) and a very tightly formed gauze bolster dressing was packed against the graft over all the involved surfaces including the helix. This bolster was then secured in place with a tie-over suture and remained in place for 1 week. At 1 week, the bolster is removed and a light gauze bandage is reapplied for the second week. For the balance of the month postoperatively, the patient is instructed to keep the delicate graft covered with a light bandage that can be changed daily. This bandage is primarily for protection from incidental bumps of the graft that could lead to partial avulsion. The 3-month follow-up photographs show a nicely reconstructed and proportioned ear with preservation of the helix and minimal distortion of the helical rim from scarring due to excellent survival of the FTSG (▶ Fig. 8.8e, f).

This case (DSC 003–2A) shows a full-thickness defect through the midportion of the helical rim but involving at least one-third of the posterior ear (▶ Fig. 8.9a, b). The posterior ear portion of the defect does not extend through the cartilage, meaning that the structural compromise is limited to the helical rim. In this situation, one could consider closing the helical rim portion of the defect separate from the posterior ear using, for example, helical advancement flap utilizing the laxity of tissue in the earlobe. The remaining defect on the posterior ear could be allowed to heal by second intention or closed with an STSG or an FTSG.

Alternatively, a retroauricular pedicle flap could be utilized predominantly for closure of the helical rim. The cartilaginous defect of the helical rim could be replaced with a cartilage graft harvested from the conchal bowl at the location of maximum curvature in order to simulate the missing helical cartilage. This cartilage is visible at the base of the defect on the posterior ear, which provides excellent access to this donor site (▶ Fig. 8.9b). Upon takedown of the retroauricular pedicle flap, the pedicle would be used to resurface as much of the remaining defect on the posterior ear as possible. Any residual defect is usually allowed to heal by second intention. Upon inspection and manipulation of the defect, it was noted that a wedge closure could be performed under modest tension with a complete recapitulation of the helix. This is due in part to an ample earlobe and excellent elasticity of the posterior ear skin.

The execution of this flap entails the full-thickness excision of the skin of the antihelix and cartilage in a V-shaped configuration extending over the conchal rim into the conchal bowl. One of the substantial disadvantages of wedge closure is the "cupping" that occurs during the approximation of the upper and lower edges of the auricular cartilage to close the wedge. Conceptually, this is due to the fact that the curvature length of the helix is now less than the remainder of the auricular cartilage resulting in tension upon closure which manifests as forward movement of the helical rim. This cupping can be addressed by several methods. Surgically, the use of a "stellate" wedge configuration excises triangles not only in the horizontal direction but also in the superior and inferior direction along the antihelix. This decreases the "reach" necessary for the superior and inferior aspects of the helical rim to be sutured together. Another tactic is through the use of retention sutures, which are left in place for at least 2 weeks with the intent to counteract the tendency for the helix to

undergo cupping. This technique was used in this case because the total amount of cupping was moderate. If the cupping tendency is more severe, the "stellate wedge" closure is a better option. As shown in ▶ Fig. 8.9c, nylon sutures are placed through the sutured ear within the helical groove and will be sutured to the postauricular skin holding the auricle in the desired anatomic position. These sutures can remain for 2 to 4 weeks before being removed, which results in slight reconfiguration of the cartilage and desirable positioning of the ear relative to the head. At 3 months (▶ Fig. 8.9d, e), the final result is seen. The aesthetics are excellent with good retention of the form of the helix and in the absence of cupping. The only notable change is the diminished size of the conchal bowl, which is functionally and aesthetically inconsequential.

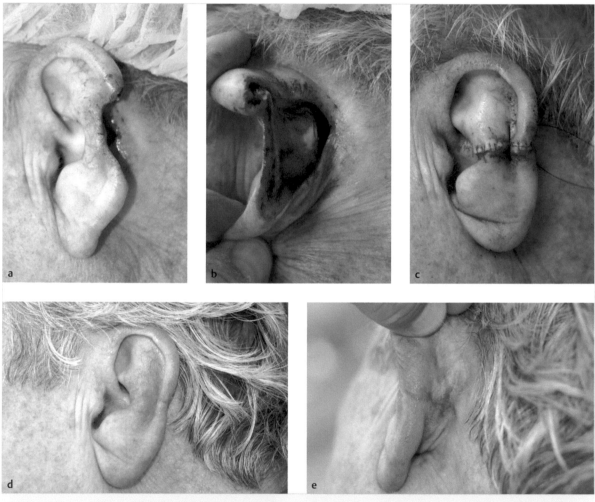

Fig. 8.9 (a) Large defect involving the full-thickness loss of the mid helix and extensively involving the posterior surface of the ear. (b) View of the posterior extent of the defect. (c) Closure following full-thickness wedge excision of skin and cartilage extending into the conchal bowl with advancement of residual inferior and superior helix. Note accentuated eversion of sutures over the curvature of the helix. A through and through nylon suture is placed in the helical groove and will be sutured to the postauricular skin as a retention suture to avoid cupping and maintain appropriate positioning and projection of the ear. The nylon suture was removed 4 weeks later once ear projection had been established and stabilized. (d) Lateral view 3 months postoperatively. (e) Postauricular view 3 months postoperatively.

Key Points

- When defects extend from the ear onto surrounding skin, always assess whether these portions of the wound can be reconstructed separately following the principle of cosmetic subunit closure.
- FTSGs are effective at providing soft-tissue replacement, matching texture for the helix and posterior ear and for inhibiting scar contraction (▶ Table 8.1).

- When wedge closures are considered, careful consideration of the degree of "cupping" is necessary as this is the most problematic challenge of wedge closures.
- Cupping can be attenuated by the use of the stellate wedge pattern, which will significantly reduce the size of the ear. Alternatively, retention sutures can provide variable correction of cupping, but they need to be left in place for 2 to 4 weeks.

9 Reconstruction of the Neck Unit

Merrick A. Brodsky, Saud Aleissa, and Anthony Rossi

Summary

Reconstruction of cutaneous surgical wounds of the neck requires understanding the anatomy and dynamics of movement. Although the neck can be a forgiving cosmetic subunit in comparison to other anatomic locations for reconstruction after cutaneous surgery, there are potential danger zones and complexities that one should be aware of. In patients with advancing age, the neck contains the largest tissue reservoir with increased tissue laxity allowing for direct repairs. However, before performing a cutaneous surgery in the neck, it is imperative to understand and master the superficial anatomy of the neck including the vascular supply, motor and sensory innervation, musculature, and danger zones.

Keywords: superficial anatomy of the neck, anterior cervical triangle, posterior cervical triangle, Erb's point, neck reconstruction

9.1 Anatomy of the Neck

The basis of superficial anatomy of the neck hinges on anatomic landmarks and the creation of the well-defined triangles of the neck.

The hyoid bone is located in the midline of the anterior neck and is approximately 2.5 to 3 cm below the chin. As you continue inferiorly, one will encounter the thyroid cartilage, followed by the anterior lamina of the cricoid cartilage, and finally the cartilaginous rings of the trachea. Laterally, the two most identifiable structures include the mastoid process superiorly and the sternocleidomastoid muscle (SCM). Posteriorly, the external occipital protuberance is the most superior prominence with each of the cervical vertebral spinous process following inferiorly in the midline of the posterior neck.

The regions of the neck are divided topographically into anterior and posterior cervical triangles by the SCM, which courses obliquely from the mastoid process of the temporal bone to the manubrium of the sternum. Each triangle possesses distinct borders and anatomic structures within their boundaries (▶ Fig. 9.1).

9.1.1 Anterior Cervical Triangle

The anterior cervical triangle is formed superiorly by the inferior border of the mandible, posteriorly by the SCM, and anteriorly by the anterior midline of the neck. The anterior cervical triangle can be further subdivided into four smaller triangles by the anterior and posterior bellies of the digastric muscle, omohyoid muscle, and hyoid bone.

The first of these triangles is the submental triangle. This triangle is formed inferiorly by the body of the hyoid bone, laterally by the anterior belly of the digastric muscle and the floor is formed by the mylohyoid muscle. Only one segmental triangle is present in the midline and its contents include submental lymph nodes, mylohyoid muscle, and nerve and veins that unite the anterior jugular veins.

The submandibular triangle is bounded by the inferior border of the mandible and the anterior and posterior bellies of the digastric muscle. Contents of this triangle include the submandibular gland and lymph nodes, facial artery and vein, hypoglossal nerve, and mylohyoid nerve.

The muscular triangle is bounded by the superior belly of the omohyoid muscle, SCM, and the midline of the neck. This triangle, as the name suggests, contains the infrahyoid or "strap" muscles such as the sternohyoid, omohyoid, sternothyroid, and thyrohyoid muscles. Additionally, below the level of the "strap" muscles lie the thyroid gland, parathyroid glands, anterior jugular veins, recurrent laryngeal nerves, larynx, and trachea, which will rarely be encountered during a cutaneous surgery and reconstruction.

Finally, the carotid triangle is formed by the superior belly of the omohyoid muscle, SCM, and posterior belly of the digastric muscle. This triangle contains the carotid sheath structures (internal jugular vein, vagus nerve, and common carotid artery), external carotid artery, superior laryngeal nerve, spinal accessory nerve, hypoglossal nerve, and ansa cervicalis.

9.1.2 Posterior Cervical Triangle

The posterior cervical triangle of the neck is bounded by the mastoid process, posterior edge of the SCM, clavicle, and anterior edge of the trapezius muscle. This triangle can be further subdivided by the inferior belly of the omohyoid muscle into the occipital triangle superiorly and the subclavian triangle inferiorly. Important structures in the posterior cervical triangle include the emergence of multiple branches of the cervical plexus and the spinal accessory nerve.

Classically, the posterior cervical triangle of the neck represents one of the major anatomic danger zones in cutaneous surgery of the head and neck. Erb's point is classically described as the point on the posterior aspect of the SCM where the bundle of four superficial branches of the cervical plexus emerges. These nerves include the greater auricular, lesser occipital, transverse cervical, and supraclavicular nerves. This point is approximately at the junction of the upper and middle thirds of this muscle. The presence and superficial nature of these nerves coursing through the posterior cervical triangle warrants extra caution during cutaneous surgery and reconstruction. The

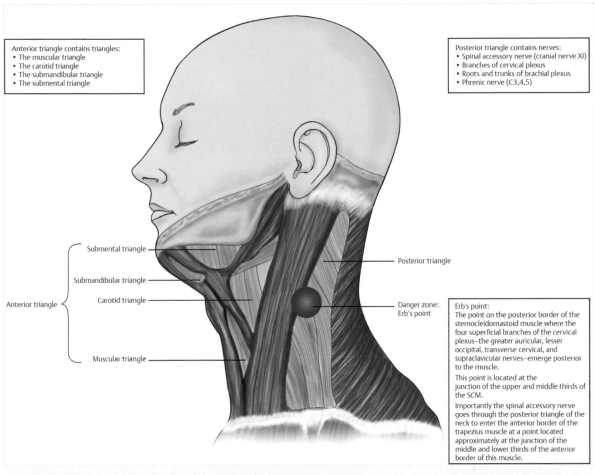

Anterior triangle contains triangles:
• The muscular triangle
• The carotid triangle
• The submandibular triangle
• The submental triangle

Posterior triangle contains nerves:
• Spinal accessory nerve (cranial nerve XI)
• Branches of cervical plexus
• Roots and trunks of brachial plexus
• Phrenic nerve (C3,4,5)

Submental triangle

Submandibular triangle

Carotid triangle

Anterior triangle

Muscular triangle

Posterior triangle

Danger zone:
Erb's point

Erb's point:
The point on the posterior border of the sternocleidomastoid muscle where the four superficial branches of the cervical plexus–the greater auricular, lesser occipital, transverse cervical, and supraclavicular nerves–emerge posterior to the muscle.
This point is located at the junction of the upper and middle thirds of the SCM.
Importantly the spinal accessory nerve goes through the posterior triangle of the neck to enter the anterior border of the trapezius muscle at a point located approximately at the junction of the middle and lower thirds of the anterior border of this muscle.

Fig. 9.1 Anterior and posterior triangles of the neck and Erb's point.

true danger zone is classically centered on the middle of the SCM muscle with a diameter of 6 cm approximately 6.5 cm inferior to the external auditory canal.[1,2] These nerves run in the investing fascia on the superficial surface of the SCM. Injury to greater auricular nerve may result in anesthesia, paresthesia, or dysesthesia of the surrounding skin of the neck, cheek, and ear.

Injury to the spinal accessory nerve is the most commonly reported complication of surgical procedures in the posterior cervical triangle of the neck. However, the majority of literature describes encountering the nerve with more invasive procedures such as cervical lymph node biopsies and open dissections of the neck.[3] The spinal accessory nerve is usually found about 1 cm superior to Erb's point but courses inferoposteriorly deep to the superficial cervical fascia across the posterior triangle until entering the anterior border of the trapezius muscle between the middle and lower thirds.[4] Injury to the spinal accessory nerve may result in chronic pain and impaired muscular function of the trapezius and SCM muscles, and may require immediate nerve repair. Clinically, the patient may present with a

drooping shoulder and wasting of the trapezius muscle on the affected side.

During skin cancer excisions and reconstructions, dissection should take place in the upper subcutaneous tissue and above the SCM, if possible, to avoid encountering these sensory and motor nerves.[5]

9.1.3 Platysma

Another important consideration in the neck is the platysma muscle. The platysma is a superficial, broad, extremely thin muscle that drapes the anterior portion of the neck. It originates from the subcutaneous tissue and fascia of the upper pectoral region of the chest. It fans across the neck until it inserts into the skin of the lower portion of the face, where it intercalates with the base of the mandible, angles of the mouth, and orbicularis oris. The platysma covers the medial part of the SCM, nerves including the greater auricular nerves, cervical branch of the facial nerve, the facial vessels, the submandibular gland, and the inferior part of the parotid gland. It is innervated by the cervical branch of the facial nerve,

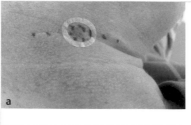
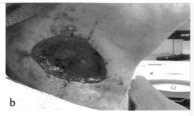
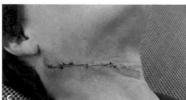
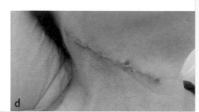

Fig. 9.2 **(a)** Example of a biopsy-proven melanoma in situ on the right lateral neck. **(b)** Surgical defect after staged excision and obtaining clear margins. **(c)** Linear surgical repair, involving the anterior and posterior triangles, underlying the laxity of the neck subunit. **(d)** Appearance of the scar 2 weeks postoperatively.

which enters the platysma on its deep surface near the angle of the mandible. the platysma serves an important mimetic function as it draws the corners of the mouth inferiorly and widens as in expressions of sadness and fright.[6,7] Platysmal banding can be quite prominent in certain individuals, and this can be elicited by asking the patient to contract their platysma muscle. Although the relaxed skin tension lines run horizontally on the neck and incision placed within these may heal more favorably, it is important to take note of competing tension vectors, such as with rotation of the neck and contraction of the platysma.

9.2 Reconstruction

Once the tumor has been fully excised, surgeons are faced with the challenge of reconstructing the defect. Factors that are important to consider when assessing each step of the reconstructive ladder include location of the defect, size of the defect, age of the patient, redundancy of tissue available, patient preference, and surgeon expertise. To date, there are no well-defined guidelines to neck reconstruction after cutaneous surgery. The majority of textbooks and journal articles focus on the defects of the cosmetic subunits of the face such as the scalp, forehead, cheek, nose, eyelid, chin, lip, and ear, and may overlook the neck.[8] Our approach will focus on defining a stepwise approach for neck reconstruction. Goals of neck reconstruction will focus on restoring form and function of the neck, and placing scars in relaxed skin tension lines, natural creases, and respecting anatomic borders.

9.2.1 Primary Closure

Primary linear closures are the workhorse of cutaneous neck reconstruction. Due to local skin laxity and the amount of tissue reservoir within the cutaneous neck, many repairs of this nature will work well within this

cosmetic subunit. Focus should be placed to orient this primary closure in the same orientation as the relaxed skin tension lines. On the anterior neck, the relaxed skin tension lines lie horizontally, which is perpendicular to the axis of contraction of the platysma muscle (▶ Fig. 9.2).

9.2.2 Secondary Intention Healing

Healing by secondary intention was historically adopted for concave sites such as the temple, periocular, periauricular, and perinasal regions.[9,10]

However, more recently, healing by secondary intention has become more widely accepted according to a recent survey of Mohs micrographic surgeons performed by Vedvyas et al in 2017. They learned that this technique may also be appropriate for convex sites, deep wounds, large wounds, and wounds complicated by dehiscence, flap necrosis, or infection.[11] With regard to defects of the neck, there is a paucity of knowledge and data suggesting which defects would be more amenable to healing by secondary intention. The neck as a cosmetic subunit has largely been overlooked, on healing by secondary intention. In our experience, healing by secondary intention should not be overlooked as a viable reconstructive method. Patients who have surgical defects that are wide but limited to the dermis or superficial subcutaneous tissue where primary closures or other reconstructive techniques would be extensive, not tolerated by the patient or patient preference. Disadvantages may include increased healing times, increased wound care, hypopigmentation in the scar (may not be ideal for more darkly pigmented patients), and contraction of the skin that can potentially limit motility.[12]

9.2.3 Skin Grafts

Skin grafts are defined as an intact piece of skin that has been completely removed from a donor site and then is

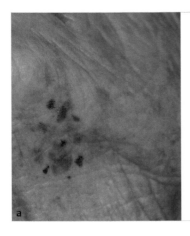
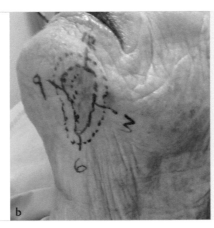

Fig. 9.3 (a) Large melanoma in situ involving the left neck and chin area in a patient with history of Merkel's cell carcinoma on the right side treated with radiation.
(b) Showing the clinical outline and the surgical margins.

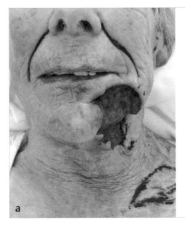
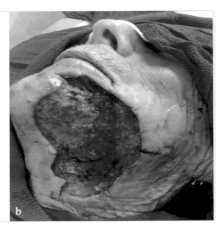

Fig. 9.4 (a,b) Final defect after staged excision and obtaining clear margins.

reattached to a recipient site. Full-thickness skin grafts (FTSGs) are comprised of the entire thickness of both the epidermis and dermis in contrast to split-thickness skin grafts (STSGs), which has a varying degree of dermal thickness along with the entire thickness of the epidermis. In dermatologic surgery, FTSGs are more desirable over split-thickness skin grafts due to improved color match, contour, and textures, and decreased contracture.[13] Skin grafting may be a viable option for complex neck repairs; however, caution is advised on highly mobile areas or tension points when rotating the head from side to side (▶ Fig. 9.3, ▶ Fig. 9.4, ▶ Fig. 9.5, ▶ Fig. 9.6).

9.2.4 Skin Substitutes

In comparison to skin grafting that uses native tissue, skin substitutes are made of synthetic or biologically derived materials. In dermatologic surgery, these skin substitutes may be used in a variety of fashions depending on the wound type and surgeon preference. We will focus mainly on their use as a temporary repair, permanent repair, or in conjunction with another reconstruction technique. Broadly, skin substitutes can be divided into four main categories based on how they are derived, including

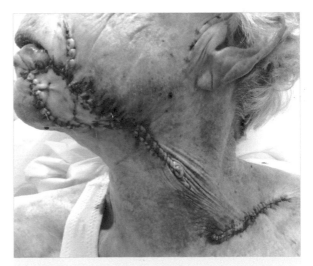

Fig. 9.5 Reconstruction by combining a linear closure with burow's full-thickness skin graft (FTSG) from the left clavicle.

xenografts, synthetic grafts, allogeneic grafts, and autologous grafts.[14] Xenografts are a source of exogenous collagen and less commonly other dermal components. These

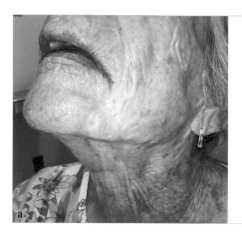
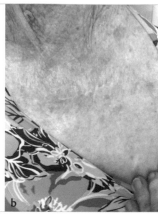

Fig. 9.6 (a,b) Final appearance of the scar and donor site 1 year postoperatively.

are derived from either porcine or bovine sources depending on the specific manufacturer. In the setting of dermatologic surgery, these may be used as a temporary solution before definitive closure or be applied to augment secondary intention healing. Synthetic grafts are manufactured as a bilayer graft. The inferior portion of the graft is comprised of collagen and other extracellular matrix elements, whereas the superior portion is composed of silicone. Synthetic bilayers serve a similar purpose to xenografts. Allogeneic grafts or allografts are further stratified into many distinct categories. The first branching point is that grafts may be acellular, meaning they consist of decellularized human tissue or are composed of cellular components. The next branching point is whether the graft is comprised of epidermal, dermal, or composite human tissue. Finally, we have the option of autologous skin grafts. Currently, autologous skin substitutes are created by culturing various epidermal and dermal components, including keratinocytes and fibroblasts, and then applying them back onto the patient's wounds most often as a suspension or spray. Currently, this is the least utilized form of skin substitute in dermatologic surgery due to a multitude of factors including cost and time to develop the graft.

9.2.5 Skin Flaps

The recruitment of adjacent tissue with local flaps provides an excellent result for defects that are not amenable to primary closure or any of the above reconstruction techniques.[15] Local flaps are defined by originating from within the same or adjacent cosmetic subunit. These flaps are then further subdivided based on their axis or type of movement. Commonly used local flaps include rotational, advancement, and transposition flaps. When dealing with defects in the cosmetic subunit of the neck, these flaps are largely comprised of advancement and rotational flaps. These types of flaps are considered random pattern flaps since they are not based on any specific arterial supply.

9.2.6 Complications

Complications following skin cancer surgery and reconstruction of the neck pose a unique array of challenges compared to other anatomic subunits of the head and neck. The neck is a highly mobile anatomic site which has musculature that extends, flexes, and rotates. The surgeon must be cognizant of these movements when designing the reconstruction and during postoperative counseling to optimize restoring form, function, and cosmesis. Postoperative complications such as hematoma, seroma, dehiscence, and abnormal or poor scar appearance may be exacerbated by the increase in mobility of this cosmetic subunit. Diligence must be taken to ensure there is no evidence of bleeding, oozing, or potential dead space when performing the closure. Due to the mobility, scars often have a less desirable outcome compared to areas of reconstruction that are not under tension related to movement such as the lateral cheek, superior forehead, or nasal tip. Surgeons across multiple specialties most often counsel patients to refrain from excessive or forceful movement to limit tensile forces on the wound, but this may prove difficult given the functionality of the neck in daily activities of living. Recently, there has been a randomized clinical trial that studied the effects of botulinum toxin in the early postoperative setting for thyroidectomies to evaluate the improvement in scar appearance.[16] This has also been studied in other facial surgical scars relating to treatment of congenital melanocytic nevi, port wine stains, arteriovenous malformations, and scar revision surgery.[17] Their conclusions showed that botulinum toxin was safe and effective in producing cosmetically superior scars. Botulinum toxin in the perioperative or early postoperative period, to our knowledge, has not been well described in the literature relating to skin cancer reconstruction and subsequent improved scar cosmesis; however, this needs to be investigated. One can postulate that temporary chemodenervation of the platysma with botulinum toxin would likely reduce tension on the surgical scar–related muscular contraction and movement. Another important complication related to neck construction is related to the potential for nerve injury. This was discussed in detail in the anatomy section of this chapter.

References

[1] Monsen H. Anatomy of the anterior and lateral triangles of the neck. In: Nyhus LM, Baker RJ, eds. Mastery of Surgery. 2nd ed. Boston, MA: Little, Brown and Company; 1992

[2] Salasche SJ, Bernstein G. Surgical Anatomy of the Skin. Norwalk, CT: Appleton & Lange; 1988

[3] Nason RW, Abdulrauf BM, Stranc MF. The anatomy of the accessory nerve and cervical lymph node biopsy. Am J Surg. 2000; 180(3): 241–243

[4] Soo KC, Hamlyn PJ, Pegington J, Westbury G. Anatomy of the accessory nerve and its cervical contributions in the neck. Head Neck Surg. 1986; 9(2):111–115

[5] Bernstein G. Surface landmarks for the identification of key anatomic structures of the face and neck. J Dermatol Surg Oncol. 1986; 12(7): 722–726

[6] de Castro CC. The anatomy of the platysma muscle. Plast Reconstr Surg. 1980; 66(5):680–683

[7] Hwang K, Kim JY, Lim JH. Anatomy of the platysma muscle. J Craniofac Surg. 2017; 28(2):539–542

[8] Ibrahim AM, Rabie AN, Borud L, Tobias AM, Lee BT, Lin SJ. Common patterns of reconstruction for Mohs defects in the head and neck. J Craniofac Surg. 2014; 25(1):87–92

[9] van der Eerden PA, Lohuis PJFM, Hart AAM, Mulder WC, Vuyk H. Secondary intention healing after excision of nonmelanoma skin cancer of the head and neck: statistical evaluation of prognostic values of wound characteristics and final cosmetic results. Plast Reconstr Surg. 2008; 122(6):1747–1755

[10] Zitelli JA. Secondary intention healing: an alternative to surgical repair. Clin Dermatol. 1984; 2(3):92–106

[11] Vedvyas C, Cummings PL, Geronemus RG, Brauer JA. Broader practice indications for Mohs surgical defect healing by secondary intention: a survey study. Dermatol Surg. 2017; 43(3):415–423

[12] Zitelli JA. Wound healing by secondary intention. A cosmetic appraisal. J Am Acad Dermatol. 1983; 9(3):407–415

[13] Brenner MJ, Moyer JS. Skin and composite grafting techniques in facial reconstruction for skin cancer. Facial Plast Surg Clin North Am. 2017; 25(3):347–363

[14] Nathoo R, Howe N, Cohen G. Skin substitutes: an overview of the key players in wound management. J Clin Aesthet Dermatol. 2014; 7(10): 44–48

[15] Starkman SJ, Williams CT, Sherris DA. Flap basics I: rotation and transposition flaps. Facial Plast Surg Clin North Am. 2017; 25(3): 313–321

[16] Kim YS, Lee HJ, Cho SH, Lee JD, Kim HS. Early postoperative treatment of thyroidectomy scars using botulinum toxin: a split-scar, double-blind randomized controlled trial. Wound Repair Regen. 2014; 22(5):605–612

[17] Hu L, Zou Y, Chang SJ, et al. Effects of botulinum toxin on improving facial surgical scars: a prospective, split-scar, double-blind, randomized controlled trial. Plast Reconstr Surg. 2018; 141(3):646–650

10 Reconstruction of the Scalp

Adam J. Tinklepaugh and Rachel Westbay

Summary

The scalp is a common site for cutaneous malignancy and poses unique reconstructive challenges. The scalp is a hair-bearing and relatively inelastic area of the body and, along with the galea aponeurotica, provides the tissue covering for the skull. The scalp is anatomically homogenous and is not divided by cosmetic subunits. Second intention healing, primary closure, and cutaneous flaps and grafts can be utilized for scalp reconstruction. This chapter will provide the surgeon with a thorough review of relevant scalp anatomy as it pertains to cutaneous reconstruction and various reconstructive techniques.

Keywords: scalp, scalp reconstruction, scalp anatomy, galeotomy, pinwheel, Orticochea, O-Z, free tissue transfer, regional flap, tissue expansion

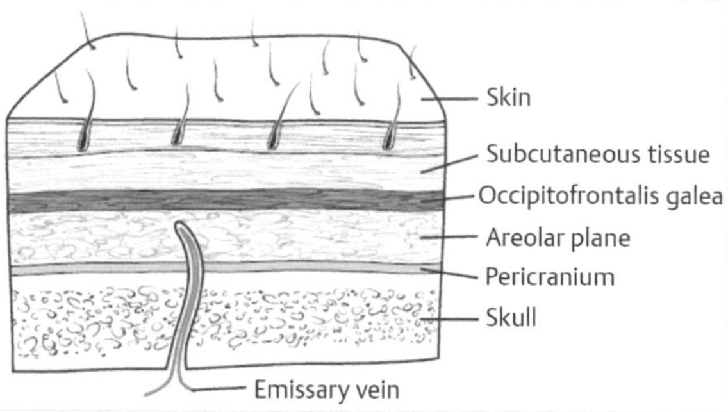

Fig. 10.1 The scalp layers as seen on the sagittal section. The loose areolar tissue plane below the galea allows mobilization of the scalp. (Reproduced from Scalp. In: Marcus J, Erdmann D, Rodriguez E, ed. Essentials of Craniomaxillofacial Trauma. 1st Edition. New York: Thieme; 2012.)

10.1 Scalp Anatomy

It requires detailed knowledge of relevant anatomy to design and execute a successful scalp reconstruction. The scalp presents distinct reconstructive challenges due to its unique structure. The cutaneous tissue of the scalp is thick and variably mobile; the latter relates to the inelastic galea aponeurotica overlying the skull. In certain patients, the immobility this confers is so significant that it complicates wound closure.[1] Familiarity with the scalp's more delicate structures is also critical. Should the surgeon raise a flap superficial to the galea, where the scalp's blood vessels, lymphatic system, and nerves exist, its vascularity may be compromised, rendering it nonviable.[2] Additionally, an aesthetically pleasing reconstruction of the scalp requires the surgeon to appreciate its hair-bearing nature, which in and of itself poses unique reconstructive challenges.[3]

10.1.1 Soft-Tissue Layers

The scalp is organized in a layered structure. "SCALP" is a mnemonic used to remember the layers of the scalp. It stands for Skin, subCutaneous tissue, galea Aponeurotica, Loose areolar tissue, and Pericranium.[4] An illustration of these layers can be seen in ▶ Fig. 10.1. Scalp skin is comprised of the epidermis and dermis and measures between 3 and 8 mm in depth.[4] This thickness makes it an excellent donor site for split-thickness skin grafts (STSGs).[4] A reflection of its terminal hair-bearing nature, it is thickest in areas of dense hair growth and thins with both pathologic and physiologic alopecia.[3] The abundant terminal hairs that characterize the scalp histologically

reside in the subcutaneous fat layer, as do other adnexal structures, such as sweat and sebaceous glands.

Deep to scalp adnexal structures lie the occipitofrontalis muscle and its connecting galea aponeurosis. The primary function of the galea aponeurotica is to strengthen the overlying integument. It is intimately connected to other anatomic structures and becomes discontiguous with the frontalis muscle fascia anteriorly, the temporoparietal fascia laterally, and the occipitalis muscle fascia posteriorly.[2] These connections underlie the so-called tight and loose portions of the scalp. Where the galea connects to the fascia and, ultimately, to muscle, tissue thickness decreases and the skin is relatively mobile.[1] These "loose" portions of the scalp are easily noted on manipulation of skin in the frontal, temporal, and occipital regions. Conversely, at the midline scalp, from vertex extending caudally to the frontal hairline, the galea is fully formed with no overlying muscle, and thus the skin is relatively inelastic.[2] Given the inability of this area to easily stretch, primary closure of large defects can be challenging. Deep to the galea is the subgaleal plane, which contains loosely arranged alveolar tissue and is largely responsible for the mobility of the overlying tissue.[5] Being an avascular space, the subgaleal plane is highly conducive to blunt dissection and is therefore optimal for wide undermining.[6] Beneath the subgaleal plane is the pericranium. The deepest of the soft-tissue layers of the scalp, the pericranium is tightly adherent to the underlying skull. In the majority of cases, the pericranium is left intact during scalp reconstruction, as it can serve as a vascularized surface for skin grafting and also allows for "back-grafting" of the donor site, if necessary.[2,3]

10.1.2 Vascular Supply and Lymphatics

Vascular Supply

The blood supply to the scalp is robust and exhibits an extensive network of anastomosing vascular plexuses, which predominantly lie in the subcutaneous plane just superficial to the galea.[2,5] This benefits the surgeon because the ample collateral circulation of most areas of the scalp promotes tissue survival even if the axial blood supply is compromised.[2] This provides significant utility as scalp anatomy often impedes primary closure. A notable exception to this is the midline scalp, which contains limited anastomotic connections and within which flaps extending a considerable distance may be compromised.[4,7]

Most of the large primary cutaneous arteries from which the smaller vascular plexuses are derived are located within the galea and temporoparietal fascia and are themselves derived from both the external carotid and internal carotid systems.[2,4] The external carotid artery supplies the majority of the scalp via three primary branching vessels: the superficial temporal, posterior auricular, and occipital arteries (▶ Fig. 10.2a). More specifically, the superficial temporal arteries supply the temporoparietal scalp, the posterior auricular arteries supply the relatively small posterolateral scalp, and the occipital arteries supply the posterior scalp above the nuchal line. Below the nuchal line, perforating musculocutaneous branches, which perforate through the trapezius and splenius capitis muscles, provide the blood supply.[2] Though a comparatively smaller contribution, the internal carotid system is significant in that it is the primary blood supply to the anterior scalp via the supraorbital and supratrochlear arteries.[4]

It is critical for the surgeon to consider the locations and typical trajectories of the primary vessels during preoperative planning. As a general rule, local flaps used for scalp reconstruction should incorporate at least one of the major scalp arteries in order to maintain axial blood supply.[3] Because larger arteries run within the galea and the temporoparietal fascia, dissection and raising of flaps in the subcutaneous plane risk vessel injury and tissue ischemia. Dissection of the subcutaneous fat poses significant risk of injury to terminal hair follicles, which may cause irreversible alopecia and thus an unacceptable aesthetic result.[4] Scalp flaps should be dissected and raised in the avascular subgaleal plane, so as to preserve the vascular supply and adnexae.[3] Although including the galeal layer renders flaps overall less elastic and distensible, this is generally considered insignificant given that the overall risk of flap failure is substantially reduced.[4]

Lymphatics

The lymphatic drainage of the scalp runs in the subcutaneous plane and parallels its venous drainage.[2] Like the forehead, lymph drains through lymphatic channels directly into basins within the parotid, anterior and posterior auricular chains, and occipital regions. Of note, there is an absence of lymph nodes, an important consideration when treating malignant scalp tumors.[1]

Innervation

The trigeminal nerve provides the majority of sensory innervation to the scalp. Its supraorbital branch, which passes through an often-palpable foramen on the bony supraorbital rim, extends superiorly across the forehead to innervate the anterior scalp. After traversing the corrugator muscle, its supratrochlear branch innervates the central scalp. Sensory innervation to the lateral and posterior scalp is provided by branches of the temporal,

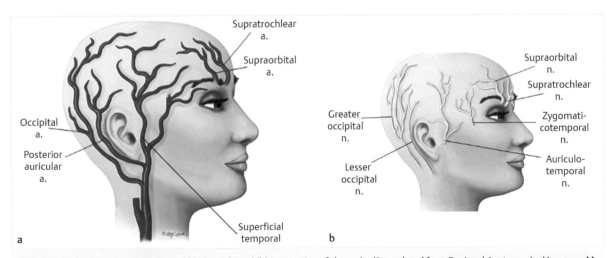

Fig. 10.2 Illustration of the (a) primary blood supply and (b) innervation of the scalp. (Reproduced from Regional Anatomy. In: Hanasono M, Robb G, Skoracki R, Yu P, ed. Reconstructive Plastic Surgery of the Head and Neck: Current Techniques and Flap Atlas. 1st Edition. New York: Thieme; 2016.)

auricular, and occipital sensory nerves (▶ Fig. 10.2b). Of note, all of the sensory nerves of the scalp traverse its periphery. Thus, the surgeon can use this to his or her advantage by infiltrating local anesthetic around the scalp periphery as a means of producing total scalp anesthesia.[7]

The temporal branch of the facial nerve is the most significant motor nerve with regard to surgical scalp anatomy. There is a risk of injury to it with superficial dissection in the temple region, where it runs within the temporoparietal fascia before terminating distally on the deep surfaces of the frontalis and corrugator muscles.[4] In most areas, dissecting deep to the galea significantly reduces risk of injury to this branch and, by extension, minimizes the likelihood of motor dysfunction. An exception to this is within the vicinity of the zygomatic arch, where dissection should be performed just beneath the superficial layer of the temporal fascia and periosteum.

10.2 Preoperative Evaluation

10.2.1 Evaluating the Patient

The initial step when approaching cutaneous reconstructive surgery is to consider patient-related factors, both intrinsic and extrinsic, which should take place before evaluation of the surgical site. The patient's medical and functional status should be considered, as the latter may affect one's ability to perform adequate postoperative wound care. Particular attention should be given to medical comorbidities and/or medications known to impede wound healing. Also, it is important to note the presence of any dermatologic conditions that may affect tissue quality and/or the overall likelihood of successful reconstruction. These include, but are not limited to, scarring alopecia, erosive pustular dermatosis of the scalp, extensive actinic damage, and any concurrent benign or malignant neoplasms. In a retrospective review of scalp reconstruction cases over a 15-year period, Newman et al found preoperative scalp radiation to be a statistically significant risk factor for developing major complications.[8] Finally, it is important to thoroughly understand and manage the patient's expectations for the postoperative course, wound care, potential complications, and anticipated outcome.

10.2.2 Evaluating the Defect

After an appropriate patient evaluation has been performed, consideration must be given to site-specific factors related to the anatomy of the surgical defect. These include the defect size and depth, whether the site is hair bearing or glabrous, and its specific location on the scalp, which may correlate to the degree of tissue laxity.

Depth

Depth of the surgical defect should be considered when selecting a reconstructive approach for the scalp. Defects on the scalp that are superficial to the hair follicle bulb and in non-hair-bearing areas heal well by second intention. For full-thickness defects, it is important to appreciate that extensive undermining in the subgaleal plane will be necessary to facilitate the tissue movement required for a successful repair. Skin grafts are unlikely to survive when the periosteum is not intact and a defect of this depth often requires bur holes to induce pinpoint bleeding.[7]

Hair Density

Also relevant to consider is whether the site of the defect is hair bearing or glabrous. On a hairless scalp, superficial defects left to heal by second intention leave a relatively inconspicuous scar. Conversely, when the defect is located in an area of dense terminal hair, these approaches tend to create aesthetically undesirable results.

Tissue Laxity

The scalp has both "tight" and "loose" areas due to the presence of the galea aponeurotica and its connections to fascia at the scalp periphery. Because of reduced tissue laxity in the "tight" portions, such as at the scalp vertex, large surgical defects in these areas are often not amenable to primary closure. Closure of large defects may require extensive undermining, scoring the galea aponeurotica, partial closure, delayed repair, and/or creation of a large local cutaneous flap.

10.3 Essential Concepts in Scalp Reconstruction

10.3.1 Reconstructive Goals

When approaching cutaneous scalp reconstruction, the surgeon should have two goals: functional preservation and cosmesis. The primary functional consideration is to preserve the scalp's viability and durability, which requires that it be both intact and adequately vascularized. This ensures the underlying calvarium remains sufficiently protected, and thereby avoids complications such as desiccation and infection. The primary cosmetic considerations include preserving the hairline and scalp contour as well as minimizing alopecia and scar appearance. This is accomplished primarily with attention to patterns of hair growth and aesthetically placed incisions.

10.3.2 Surgical Principles

Proficiency in several surgical concepts is essential for a successful scalp reconstruction. An important principle is accessing the subgaleal space. Being relatively avascular, it is an excellent plane for atraumatic, blunt undermining (▶ Fig. 10.3).

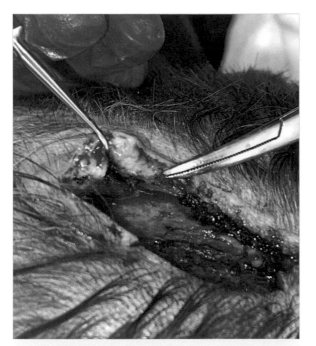

Fig. 10.3 Subgaleal space dissection.

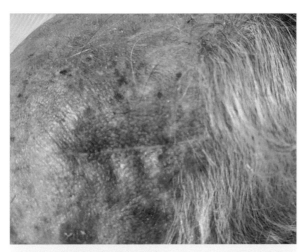

Fig. 10.4 Inverted scar.

A second principle is the importance of reapproximating the galea at the time of closure. If the galea is not reapproximated, the skin must be stretched significantly and the resulting tension placed on the epidermal edges may result in an inverted scar or wound dehiscence (► Fig. 10.4). By taking a large bite of the galea with the suture needle at the leading edge of the defect, however, the galea becomes reapproximated and absorbs the tension from the epidermal margins, resulting in a more aesthetically pleasing scar (► Fig. 10.5a, b).

A third principle is knowing when and how to perform a galeotomy for an immobile scalp. In order to enhance tissue laxity, a galeotomy can be performed to allow the skin to stretch. The technique is relatively simple and performed in the subgaleal space. Linear incisions are made through the galea and are oriented parallel to the wound edge (► Fig. 10.6). Ideally and if possible, the incisions should also be made parallel to the underlying vascular supply. Galeotomies are simple to perform on large flaps, which allow reflection of the flap to expose the galea for incision. They can be more challenging during a primary closure, where skin reflection and galea visualization are more difficult to perform.

10.4 Choosing the Reconstructive Approach

10.4.1 Second Intention

In certain situations, wound healing by second intention is appropriate. Second intention is suitable in patients who cannot tolerate or do not desire extensive reconstructive surgery. Second intention healing may be the most appropriate reconstructive option in patients with alopecic scalps, where the resulting scar is often more aesthetically acceptable than on hair-bearing skin. Patients with lighter skin types have improved aesthetic outcomes, as their surgical scar becomes pale due to an increase in collagen density and a decrease in tissue vascularity. Intact periosteum is necessary for granulation tissue formation. When present, even deep surgical wound healing by second intention will re-epithelialize in time (► Fig. 10.7).

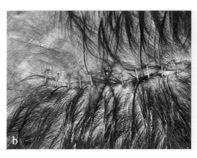

Fig. 10.5 (a,b) Galeal approximation and resulting scar. (Photograph courtesy of Dr. David H. Ciocon.)

Second intention healing has several notable disadvantages. Delayed wound healing is common on the scalp due to minimal wound contraction. Delayed healing is significant for patients planning to undergo adjuvant treatment postoperatively, such as radiation therapy, which may delay treatment initiation. Also, second intention healing carries a high probability of alopecia within the scar.

10.4.2 Primary Closure

Primary linear repair is the preferred reconstructive option on the scalp. It is often a technically simple procedure that produces minimal scarring, tissue displacement, and alopecia. Additionally, tumor recurrence surveillance is easier compared to local flaps and grafts.

The convexity of the scalp requires a longer fusiform ellipse with a length-to-width ratio of 4:1 or greater for primary closure. Whether or not a defect can be repaired primarily is largely determined by two factors: defect size and location. As a general rule, defects less than 3 cm in diameter on "loose" areas of the scalp can be closed primarily

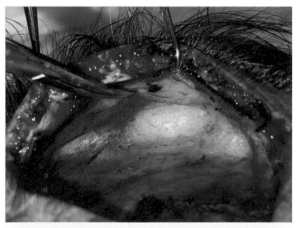

Fig. 10.6 Galeotomy technique.

(▶ Fig. 10.8). Larger defects may be closed primarily and is most successful when the defect is in a "loose" region. A helpful tool to assess whether primary closure is likely to be successful is to first attempt to manually close the defect. If the defect will not close manually, it is often unlikely to close completely with primary repair and may require partial closure.

Primary linear repair has several disadvantages. Primary repair can distort the position of the hairline and produce standing cutaneous cones, the latter of which typically resolve without the need for scar revision. Scar spread may occur with inadequate subgaleal undermining, which can result in areas of alopecia. The likelihood of alopecia can be reduced by orienting the repair in the direction of hair growth to minimize transection of hair follicles.

There are several surgical techniques that can be employed during primary repair to minimize tension on the wound edges. If a defect involves only skin, it should be deepened by removing the galea before any attempt at closure is made. This is necessary to allow access to the subgaleal space, where undermining is performed. Because the convexity of the scalp often limits the mobility that can be gained from undermining alone, galeotomy is particularly useful for primary repairs. Alternatively, some authors advocate for intraoperative tissue expansion (ITE). When closing the defect, the galea should be reapproximated first, as this allows the galea to bear the majority of the wound tension, thereby reducing tension on overlying skin. The needle should be placed through the galea only. Including the dermis with galea during suturing may increase the risk of an inverted scar. Galeal closure should be performed from the edges to the center with buried interrupted sutures. If a point is reached at which the galea will not reapproximate, the remainder of the defect can be closed with dermal sutures and horizontal mattress surface sutures, though this may result in focal scar inversion. Alternatively, the unapproximated area can be left to heal by second intention, that is, a partial closure.

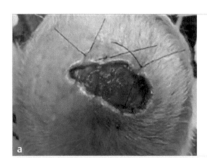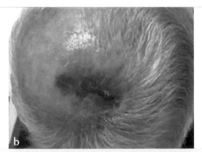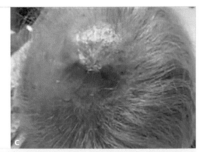

Fig. 10.7 Healing by second intention. (**a**) A patient with an open scalp wound referred for closure. (**b**) One month after treatment with a topical antimicrobial. (**c**) After 3 months. (Reproduced from Secondary Intention. In: Cohen M, Thaller S, ed. The Unfavorable Result in Plastic Surgery: Avoidance and Treatment. 4th Edition. New York: Thieme; 2018.)

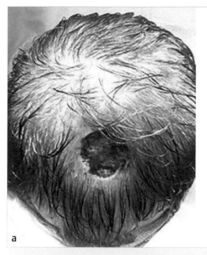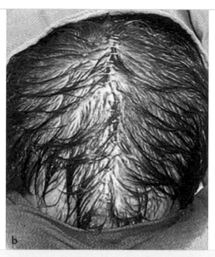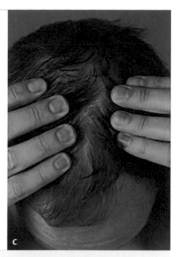

Fig. 10.8 A 36-year-old white male status post 4 × 3.5 cm Mohs excision for basal cell carcinoma on the scalp vertex. Wound was repaired with primary closure with standing cone excision. Postoperative results shown at 7 months. (Reproduced from Direct Closure. In: Thornton J, Carboy J, ed. Facial Reconstruction After Mohs Surgery. 1st Edition. New York: Thieme; 2018.)

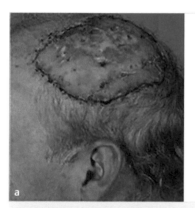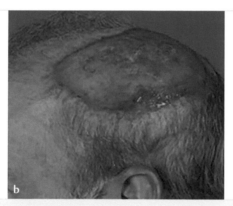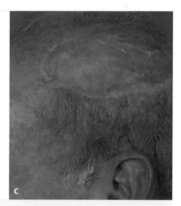

Fig. 10.9 (a–c) A 54-year-old man status post Mohs excision of multifocal squamous cell carcinoma. Mohs defect closed with Integra and color-matched split-thickness skin graft. Postoperative results shown at 5 months. (Reproduced from Integra and Split-Thickness Skin Grafting. In: Thornton J, Carboy J, ed. Facial Reconstruction After Mohs Surgery. 1st Edition. New York: Thieme; 2018.)

10.4.3 Skin Grafting

Types

Split-Thickness Skin Grafts

When faced with a medium to large scalp defect, particularly in a patient who cannot otherwise tolerate a more complex repair, an STSG is a reasonable choice. Most often, STSGs are placed to provide temporary closure of a defect in anticipation of a more definitive repair, such as an advanced local or free flap. They are also used to close secondary defects. In general, they tend to work best for defects on the vertex of an alopecic scalp and on the forehead.

STSGs should be chosen only when cosmesis is not a concern. Once healed, they fail to match the surrounding skin and result in a scar that is shiny, depressed, and alopecic (▶ Fig. 10.9). STSGs lack hair follicles and are thinner than full-thickness skin grafts (FTSGs). An additional disadvantage is that the grafted area is much less able to withstand shearing forces, rendering it fragile and susceptible to trauma. STSGs are not well suited for patients who will receive postoperative radiation therapy. STSGs offer several advantages such as being quick and faster to heal than a second intention wound. Compared to flaps, STSGs offer easier surveillance for tumor recurrence.

Full-Thickness Skin Grafts

FTSGs have been described for scalp reconstruction, but they have limited utility due to several factors. There are few suitable donor sites with sufficient terminal hair growth and, when found, generally have high metabolic demands that risk ischemic necrosis of the FTSG. FTSGs

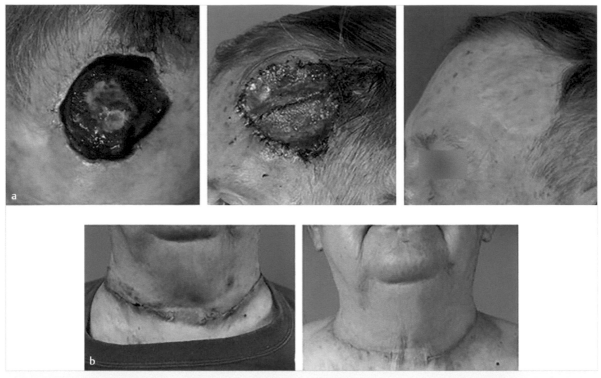

Fig. 10.10 (a) A 73-year-old man status post 7 × 7 cm Mohs excision for basal cell carcinoma at the upper left forehead/scalp. Wound treated with color-matched full-thickness skin graft. Postoperative results of the scalp shown at 7 months. **(b)** Note graft bisected and taken from neck bilaterally due to dimensions of the defect. Donor site pictured 1 week postoperatively and again 2 months postoperatively. (Reproduced from Full-Thickness Skin Grafts. In: Thornton J, Carboy J, ed. Facial Reconstruction After Mohs Surgery. 1st Edition. New York: Thieme; 2018.)

offer several advantages, such as rapid healing of the donor site and ability to close it primarily, which can be favorable in elderly or debilitated patients for whom minimal donor site care is ideal. Other scenarios in which FSTGs are useful include grafting of the donor site in large rotational advancement flaps or to provide coverage of the defect when tissue expansion is a temporary measure. FTSGs also offer more acceptable cosmetic results for both donor and recipient sites when compared to STSGs (► Fig. 10.10).

A common FTSG performed on the scalp is the Burow's graft. The graft donor site is a single Burow's triangle excised when a circular defect is converted into a fusiform ellipse. The two apices of the ellipse are closed from the periphery inward until the tension is too great in the center to withstand primary closure. The small, residual central defect can then be covered with the Burow's graft. Because the defect and graft are small, terminal hairs contained within the graft typically survive and, therefore, the cosmetic appearance is relatively well preserved. Given that tension on the scalp often prevents primary closure, a Burow's graft is especially useful because it allows medium-sized defects, which could otherwise not be primarily closed along their length, to be closed without the use of a larger flap.

Considerations

STSGs and FTSGs require an intact periosteum because graft survival is highly dependent on the presence of a sufficient vascular supply. If the periosteum is absent, bleeding can be induced by burring into the outer cortex of the cranium to expose the diploic space. One of several instruments can be used for this purpose, including a chisel and hammer or a high-speed drill.[7] However, some consider this method to result in poor wound healing and to carry the risk of intracranial complications. An alternative option is to cover the exposed bone with a regional flap. Delayed graft placement is often advantageous, as the site can partially heal by second intention, increasing the likelihood of graft survival. When using a delayed graft for a large defect, a purse-string closure can be performed to reduce its diameter anywhere from 10 to 30% (► Fig. 10.11).[7] This is done by taking small bites of the galea circumferentially around the defect and then tying the sutures off within the wound so they do not need to be removed at a later time. The graft is then placed centrally within the final defect.

An alternative method to skin grafting is the use of artificial dermal regeneration products to promote

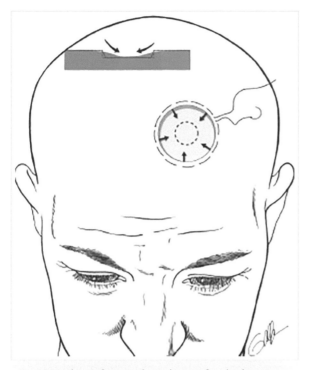

Fig. 10.11 Skin grafting on the scalp can often lead to a canyonlike step-off that is not aesthetically pleasing. The purse-string technique achieves two goals. First, the adjacent tissue advancement typically decreases the surface area of the defect by approximately 40%. The second effect of the purse-string technique is to create a gentler slope that will prevent the large step-off. (Reproduced from Skin Grafts. In: Cheney M, Hadlock T, ed. Facial Surgery: Plastic and Reconstructive. 1st Edition. New York: Thieme; 2014.)

cellular ingrowth. These include Integra, acellular human dermis (AlloDerm), and bovine collagen construct. These products can be placed immediately over the defect prior to placing the skin graft (▶ Fig. 10.12). Traditionally, artificial dermal regeneration products are left in place for 14 to 21 days, at which time granulation occurs, and are then removed. Compared to STSGs placed immediately after skin cancer removal, delayed grafts following dermal regeneration products have been shown to result in scars that are more aesthetically pleasing, with less contraction and improved pliability.[9]

10.4.4 Local Flaps

Introduction and Terminology

Local flaps are the preferred repair method for defects on the scalp that cannot be closed primarily. They have good survival rates with minimal risk of necrosis and are considered safe with minimal complication risk.[10] When approaching local flap design, there are several important considerations. General tenets for success include designing large flaps with wide bases, creating as few flaps as possible, and avoiding critical suture lines. Also important to consider is that the scalp lacks relaxed skin tension lines. Therefore, unlike on other areas of the body such as the face, incisions should be made to maximize tissue recruitment and optimize vascular supply. Reconstruction should be parallel to the direction of hair growth in order to minimize hair follicle trauma. Additionally, the surgeon should always consider the anterior hairline as the primary anatomic landmark and aim to preserve it.

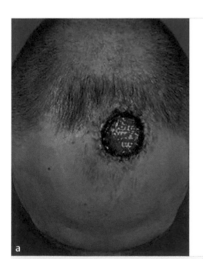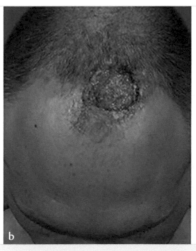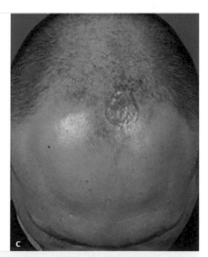

Fig. 10.12 (a–c) A 32-year-old man status post wide local excision of 0.5-mm-thick cutaneous melanoma on the vertex of the scalp. Wound treated with Integra and subsequent split-thickness skin graft. Postoperative results shown at 4 months. (Reproduced from Integra and Split-Thickness Skin Grafting. In: Thornton J, Carboy J, ed. Facial Reconstruction After Mohs Surgery. 1st Edition. New York: Thieme; 2018.)

Types

Advancement Flaps

Advancement flaps are infrequently performed on the scalp because they require significant tissue laxity. Defects that cannot be closed primarily will not be amenable to a unidirectional advancement flap with essentially identical tension direction and magnitude. As a result, advancement flaps on the scalp are often combined with rotation flaps, which are better suited to the scalp's natural convexity.

Despite their limited use, pure advancement flaps are used for small defects on the temporoparietal scalp. They can also be used for defects on the frontal scalp, where the incision can be easily hidden in the anterior hairline. In these cases, the O-T advancement flap works well. This flap is performed by making bilateral incisions along the hairline and elevating the flap just underneath the frontalis muscle in the subgaleal space. The redundant tissue at the inferior margin of the defect, which is created when the flap is advanced, is then removed in a vertical direction to form the shape of a "T" (▶ Fig. 10.13). For the O-T advancement flap to be successful in this area, extensive undermining is required.

A galeotomy may also be necessary to reduce tension sufficiently.[11] Island pedicle advancement flaps can be used to close large operative wounds based on a known vascular supply. To repair scalp defects, island pedicle advancement flaps with a lateral arterial supply, such as the temporal or occipital artery and their tributaries, can be lifted and advanced a large distance because the galea is severed prior to advancement of the flap (▶ Fig. 10.14).

Several rules can be applied to increase the likelihood of success and for a good cosmetic outcome for advancement flaps. Because tissue advancement generates standing cutaneous deformities, advancement flap incisions need to be long in order to reduce "dog-ear" protrusions. Although these redundant Burow's triangles can be removed, doing so requires them to be excised vertically and thus perpendicular to the horizontal incisions ideal for advancement flaps.

Rotation Flaps

As the convexity of the scalp is well suited to curvilinear incisions, rotation flaps are commonly utilized in scalp reconstruction. Rotation flaps can be used to repair medium to large defects that cannot be easily repaired primarily.

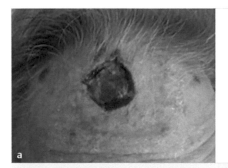
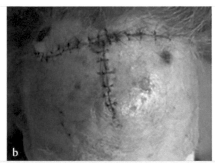
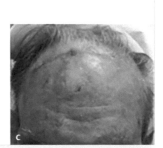

Fig. 10.13 (a–c) Photo of O-T advancement flap steps. (Photograph courtesy of Dr. David H. Ciocon.)

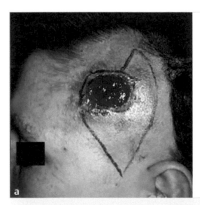
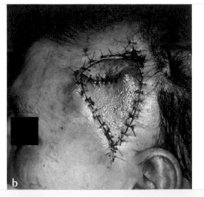
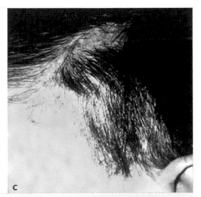

Fig. 10.14 Extended V-Y flap. (a) An extended V-Y advancement flap design. (b) A double extended V-Y advancement flap design with two extension limb flaps. (c) An extended V-Y advancement flap design for coverage of a right temporal scalp defect. The immediate and long-term postoperative results. The direction of hair growth is changed by the extension limb of the flap. (Reproduced from V-Y Flaps. In: Neligan P, Wei F, ed. Microsurgical Reconstruction of the Head and Neck. 1st Edition. New York: Thieme; 2009.)

Rotation flaps are particularly advantageous when faced with large defects because they generate motion in multiple vectors. The use of a double-rotation flap, such as the O-Z, or multiple-rotation flaps, such as a "pinwheel flap" or "hurricane flap," can be utilized when defects cannot be repaired with single-rotation flaps.

Technical considerations for rotation flaps are similar to those for other local flaps. Rotation flap incisions must be long. As a rule, rotational incisions should be four to six times as long as width of the defect.[4] If the incisions are made too short, they are likely to require too much tension for complete closure and attempting to do so carries a significant risk of necrosis. Residual tension within a short incision can result in partial closure, which requires a portion to heal secondarily. As with all flaps, rotation flaps should be undermined widely in the subgaleal plane.

Although rotation flaps are considered most optimal for repair for large defects on the scalp, they are an excellent choice for small to medium-sized defects. In these cases, a single-rotation flap, rather than bilateral or multiple-rotation flaps, typically suffices. A single-rotation flap is performed by making a curvilinear incision from the edge of the defect and extending outward. This ensures that it incorporates the galea and the flap is undermined in the subgaleal space. Once the appropriate incision is made, the resulting flap is rotated 180 degrees from the incision point on the defect and closed (▶ Fig. 10.15). If the incision results in a curve that is either too shallow or too deep, it creates excess tension at the pivot point that is difficult to overcome and significantly hinders flap motion. To generate an appropriately curved flap, it is best to make the incision first in a linear fashion by extending the leading edge. Then, carefully arc the blade when approaching the end of the incision. Redundant tissue will form when the flap is rotated into the primary defect, usually at the pivot point. To remove this, a "dog-ear" excision can be performed. For larger flaps, a "dog-ear" excision can be performed anywhere along the flap's motion. This may be preferential if an alternative site distant from the pivot point allows the necessary incisions to be more easily concealed for a better cosmetic outcome.

There are some instances where a defect is too large to be repaired using a single-rotation flap. In these cases, bilateral or multiple-rotation flaps provide greater tissue surface area and allow tension to be distributed across several incision lines. In particular, multiple-rotation flaps are very well suited for repair of large defects at the vertex and crown. The O-Z closure, a type of double-rotation flap, is commonly performed for this purpose. This type of repair is done by making two curvilinear incisions, one on either side of the defect, to create two rotation flaps. Each flap is then lifted and both are pivoted in the same direction (clockwise or counterclockwise) to close a centrally located defect. The resulting formation is similar to the shape of a "Z," newly formed from the defect (the "O"; ▶ Fig. 10.16). If the tissue on the vertex or crown is particularly inelastic, a commonly employed multiple-rotation flap called a "pinwheel" or "hurricane" may be required. This is also useful in repair of central defects of the anterior and posterior scalps. To perform this repair, three to six equidistant incisions are made along the circumference of the defect to generate three to six individual flaps.

All of the incisions are arced in the same direction (▶ Fig. 10.17a). This allows every flap to be lifted and rotated clockwise or counterclockwise, analogous to the motion of a pinwheel, to fill the defect (▶ Fig. 10.17b). Because multiple incisions are required for this type of repair, the major disadvantage is that each incision has the potential to develop alopecia.

Transposition Flaps

Although they are not as frequently performed on the scalp as rotation flaps, transposition flaps are of particular use because they allow the surgeon to borrow tissue from "loose" areas in order to cover a defect in a "tight" area, such as the vertex and crown. Because single-transposition flaps infrequently offer much benefit over primary closure, their use on the scalp is limited. The unidirectional motion of single-transposition flaps makes redistributing tension difficult. Transposition flaps lifted from the peripheral scalp can be positioned to close

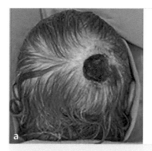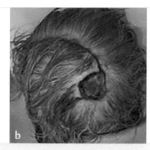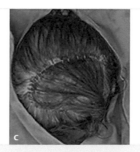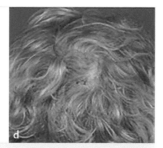

Fig. 10.15 (a–d) A 65-year-old woman status post 3 × 3 cm Mohs excision of basal cell carcinoma on the posterior scalp. Wound closed with rotation advancement flap. Postoperative results shown at 7 months. (Reproduced from Rotation Flaps. In: Thornton J, Carboy J, ed. Facial Reconstruction After Mohs Surgery. 1st Edition. New York: Thieme; 2018.)

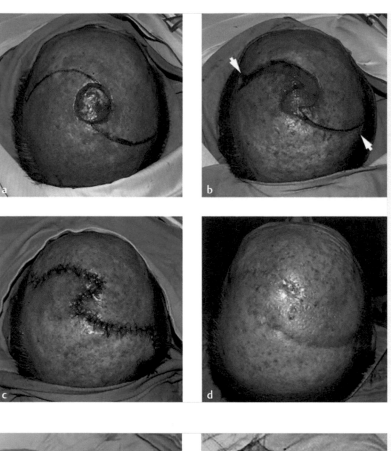

Fig. 10.16 (a) Scalp defect following resection of a cutaneous malignancy. **(b)** Design of double opposing rotation flaps. The arrows indicate Burow's triangles excised away from the base of the flap, to avoid a standing cone or "dog-ear" deformity while preserving maximum blood supply to the flaps. **(c)** Immediate and **(d)** late postoperative results. (Reproduced from Local Flaps. In: Hanasono M, Robb G, Skoracki R, Yu P, ed. Reconstructive Plastic Surgery of the Head and Neck: Current Techniques and Flap Atlas. 1st Edition. New York: Thieme; 2016.)

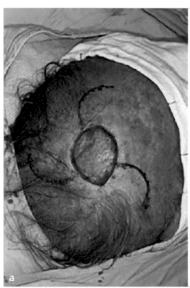
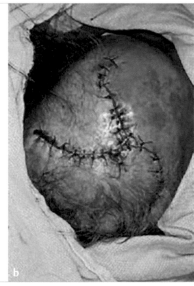

Fig. 10.17 (a) Medium-sized scalp defect with planned pinwheel closure. **(b)** Wide undermining of the scalp allows for a pinwheel closure of the defect. (Reproduced from Options for Reconstruction. In: Genden E, ed. Reconstruction of the Head and Neck. A Defect-Oriented Approach. 1st Edition. New York: Thieme; 2012.)

defects of the vertex and crown. They allow easier closure by borrowing laxity from "loose" areas while simultaneously redirecting tension toward them. Examples include lifting a flap from the occiput to close a defect at the posterior vertex and lifting from the lateral scalp to cover a defect on the crown or temporal scalp (▶ Fig. 10.18). A significant advantage of transposition flaps is that hair-bearing skin can be transferred to visible areas, such as

the anterior and temporal scalps, and posterior donor sites can be covered with a skin graft.

Multiple-transposition flaps can be used to cover a single, large defect.[12] Similar to the pinwheel technique, the contribution of multiple flaps allows tension to be redistributed across multiple vectors. This is especially helpful on areas of limited motion, such as the vertex. Multiple-transposition flaps are also an excellent choice for repair

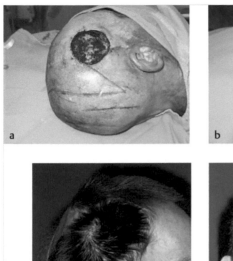
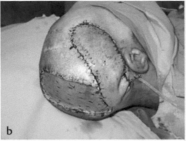
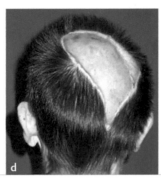

Fig. 10.18 (a) A 66-year-old patient with a chronic wound after squamous cell carcinoma resection and irradiation. A transposition of scalp is planned on the occipital artery, which is located by Doppler examination and marked. **(b)** Tension-free rotation and inset of the flap are performed and the rotational dog-ear is left for future revision if needed. A skin graft will take well in the nonirradiated bed of the donor site. **(c)** Lateral view of flap at 6 months. **(d)** Posterior view of donor site skin graft at 6 months. (Reproduced from Case Examples. In: Hanasono M, Robb G, Skoracki R, Yu P, ed. Reconstructive Plastic Surgery of the Head and Neck: Current Techniques and Flap Atlas. 1st Edition. New York: Thieme; 2016.)

of defects on the anterior scalp and hairline. The most common repair of this type is the Orticochea technique, which is composed of three rhombic flaps. An illustration of this technique is shown in ▶ Fig. 10.19. A technically challenging repair, it is particularly useful in select patients. Patients who wish for an aesthetically optimal result with hair-bearing flaps but are unwilling to undergo prolonged tissue expansion are good candidates. The Orticochea technique is also appropriate in those unable to tolerate the prolonged anesthesia required for microsurgical flaps. As is standard for scalp reconstruction, undermining must be extensive. In the majority of cases, the entire scalp must be undermined during the course of flap dissection and transfer. It is important for the surgeon to be absolutely certain that all margins are tumor free before this type of repair is attempted, as monitoring for recurrence is particularly challenging.

When executing a transposition flap, the flap should be lifted from within the area of maximal tissue laxity to optimize closure of the primary defect. In contrast to advancement and rotation flaps, the secondary defect should be closed first to facilitate movement of the flap into the primary defect with minimal tension. Rhombic transposition flaps can be considered for scalp reconstruction. Because of the 120-degree transposition angle inherent to standard rhombic flaps, a large dog-ear is expected and should be excised opposite the secondary defect. An additional disadvantage of rhombic flaps is the increased likelihood of a "trapdoor" deformity. This can be mitigated, in part, by wide undermining of the defect. It is also helpful to extensively undermine the recipient site. Along with placing buried sutures around the flap, this helps the scar contract. In doing

so, it reduces the risk of flap protrusion as the wound heals is reduced.

10.4.5 Regional Flaps

In some instances, regional musculocutaneous or muscle flaps are indicated for the repair of very large scalp defects. These flaps are best suited for defects on the temporal and inferior occipital scalp, as these are the only regions within reach of the flap's vascular pedicle. Appropriate indications for regional flaps include patients with poor wound healing and/or patients with a history of radiation who are not optimal candidates for free tissue transfer (FTT) despite requiring a large amount of vascularized tissue. Regional flaps can also be appropriate as a palliative care measure.

Despite their utility in certain clinical scenarios, regional flaps are associated with significant donor site morbidity. Because the tissue is heavy and so results in significant gravitational pull parallel to the pedicle, there is a great risk of ischemic necrosis distally. In addition, regional flaps do not provide hair-bearing tissue to the recipient site. Consequently, with the exception of the temporoparietal fascia flap (TPFF), regional flaps are infrequently preferred over FTT.

The TPFF can be designed in several forms, including a local pedicled flap, a microsurgical flap, or as a composite flap that incorporates underlying bone or overlying hair-bearing scalp. It is particularly useful for large defects that involve the frontal or temporal hairline (▶ Fig. 10.20). As a pedicled flap, it can be raised as large as 14 × 17 cm.[4] The TPFF is supplied by the superficial temporal artery and vein, both of which must be incorporated into the pedicle.

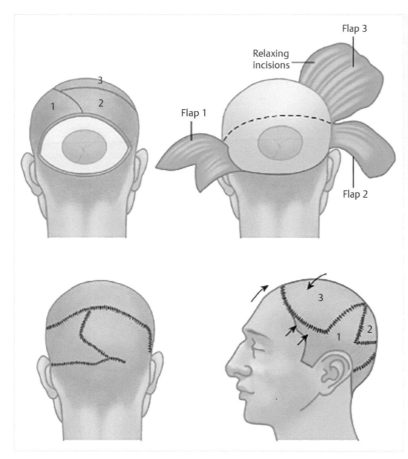

Fig. 10.19 Orticochea three-flap technique for coverage of large defects of the scalp. (Reproduced from Reconstruction by region. In: Woo A, Shahzad F, Snyder-Warwick A, ed. Plastic Surgery Case Review: Oral Board Study Guide. 1st Edition. New York: Thieme; 2014.)

Either the anterior or the posterior branches of the temporal artery can be contained within the flap. Given the significant anatomic variability in the course of the temporal artery, it is critical to map it preoperatively with a Doppler probe before designing a TPFF. In some instances when the flap is hair bearing, the adjacent skin may require controlled tissue expansion (CTE) in order to facilitate closure of the secondary defect.

10.4.6 Microsurgical Free Tissue Transfer

Medium and large defects of the scalp can also be repaired with FTT. This procedure involves the transfer of very large flaps of skin and soft tissue from distant anatomic sites, with the superficial temporal artery and vein serving as the recipient vessels for anastomosis in the majority of cases. FTT is particularly well suited to repair of extensive defects involving exposed neurocranial structures, difficult cases with a history of prior radiation therapy, and patients with a history of chronic infections. They are also advantageous in patients planned for postoperative radiation therapy because they are highly resilient to breakdown.[13] Flaps lifted as FTT offer a large bulk of highly vascularized tissue that serves as an excellent recipient site for skin grafts and also contours nicely to the calvarium. Even muscle flaps, which are initially bulky, atrophy over time to a thickness and contour that replicates the normal scalp nicely. Though typically minor in comparison to the extensive defects for which FTT is indicated, the major disadvantage is the lack of hair replacement and lack of color match.

The most common free flaps for scalp reconstruction are the latissimus dorsi, rectus abdominis, radial forearm, and scapula. The anterolateral thigh and gracilis muscle are used less often. Overall, however, the choice of flap is a decision highly dependent on the surgeon's comfort level and experience. In dermatologic reconstructive surgery, the latissimus dorsi flap is performed most frequently.[4] This is because it offers a large surface area of transferrable tissue despite low donor site morbidity, is flexible, and possesses a large-caliber vascular pedicle. When lifting this flap, only the muscle is taken and not the overlying skin, as the bulk of the subcutaneous fat prevents good scalp contour (▶ Fig. 10.20). It is for this reason that the latissimus dorsi flap is almost always followed by placement of an overlying skin graft. In comparison, radial forearm and anterolateral thigh flaps do not require a skin graft. Because these flaps lack substantial subcutaneous fat, good scalp contour is easily achieved when placed.

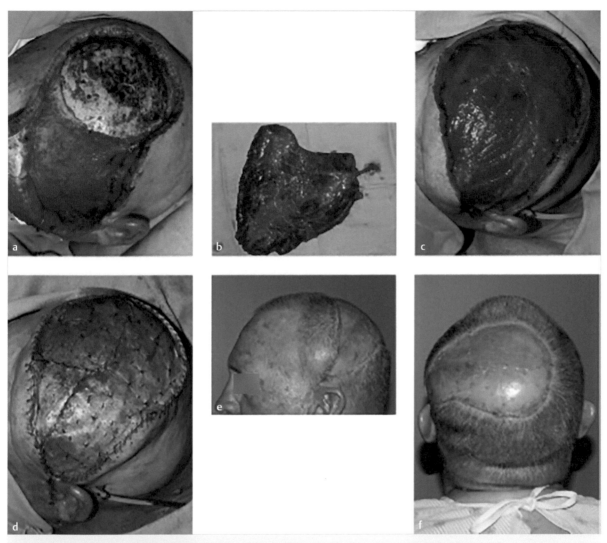

Fig. 10.20 (a) Large scalp defect requiring free flap reconstruction. **(b)** A latissimus dorsi muscle free flap. **(c)** Flap inset with anastomosis to the left superficial temporal blood vessels. **(d)** Coverage with an unmeshed split-thickness skin graft. **(e,f)** Postoperative result. (Reproduced from Latissimus Dorsi Flap. In: Hanasono M, Robb G, Skoracki R, Yu P, ed. Reconstructive Plastic Surgery of the Head and Neck: Current Techniques and Flap Atlas. 1st Edition. New York: Thieme; 2016.)

10.4.7 Piecemeal Closure

In patients with moderate to high cosmetic expectations who want to preserve hair, yet do not want or will not tolerate extensive surgical excisions, piecemeal closure should be considered. This type of repair attempts to close the defect as much as possible with a combination of small local flaps and partial linear closures. The portion of the defect that cannot be closed is then left to heal secondarily. Though this area is likely to be alopecic, the surrounding flaps often preserve hair-bearing scalp sufficient to mask the appearance in a way that is cosmetically acceptable. This is particularly true if the portion left to heal by second intention is small. This is because wounds heal better by second intention when they are part of a partial closure and contract significantly.

10.5 Adjuvant Surgical Techniques

10.5.1 Tissue Expansion

Tissue expansion is an adjuvant surgical technique of particular use in scalp reconstruction. The limited mobility of the scalp can detrimentally impact closure, but the scalp benefits substantially from tissue expansion and it is employed more frequently than for other anatomic sites. There are two primary types of tissue expansion surgeons should be familiar with: CTE and ITE.

Controlled Tissue Expansion

CTE involves placing a tissue expander under the galea and on top of periosteum. It is left in place for weeks to months and inflated once or twice per week until tissue expansion is considered sufficient, at which time the expanders are removed and the defect is closed (▶ Fig. 10.20). This induces significant metabolic and physical stress on the wound margins in the form of tension, which generates large, vascularized hair-bearing flaps. Though comparable flaps can be created from FTT, they are not hair bearing and do not offer comparable tissue match to CTE. Hair follicles can be traumatized during expansion; however, they generally recover and alopecia is rarely permanent.

CTE is suitable in select situations only. The first is for wounds that are fully healed and the second is for preoperative wounds prior to resection. The latter is inappropriate in cases of cutaneous malignancy because the time needed for expansion significantly delays time to tumor removal. Ultimately, the major disadvantages of CTE are the time it requires, the need for multiple office visits, and the associated discomfort.

Intraoperative Tissue Expansion

As its name suggests, ITE is a fast expansion process that occurs intraoperatively. It is performed just before placing a flap or closing a defect primarily. ITE continues to be a somewhat controversial technique. Some are strong advocates, while others believe it offers little other than to facilitate undermining, and its overall benefit continues to be questioned. Standard ITE procedures involve three sequential inflations lasting 3 minutes each, on average.[4] The expander is inflated until the surrounding tissue blanches. The advantage of ITE compared to CTE is that it can be performed quickly and on fresh wounds. This is a reflection of the fact that ITE does not place the same metabolic and physiologic demands on tissue as CTE.

10.6 Algorithm for Scalp Reconstruction

Several algorithms have been proposed to assist the reconstructive surgeon with deciding on the best approach to scalp defects. The algorithms vary with respect to considering the following primary factors: defect size, defect location, and ability to preserve the hairline. Some algorithms also account for secondary factors, such as tissue quality and radiation history. The decision as to which algorithm to follow, or to follow one at all, lies with the reconstructive surgeon, his or her preferences and comfort level.

One algorithm was outlined by Leedy et al and begins with the defect location as on the anterior, parietal, occipital, or vertex scalp.[3] The primary consideration that drives decision-making in this algorithm is preservation of the hairline. With the exception of defects located on the vertex, they propose considering first whether or not primary closure can be performed without distorting the respective hairline. If it can be done, primary closure should be the chosen repair. If not, they recommend considering whether local tissue rearrangement would allow hairline preservation and selecting local flaps or tissue expansion. For vertex defects, they recommend always closing primarily, if possible. If not, the primary question is not whether the hairline can be preserved, but rather whether the defect is less than or greater than 4 cm in width. If greater than 4 cm, they propose primary closure with galeal scoring or pinwheel flaps. If less than 4 cm, they propose local tissue rearrangement with large rotation/advancement flaps, possible back-grating and tissue expansion. Notably, this algorithm does not consider the quality of the local tissue or a history, such as radiation, known to alter the wound environment.

Several other algorithms exist, as well. Beasley et al proposed a bimodal algorithm for reconstruction, which considers defect size, tissue quality, and location as either scalp or forehead.[13] It does not account for tissue quality and is limited in large part by failing to subdivide scalp defects by their particular location as either anterior, parietal, occipital, or vertex. Iblher et al outlined an approach for oncologic scalp reconstruction that emphasizes clear surgical margins in addition to defect size, but does not consider location, tissue quality, or hairline preservation.[14]

The simplest algorithm was proposed by Newman et al. This approach is based first and foremost on size and classifies defects as small ($<10\,cm^2$), medium ($10–50\,cm^2$), or large ($>50\,cm^2$) before then factoring in the quality of tissue as good or poor.[8] We suggest a very similar, equally simple algorithm outlined by Hanasono et al, which is shown in ▶ Fig. 10.21.[15] It also classifies the defect size as small, moderate, or large, but defines them as less than 3, 3 to 5, and greater than 5 cm, respectively. Within each category, there are several potential reconstructive methods. As with Newman et al's algorithm, choosing the most appropriate method is dependent solely on tissue quality.

Ultimately, the most appropriate algorithm is one the surgeon finds easy to implement. It should be adjusted, as necessary, in accordance with individual variations in experience and expertise. Because of the difficulty in dividing the scalp into cosmetic units, we find an algorithmic approach to be of particular use early in training and practice. However, with experience, this may become less necessary. For those who prefer a more comprehensive approach, a thorough review of reconstructive options for the scalp, including advantages, disadvantages, and optimal indications, can be found in ▶ Table 10.1.

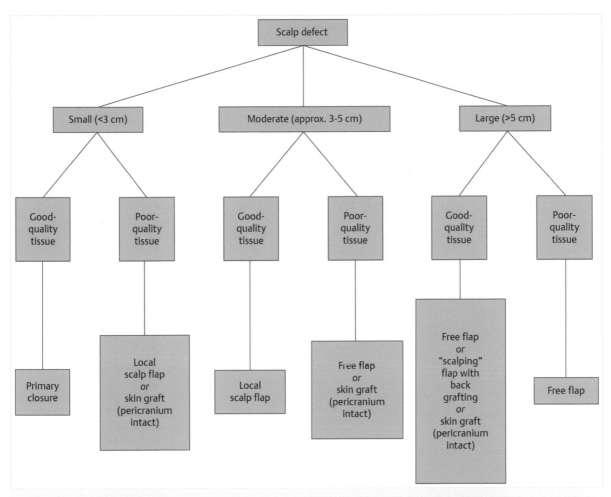

Fig. 10.21 Scalp reconstruction algorithm outlined by Hanasono et al. (Reproduced from Algorithm. In: Hanasono M, Robb G, Skoracki R, Yu P, ed. Reconstructive Plastic Surgery of the Head and Neck: Current Techniques and Flap Atlas. 1st Edition. New York: Thieme; 2016.)

Table 10.1 Reconstructive options for repair of scalp defects

Repair type	Advantages	Disadvantages	Considerations	When to use
Second intention	• Does not require extensive reconstructive surgery	• Delayed wound healing • Prolonged wound care • Results in alopecia	• Requires intact periosteum • May not be appropriate for patients requiring postoperative adjuvant RXT • Best cosmesis in FST1–3 • Poor wound healing probable in diabetics, pharmacologic and physiologic immunosuppression, history of RXT	• Can be employed anywhere on the scalp • Glabrous skin
Primary closure	• Technically simple • Minimal scarring • Minimal alopecia • Easier to monitor for tumor recurrence compared to both flaps and grafts	• May distort hairline	• Requires fusiform ellipse length-to-width ratio of 4:1 • Extensive undermining required to minimize scar spread • Galeotomies often helpful	• Defects < 3 cm in diameter on "loose" areas

(Continued)

143

Table 10.1 (*Continued*) Reconstructive options for repair of scalp defects

Repair type	Advantages	Disadvantages	Considerations	When to use
Split-thickness skin graft	• Can be done in patients who cannot tolerate a more complex repair • Fast, relatively simple, and reliable • Easier to monitor for tumor recurrence compared to flaps	• Poor cosmesis due to poor donor to recipient tissue match • Result in alopecia • Fragile and susceptible to trauma • Poorly replicate normal scalp mobility • Donor site morbidity	• May be performed to close a secondary defect definitively or temporarily before a more definitive repair • Requires an intact periosteum • Cosmesis may be improved via serial excisions in conjunction with serial flaps or primary closure • Artificial dermal regeneration templates can improve donor/recipient mismatch	• Defects on the vertex of an alopecic scalp
Full-thickness skin graft	• Rapid healing • Can be closed primarily	• Suitable donor sites typically carry high risk of necrosis 2/2 high metabolic demand • Donor site morbidity	• Requires an intact periosteum • Useful in grafting donor sites in large rotational advancement flaps • Can provide temporary coverage of defects undergoing tissue expansion	• Overall limited utility[a] • Favored in elderly, debilitated patients
Advancement flap	• Good survival rates • Minimal complications	• Standing cutaneous deformities common • Requires significant tissue laxity • Surveillance for tumor recurrence difficult • Can distort hairline	• Often combined with rotation flaps • Incisions must be long to reduce "dog-ears" • Extensive undermining required • May necessitate galeotomy	• Overall limited utility • Small defects in temporoparietal scalp • Defects of frontal scalp
Rotation flap	• Good survival rates • Minimal complications	• Occasionally require extensive tissue manipulation • Multiple incisions needed • Surveillance for tumor recurrence difficult • Can distort hairline	• Incision must be 4–6 times as long as it is wide • Extensive undermining required • May be single or multiple, e.g., O-Z	• Most common repair method • Best for large defects anywhere on the scalp; can also be used for small and medium defects • Preferred repair for full-thickness defects unable to be closed primarily
Transposition flap	• Good survival rates • Minimal complications	• "Trapdoor" deformity • Surveillance for tumor recurrence difficult • Can distort hairline	• Extensive undermining required • May be single or multiple, e.g., Orticochea	• Defects of vertex and crown, also anterior scalp and hairline
Regional flap, e.g., TPFF	• Large amount of vascularized tissue without microvascular anastomosis	• Requires technical expertise • Results in alopecia • Donor site morbidity • High risk of ischemic necrosis	• Consider preoperative Doppler mapping for TPFF	• Defects of occipital and temporoparietal scalp • Ideal in patients with poor wound healing and/or history of RXT who are not candidates for FTT • Useful as palliative measure
Microsurgical free tissue transfer	• Large surface area of vascularized tissue • Resilient to tissue breakdown • Excellent recipient site for skin grafts • Contours well to calvarium	• Results in alopecia and poor color match		• Ideal for extensive defects involving exposed neurocranial structures • Works well in patients with RXT and/or chronic infection history • Good choice in patients planned for postoperative RXT

Abbreviations: FST, Fitzpatrick skin type; FST1-3, Fitzpatrick skin type 1-3; FTT, tree tissue transfer; RXT, radiation therapy; TPFF, temporoparietal fascia flap.
[a]Notable exception: Burow's graft.

References

[1] Olson MD, Hamilton GS, III. Scalp and forehead defects in the post-Mohs surgery patient. Facial Plast Surg Clin North Am. 2017; 25(3):365–375

[2] Desai SC, Sand JP, Sharon JD, Branham G, Nussenbaum B. Scalp reconstruction: an algorithmic approach and systematic review. JAMA Facial Plast Surg. 2015; 17(1):56–66

[3] Leedy JE, Janis JE, Rohrich RJ. Reconstruction of acquired scalp defects: an algorithmic approach. Plast Reconstr Surg. 2005; 116(4):54e–72e

[4] Hoffman JF. Reconstruction of the scalp. In: Baker, SR. Local Flaps in Facial Reconstruction. Philadelphia, PA: Elsevier; 2007:637–665

[5] Goldman GD, Dzubow LM, Yelverton CB. Scalp. In: Facial Flap Surgery. New York, NY: McGraw Hill; 2013:292–305

[6] Bradford BD, Lee JW. Reconstruction of the forehead and scalp. Facial Plast Surg Clin North Am. 2019; 27(1):85–94

[7] Leitenberger JL, Lee KK. Scalp reconstruction. In: Rohrer TE, Cook JL, Lee KK, eds. Flaps and Grafts in Dermatologic Surgery. Philadelphia, PA: Elsevier; 2018:145–155

[8] Newman MI, Hanasono MM, Disa JJ, Cordeiro PG, Mehrara BJ. Scalp reconstruction: a 15-year experience. Ann Plast Surg. 2004; 52(5):501–506, discussion 506

[9] Wilensky JS, Rosenthal AH, Bradford CR, Rees RS. The use of a bovine collagen construct for reconstruction of full-thickness scalp defects in the elderly patient with cutaneous malignancy. Ann Plast Surg. 2005; 54(3):297–301

[10] Steiner D, Hubertus A, Arkudas A, et al. Scalp reconstruction: a 10-year retrospective study. J Craniomaxillofac Surg. 2017; 45(2):319–324

[11] Barry RB, Lawrence CM, Langtry JA. The use of galeotomies to aid the closure of surgical defects on the forehead and scalp. Br J Dermatol. 2009; 160(4):875–877

[12] Frodel JL, Jr, Ahlstrom K. Reconstruction of complex scalp defects: the "banana peel" revisited. Arch Facial Plast Surg. 2004; 6(1):54–60

[13] Beasley NJ, Gilbert RW, Gullane PJ, Brown DH, Irish JC, Neligan PC. Scalp and forehead reconstruction using free revascularized tissue transfer. Arch Facial Plast Surg. 2004; 6(1):16–20

[14] Iblher N, Ziegler MC, Penna V, Eisenhardt SU, Stark GB, Bannasch H. An algorithm for oncologic scalp reconstruction. Plast Reconstr Surg. 2010; 126(2):450–459

[15] Hanasono M, Robb G, Skoracki R, et al. Algorithm. In: Reconstructive Plastic Surgery of the Head and Neck. Current Techniques and Flap Atlas. 1st ed. New York, NY: Thieme; 2016

11 Reconstruction of the Hand and Nail Unit after Mohs Surgery

Evelyn R. Reed, Thomas J. Wright, Madison E. Tattini, and Shaun D. Mendenhall

Summary

Mohs surgery is an effective treatment tool for both non-melanoma skin cancer and melanoma of the hand. The nature of the surgery yields individualized and variable defects throughout the hand, fingers, and thumb. The hand is anatomically complex and each region has different functional and aesthetic requirements, both of which should be considered in planning reconstruction. Fortunately, there are a variety of acceptable and versatile reconstructive options for each of these regions that range from simple local closures to complex free tissue transfers. Dermatologic surgeons should be familiar with these options and their indications. Many of them may choose to include some of the techniques in their own reconstructive wheelhouse; however, we recommend having a low threshold to refer to a hand or plastic surgeon whenever there is any question about providing the best outcome for the patient.

Keywords: melanoma, nonmelanoma skin cancer, squamous cell carcinoma, Mohs surgery, reconstruction, dorsum of hand, thumb, flaps, nail unit, skin substitute

11.1 Introduction

Mohs micrographic surgery (MMS) was developed for the treatment of cutaneous malignancies with the intent to reduce risk of recurrence while simultaneously minimizing the ultimate defect. Mohs surgery offers great benefit in the treatment of melanoma as well as nonmelanoma skin cancers (NMSCs), particularly in anatomically sensitive areas such as the hands and face. It has repeatedly shown to yield excellent disease-related outcomes, patients tolerate it well, and the process is cost-effective.[1] As a result of using Mohs techniques to conserve tissue and function, the standard of care has shifted from wide local excision (WLE) and amputation to tissue conservation and digit salvage. Cutaneous malignancies of the hand result in a wide variety of defects that require special considerations depending on their size, location, and impact on function. The dermatologic surgeon should not only feel comfortable with the basics of hand anatomy as it pertains to resection and reconstruction of these malignancies but also recognize when the patient may best be served by a plastic and reconstructive or hand surgeon.

11.2 Cutaneous Malignancies of the Hand

11.2.1 Nonmelanoma Skin Cancers of the Hand

Basal cell carcinoma (BCC) is the most common type of malignancy in the United States, affecting almost 3 million people per year.[2] Although ultraviolet (UV) exposure is a known risk factor for all BCCs, there is a notable underrepresentation of these malignancies on the surface of the hand in comparison to other sun-exposed regions of the body. This is thought to be attributable to the decreased number of sebaceous structures on the dorsal hand, as BCCs likely develop from pilar structures. Males are at higher risk than females, which is also likely related to their higher overall risk of sun exposure. Although the overall incidence of BCC is lower than squamous cell carcinoma (SCC), both are most common on the dorsum of the hand.[3] BCC is rarely seen in the nail unit. If BCC of the nail unit is present, it is seen most often on the thumb.[4]

SCC accounts for 90% of hand malignancies,[5] and are most commonly seen on the dorsum of the hand. Sun exposure is a major risk factor and SCC is twice as likely to be seen in males.[6] Despite often being present on the dorsal surface of the hand, SCC is not often diagnosed in the nail unit. This may in part be under-recognition due to its resemblance to other diseases. When SCC of the nail unit is present, it is more commonly seen affecting the thumb. SCC of the nail unit is found in males 70% of the time and 71% of the time it affects the nail bed itself rather than the surrounding nail folds.[5]

11.2.2 Treatment for NMSC of the Hand

Given the relatively thin soft-tissue coverage over the skeleton of the hand, radiographic imaging should be considered if there is any concern for osseous involvement. In order to remove the carcinoma, 4 to 5 mm of negative margin is required, which usually results in a sizable defect on a sensitive region of anatomy. As a result, MMS is an increasingly popular method of treatment for NMSCs, allowing for maximal conservation of uninvolved tissue and preservation of important structures.[4] However, the anatomy of the hand is precise and complex, and even defects with relatively small areas may need careful consideration of reconstructive options. These options range from primary closure or skin grafting to regional or even free flap coverage. Mohs surgeons should carefully consider what they are comfortable managing and have a low threshold to refer to a hand surgeon for assistance with reconstruction.[7] The rare cases of NMSC in the nail unit bring their own anatomic and reconstructive challenges, specifically aiming to preserve the look and function of the nail.

11.2.3 Melanoma of the Hand

Although melanoma represents less than 5% of cutaneous malignancies, it is responsible for an estimated 80% of the associated deaths. Management of melanoma will often involve a dermatologist, a surgical and medical oncologist, and a plastic surgeon as needed for reconstruction. The dorsum of the hand is most frequently affected. The rich lymphatic and vascular systems in this region are thought to contribute to its high metastatic potential. It is also seen in the fingers and nail unit complexes, and, unlike NMSCs, can less frequently be seen on the volar surface of the hand. Subungual melanoma is a rare variant that is most commonly present on the thumb. Its incidence is higher in patients with Fitzpatrick skin type greater than IV and its mortality is higher, partially due to delay in diagnosis.[8]

11.2.4 Treatment for Melanoma of the Hand

Traditional surgical treatment options for melanoma of the hand include WLE and digital amputation, often leaving significant defects with accompanying functional deficits. Management of melanoma with MMS is becoming increasingly popular and there is evidence to suggest it can help preserve hand function while still maintaining low recurrence rates, particularly with the addition of

melanoma antigen recognized by T cells 1 (MART-1), also called MelanA, staining to assist with identification. Consideration of Mohs as an option is especially important for the thumb, given its dominant role in hand function.[9]

11.3 Dorsum of Hand (▶ Fig. 11.1)

11.3.1 Anatomy

The dorsal, sun-exposed region of the hand is much more likely to develop cutaneous malignancies than the volar (palmar) surface. The skin that covers the dorsal surface of the hand is also quite distinct from the thick, glabrous skin covering the volar surface. It is thin, pliable, and connected primarily by loose areolar connective tissue with rich vascular and lymphatic channels coursing underneath. These qualities make the dorsum of the hand significantly more amenable to the creation of local flaps.

The innervation to the dorsal hand is from the superficial radial nerve on the radial side, and the dorsal branch of the ulnar nerve on the ulnar side. The dorsal surface of the hand houses extensor tendons in six distinct compartments, with variable intertendinous connections termed juncturae tendinum.

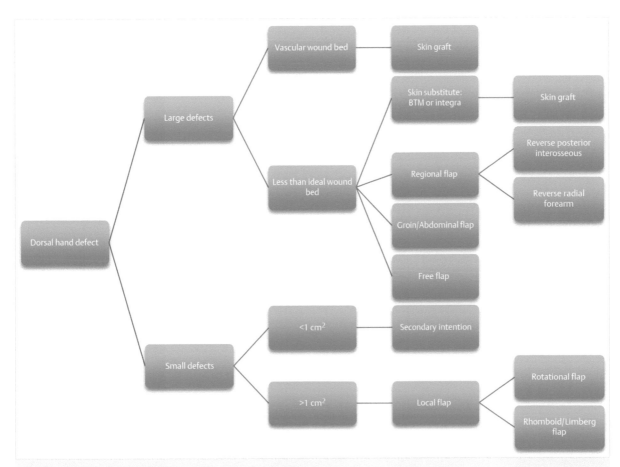

Fig. 11.1 Algorithm for reconstruction of dorsal hand defects.

The radial and ulnar arteries supply the vasculature of the hand. The ulnar artery enters the hand through Guyon's canal, where it splits into superficial and deep branches. The superficial branch forms the superficial palmar arch, whereas the deep branch joins the radial-dominant deep palmar arch. At the level of the wrist, the radial artery courses dorsally through the region known as the "anatomic snuffbox" to supply this deep palmar arch. The superficial arch lies just underneath the palmar fascia and gives off the common digital arteries, which bifurcate into the proper palmar digital arteries. The deep palmar arch lies deeper, just under the flexor tendons, where it branches into the first metacarpal artery (supplying the radial index finger) and the princeps pollicis to the thumb. The dorsal surface of the hand also contains the dorsal metacarpal arteries. These are branches of the dorsal metacarpal or basal arch, which is supplied primarily by the posterior interosseous artery (PIA). Within the dorsal hand lies a rich venous network of deep venae comitantes as well as a superficial plexus system—these ultimately contribute to the basilic and cephalic veins.

11.3.2 Reconstruction

Secondary Intention

Healing by secondary intention is a feasible option for wounds less than 1 cm² without exposed tendon or bone in the wound bed. It should be carefully considered depending on the precise location on the dorsal hand, as there is a high likelihood of contracture that could interfere with function. Children are likely to heal wounds this size robustly; however, they experience increased wound contracture. The elderly may be good candidates for healing by secondary intention as it may help them avoid prolonged immobility and stiffness.[10,11]

Skin Grafting and Skin Substitutes

For larger defects that are not directly over critical structures, skin grafting should be considered. The dorsal hand specifically is composed of thin, pliable skin that requires up to 20% stretch to accommodate full flexion of the digits. For skin grafts to survive, it is imperative that the paratenon over the tendon be intact. The paratenon carries a rich vascular supply that can support the graft and also decreases the friction of the gliding tendon beneath. Any adhesions or scarring to these tendons can significantly impair hand function. If paratenon is absent, a bilayer skin substitute such as Integra (Integra LifeSciences Corporation, Plainsboro, New Jersey, United States) or Novosorb Biodegradable Temporizing Matrix (BTM; PolyNovo, Melbourne, Australia) should be considered to improve the vascularity of the wound bed and reduce adhesion formation between the tendon and the overlying skin (▶ Fig. 11.2).

Once an appropriate wound bed has been established, the choice between full- and split-thickness skin grafts must be made. Full-thickness skin grafts are likely to give better appearance and less secondary scar contracture, but they carry a more significant donor site morbidity. Due to lower metabolic demand, split-thickness skin grafts may demonstrate increased "take" or overall survival, but they are more likely to secondarily contract.

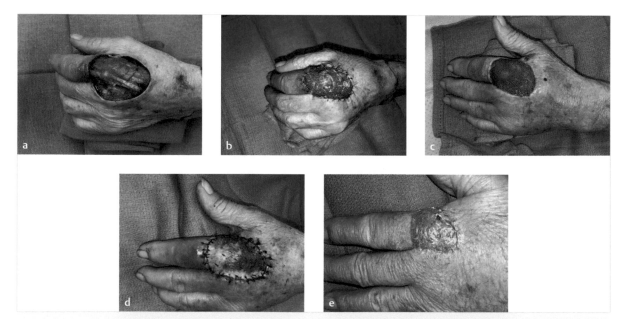

Fig. 11.2 Dorsal hand coverage with NovoSorb Biodegradable Temporizing Matrix (BTM) and subsequent skin graft. (a) Original defect after squamous cell carcinoma resection. (b) Placement of BTM in defect. (c) Integrated BTM and granulation tissue developing over 4 weeks. (d) Full-thickness skin graft inset. (e) The wound has healed with some contraction noted as expected with a skin graft.

Depending on the location of the graft, this can cause a functional hindrance; however, on the dorsal hand there may be some benefit as the overall size of the wound will be reduced. Meshing the graft will allow for improved drainage and expanded area of coverage; however, the pattern may be less aesthetically pleasing and therefore is generally avoided on the hand.

The graft/wound interface must remain stationary for a minimum of 5 days to allow for take of the graft and neo-vascularization. This is best accomplished with a compressive bolster dressing or negative pressure wound therapy coupled with a splint to prevent finger flexion/ extension, which could cause shear forces between the graft and wound, causing graft failure.[11]

Rotational Flaps

Random pattern flaps are a useful flap option in patients with sufficient skin laxity. Rotational flaps can be used to cover small defects, especially those with triangular or rhomboid shapes. The flap should be designed around a rotation point such that the arc of the rotation is more than three times the diameter of the defect. This will ensure that the wound closes without too much tension, although adjunct techniques such as Burow's triangle and back-cuts can provide small gains in rotation.[12]

Rhomboid/Limberg Flaps

Another type of random local pattern flap is the rhomboid/Limberg flap. This is an example of a transposition flap. The defect must be created in rhomboid shape. Attention should be paid to the natural relaxed skin tension lines so that the ultimate direction of closure won't have excess tension. With this in mind, a line is extended from one corner of the rhomboid that is equivalent in length to the width of the defect. An additional line is extended 60 degrees from the end of this line in parallel with the defect, creating a parallelogram shape that can then be elevated and rotated into the defect. The transposed flap can be trimmed as needed for appropriate closure.[12]

Reverse Radial Forearm Flap (Pedicled)

The pedicled radial forearm flap is a versatile coverage option for larger hand soft-tissue defects after resection with exposed vital structures such as bone, or tendons without paratenon. It can be harvested as a fasciocutaneous or fascia-only flap as needed. The flap is designed along the axis of the radial artery with an intentional pivot point at the wrist crease to allow the flap to be easily rotated into the defect without kinking its pedicle. The radial artery runs with venae comitantes that should also be taken. The flap is elevated from ulnar to radial, and care is taken to preserve perforating blood vessels between the brachioradialis and the flexor carpi radialis from the radial artery that perfuse the skin of the flap.

Perforator branches are dissected and ligated along the way as the pedicle is dissected from proximal to distal. Once the flap is elevated, the proximal end of the artery is ligated to free the flap. The flap can be inset by tunneling, or through direct incision. The donor defect is typically closed with split-thickness skin graft. If a fascia-only flap is taken, then the donor site can be closed primarily with skin, and the fascia can be skin-grafted once inset. This flap is based on blood flow through the ulnar artery, the superficial palmar arch, and retrograde through the radial artery. The venous return is also reverse and can be compromised due to venous valves. The cephalic vein can be harvested proximally and anastomosed into a recipient vein on the dorsum of the hand to restore antegrade flow and prevent venous congestion of the flap.

The cosmetic aspect of a sometimes bulky flap is not the only potential morbidity—there are certainly patients who are not a candidate for ligation of the radial artery. An Allen test should be performed to ensure adequate perforation through the ulnar artery, and patients with known peripheral vascular disease may not be appropriate candidates for this flap option.[11,13]

Reverse Posterior Interosseous Flap

Another regional fasciocutaneous flap option for dorsal hand defects is the reversed PIA flap. This flap is perfused through perforators from the PIA, which in the majority of patients communicates with the anterior interosseous artery (care should be taken to ensure this communication exists prior to flap elevation). The flap is designed over the dorsal skin of the forearm, between the radius and the ulna, with an axis along the line between the lateral epicondyle and distal radioulnar joint (DRUJ). The PIA runs between the extensor carpi ulnaris (ECU) and extensor digiti minimi (EDM), and once identified should be dissected from proximal to distal while preserving the posterior interosseous nerve. The rotation point should be approximately 2 cm proximal to the DRUJ for dorsal hand coverage. The flap is elevated in a subfascial plane to protect the septocutaneous perforators perfusing the flap. Once elevated, the proximal PIA should be ligated and retrograde flow perfusing the flap should be confirmed. The flap is inset into the dorsal hand. The donor site can be closed primarily or with a skin graft.[13,14,15]

Groin and Abdominal Flaps

Pedicled groin and abdominal flaps continue to be workhorses for distal upper extremity reconstruction, even as the microsurgical techniques of free flap construction have continued to improve. These flaps can provide a large amount of soft pliable tissue for the dorsal hand and do not require microsurgical expertise or equipment. In patients who require extensive tissue resection of the dorsal hand, a pedicled groin or abdominal flap may be considered.[16]

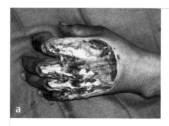
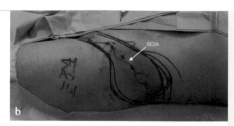
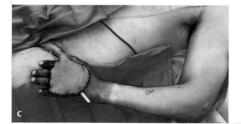
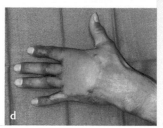

Fig. 11.3 Groin flap based on superficial circumflex iliac artery (SCIA) pedicle for dorsal hand defect. **(a)** Dorsal hand defect in need of flap reconstruction. **(b)** Preoperative markings of the flap design, including outline of the SCIA pedicle. The patient's head is toward the right. **(c)** The flap has been raised, donor site closed, flap formed into a tube proximally, and inset on the hand. **(d)** Final appearance of the hand after one debulking surgery and syndactyly releases.

The "groin flap" is a pedicled flap based on the superficial circumflex iliac artery (SCIA) in the inguinal region. The origin of the SCIA is the femoral artery about 2 cm below the inguinal ligament—it crosses over the sartorius muscle and courses toward the anterior superior iliac spine (ASIS). The flap is medially based along this course, on the ipsilateral side of injury (▶ Fig. 11.3). The lateral femoral cutaneous nerve should be carefully avoided. The donor site can usually be designed to avoid skin with significant hair growth. The flap is elevated, the donor site is closed, and the proximal portion of the flap is often sewed into a tube to protect the pedicle. The flap is then sutured on to the hand. Positioning can be somewhat awkward for the patient since they remain attached to their groin area for approximately 3 to 4 weeks after inset. At that point, the flap pedicle is divided. The flap often requires thinning and other revisions once well healed. Contraindications to this flap include patients with chronic groin infections, lack of willingness to remain attached for 3 weeks, or significant elbow or shoulder trauma that would lead to significant stiffness in those joints.

The superficial inferior epigastric artery (SIEA) can also be used to design a more superiorly oriented abdominally based flap. This artery arises from the femoral artery just inferior to the inguinal ligament, and ascends vertically and medially toward the umbilicus. This flap is often designed on the contralateral side so that the hand can be positioned more comfortably for its 3-week inset prior to division.[11]

Additional, less common flaps include the superficial external pudendal artery (SEPA) and the paraumbilical perforator (PUP) flaps. The SEPA originates from the femoral artery about 1 cm inferior to the inguinal ligament and courses medially to the pubic tubercle. The PUPs are present circumferentially around the umbilicus and originate from the deep inferior epigastric artery system.[16]

Free Flaps

The dorsal skin of the hand is thin, pliable, and also in a relatively conspicuous location on the body. Although skin grafts and local or regional flaps can certainly provide coverage for many defects, larger defects, particularly if tendon or bone is exposed, can end up being associated with significant scar contractures and wound-healing issues, which contribute to unacceptable functional and aesthetic outcomes. Distant flaps such as groin and abdominal flaps require prolonged periods of discomfort and immobility. For coverage of large defects in appropriate candidates, free flaps should be considered.

There are a variety of free flaps available for reconstruction, each with unique risks and benefits. The types of flaps typically used in reconstruction include muscle with split-thickness skin grafts, fascia with split-thickness skin grafts, and fasciocutaneous flaps. Venous flow through flaps can also be used.

Common muscle flaps used include latissimus dorsi, gracilis, and rectus abdominis. These flaps are customizable and can be harvested as partial muscle flaps to fit the exact specifications of the defect. Anterolateral thigh fascial flaps, lateral arm fascial flaps, and temporoparietal fascial flaps with split-thickness skin grafts are also commonly used.[11,17] Alternatively, anterolateral thigh and lateral arm flaps can be designed as fasciocutaneous flaps, and radial forearm flaps can also be designed as free fasciocutaneous flaps. Fasciocutaneous flaps frequently require debulking procedures to achieve acceptable aesthetic outcomes. Fasciocutaneous flaps may also have greater donor site morbidity, and there is some evidence to demonstrate they may be more prone to wound-healing complications.[18]

11.4 Dorsal Surface of Fingers (▶ Fig. 11.4)

11.4.1 Anatomy

The fingers are essential and complex components of human anatomy. Each finger contains three phalanges—proximal, middle, and distal. There are three hinged joints—the metacarpophalangeal (MCP) joint, the proximal

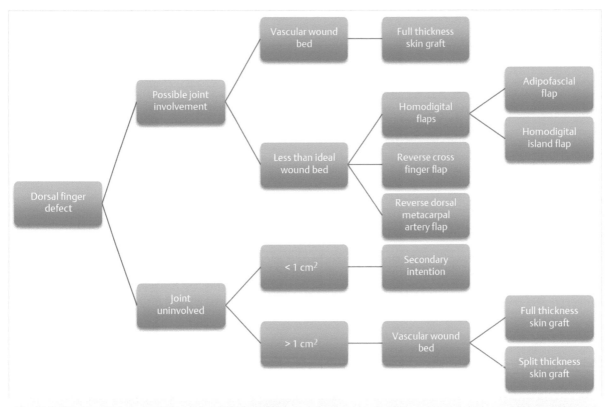

Fig. 11.4 Algorithm for reconstruction of dorsal finger defects.

interphalangeal (PIP) joint, and the distal interphalangeal (DIP) joint. Flexion of these joints is performed by the flexor tendons—the flexor digitorum superficialis (FDS) and flexor digitorum profundus (FDP). These flexor tendons are anchored by fibrous pulleys—the most important of which are the A2 pulley (continuous with proximal phalanx periosteum) and A4 pulley (over the middle phalanx). The FDS runs superficial to the FDP initially. At the level of the A1 pulley, it splits and wraps around and underneath the FDP to insert onto the middle phalanx. The FDP continues through this chiasm and inserts on the distal phalanx to provide flexion of the DIP joint.

The extensor digitorum communis (EDC) tendons, in addition to extensor indicis proprius (EIP) and extensor digit minimi (EDM), work to extend the fingers. After crossing the MCP joint on the dorsal side, they join with the tendons of the interossei and lumbrical muscles to form a broad aponeurotic sheet that covers the dorsal first phalanx termed the dorsal hood. Once this aponeurosis crosses the PIP, it splits into three pieces: one central slip and two lateral bands. The central slip inserts onto the dorsal portion of the middle phalanx, while the lateral bands extend distally to insert onto the distal phalanx, allowing for extension of the DIP joint.

The lumbrical muscles originate on the FDP and insert onto the extensor expansion—this allows for assistance with flexion at the MCP joint and extension at the PIP joint. The interossei muscles come in two sets: the palmar interossei and the dorsal interossei. The palmer interossei originate on the second, fourth, and fifth metacarpals and insert onto the proximal phalanges and extensor expansions of the index, ring, and small fingers. They provide adduction of the fingers and assistance with MCP flexion and PIP extension. The dorsal interossei are bipennate muscles that originate on the metacarpals and insert onto the index, middle, and ring finger proximal phalanges and their extensor mechanisms. They provide abduction and also assist with MCP flexion and PIP extension.

The vascular supply to the fingers arises primarily from the superficial palmar arch, which branches into common digital arteries that split into proper palmar digital arteries at the web spaces. These proper palmar digital arteries run on either side of each finger, just dorsal to their respective digital nerves. Each of these proper palmar digital arteries also gives off anastomoses to the dorsal digital arteries, which arise from the dorsal metacarpal arteries. The dominant digital artery for each finger is generally on the ulnar side of the finger, or whichever side is closest to midline. Venous networks are present throughout the digits in random patterns, concentrated axial and dorsal.

11.4.2 Reconstruction

Secondary Intention

Healing by secondary intention is a feasible option for wounds less than 1 cm² without exposed tendon or bone in the wound bed. The precise location on the dorsal surface of the finger is important, as wounds directly over joints may result in contractures that significantly impair function and mobility. Healing may also take significantly longer if allowed to happen by secondary intention. However for small defects, especially over the phalanges and not the joints, this may be appropriate and have the lowest associated morbidity for many patients.[10]

Skin Grafting and Skin Substitutes

For wounds that are unlikely to heal by secondary intention alone, skin grafts should be considered as the next step. Just like in the dorsal hand, the preservation of the paratenon is important for supporting graft survival and preserving tendon glide. If a more vascular wound bed is needed, or there is significant concern for tendon scarring, skin substitutes or dermal regenerative templates such as PolyNovo BTM or Integra may be placed prior to grafting. Split-thickness skin grafts are more likely to have full "take"; however, they are also more likely to secondarily contract. If the wound is over a joint, a full-thickness skin graft should be considered.[11]

Adipofascial Turndown Flap

The adipofascial turndown flap is a random pattern homodigital flap that is useful for covering exposures over the PIP joint. It requires incising the skin in an "H" pattern, such that the area of the flap is at most four times the area of the "base" to preserve blood supply. The dermis is elevated from the subcutaneous layer and the flaps are opened, revealing the subcutaneous layer underneath. This layer is elevated with caution to ensure the paratenon is left down and turned over and inset to cover the defect. The skin and dermal flaps are then laid back down and closed primarily. The subcutaneous tissue newly covering the defect is then skin grafted, preferably with a full-thickness skin graft.

Homodigital Island Flap

The homodigital island flap can be designed to cover both proximal and more distal defects of the fingers. The flap is designed on either the radial or ulnar palmar digital artery. For proximal defects, the flap is designed on the lateral border of the digit with a proximal base and rotated to be inset into the defect. For more distal defects, a reverse pedicle digital island flap can be performed. The flap is again designed on the lateral border of the digit; however, the dissection should be carried out from proximal to distal. The proximal end of the digital artery

should be ligated as the flap is raised. The flap can then be rotated and inset loosely into the defect. Full-thickness skin grafts are recommended to close the defects.

The digital nerve should be separated from the rest of the neurovascular bundle and preserved if possible. When elevating the flap, it is recommended to keep a cuff of fat and subcutaneous tissue to preserve the venous plexus, and therefore outflow, to reduce congestion. Candidates for this flap should not have peripheral vascular disease or any other conditions that could compromise the vascularity of the finger once it is dependent only on the digital vessels of the unaltered side.[12,17,19,20]

Reverse Cross-Finger Flap

For dorsal defects on the finger, especially over the middle phalanx, a reverse cross-finger flap should be considered. This is a similar idea to the coverage provided with a cross-finger flap for the volar surface. The skin of the donor finger is elevated at the same level as the recipient defect, such that the base of the skin flap is opposite the side of the injured finger. The subcutaneous tissue is then carefully elevated off of the paratenon, turned over, and inset into the dorsal defect of the adjacent digit. The elevated skin flap is then sutured back into place. The donor subcutaneous flap is skin grafted. The flap is divided 2 weeks later.[11,13,17,21]

Reverse Dorsal Metacarpal Artery Flap

The reverse dorsal metacarpal artery flap is another versatile option for finger coverage that provides similar thin, pliable tissue to the area. The flap is based on the dorsal metacarpal artery in reverse flow from the associated common digital artery. Depending on the precise location of the defect, the flap can be designed over various perforators near the web space or metacarpal head (▶ Fig. 11.5a). The flap is elevated in the plane of loose areolar tissue, superficial to the extensor tendons. The flap is rotated to fill the defect, and the pedicle can be managed by tunneling or by excising intervening skin and soft tissue to accommodate its pedicle for inset (▶ Fig. 11.5b).[22] The flap can also be raised as a fascia-only flap, with skin grafting to cover the inset. The donor site can often be closed primarily in small defects, or be skin grafted as well (▶ Fig. 11.5c,d).[20,23]

11.5 Thumb (▶ Fig. 11.6)

11.5.1 Anatomy

The thumb has anatomic features distinct from the fingers that allow for opposition with the other digits. Rather than three phalanges, the thumb only has two. It therefore only articulates at the MCP joint and a single interphalangeal (IP) joint. The thumb is maneuvered by both extrinsic and intrinsic musculature. There are four

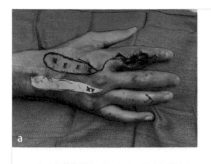
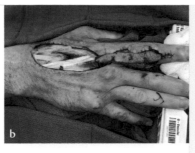
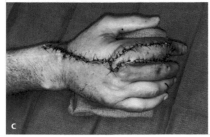
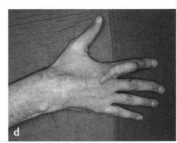

Fig. 11.5 Reverse dorsal metacarpal artery flap for dorsal finger defect. **(a)** Preoperative markings of the dorsal metacarpal artery pedicle and planned skin paddle. **(b)** Elevation and rotation of the flap into the defect, with care taken not to kink the pedicle. **(c)** Inset of the flap and primary closure of the donor site. **(d)** Follow-up after flap has healed.

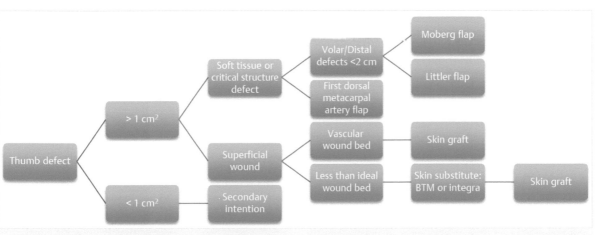

Fig. 11.6 Algorithm for reconstruction of thumb defects.

extrinsic muscles. The flexor pollicis longus (FPL) inserts onto the volar base of the distal phalanx and allows flexion of the thumb. The extensor pollicis longus (EPL) passes around Lister's tubercle on the radius and inserts onto the dorsal base of the distal phalanx. The EPL extends the thumb as well as dorsiflexes and abducts away from the hand. The extensor pollicis brevis (EPB) and abductor pollicis longus (APL) run in the first extensor compartment. The EPB inserts onto the proximal phalanx and extends and abducts the thumb, while the APL has portions that insert onto the first metacarpal and trapezium, with connection to the EPB and the abductor pollicis brevis (APB). The EPL and APL tendons mark the borders of the anatomic snuffbox, where the radial artery can be palpated.

The intrinsic muscles of the thumb include the adductor pollicis and the three thenar muscles. The adductor pollicis has two heads: the transvers originates on the third metacarpal and the oblique originates on the capitate. It inserts onto the ulnar sesamoid bone of the thumb MCP joint, where it adducts and assists in opposition and flexion. The APB originates on the scaphoid and flexor retinaculum, and inserts onto the radial sesamoid bone and proximal phalanx to assist with abduction. The flexor pollicis brevis (FPB) has a superficial head originating on the flexor retinaculum and a deep head on the carpal bones—it also inserts onto the radial sesamoid bone. This contributes to flexion, abduction, and opposition at the MCP joint. The opponens pollicis originates on the trapezium and flexor retinaculum and inserts onto the first metacarpal—it opposes and adducts the thumb.

The thumb has two proper digital arteries that arise from the princeps pollicis artery, as well as two variable dorsal digital arteries that arise from the first dorsal metacarpal artery. Both arterial systems are generally sufficient for the entire digit to survive. The digital arteries are accompanied by associated digital nerves on both the radial and ulnar side; however, unlike the fingers, the dorsal surface of the thumb is innervated by the superficial branch of the radial nerve.

11.5.2 Reconstruction

Secondary Intention

The same considerations for healing by secondary intention apply to the dorsal thumb as for dorsal fingers. This works well for wounds that are less than $1 \, cm^2$ without exposed tendon or bone in the wound bed. The location of the wounds in comparison to joints should still be evaluated for ultimate risk of contracture. The range of motion of the thumb, specifically its ability to oppose and apply pinch grip, is critically important to hand function.

Skin Grafting and Skin Substitutes

Defects of the dorsal thumb may also require skin grafting. Once again, the principles of a well-vascularized wound bed and absence of interference with underlying critical structures are important. Small sections of biologic skin substitutes may be appropriate for restoration of vascularity or protection of structures such as tendons. Both split-thickness and full-thickness skin grafts may be appropriate depending on the balance of needs, including cosmesis, concern for ability to take, risk for eventual contraction, and need for sensation.

Moberg Flap

Preservation of adequate sensation in the volar aspect of the thumb is important for normal function, and most local reconstruction options attempt to maintain this. For transverse amputations or defects up to 1.5 cm of the distal thumb, the volar neurovascular advancement (Moberg) flap is an option. Longitudinal incisions are made on either side of the thumb, just dorsal to the neurovascular bundles. The flap is elevated on the volar side of the flexor tendon sheath, all the way down to the MCP skin crease. It is then advanced distally and inset. Some patients may require splinting in flexion in order to reduce tension sufficiently. The flap can be incised across the proximal base to gain distal coverage, but the donor site proximally must then be skin grafted.[11,13]

Littler/Neurovascular Island Flap

The volar aspect of the thumb can also be reconstructed using a neurovascular island/Littler flap. This flap is taken from the dorsoulnar aspect of either the middle or ring finger and raised on the neurovascular bundle of that aspect. To obtain the necessary pedicle length, the artery

and nerve are dissected down to their origins at the palmar arch and common digital nerve, respectively. The flap is then rotated across the palm to be inset into the volar thumb defect, with the pedicle tunneled under the palm and volar surface of the thumb. The donor defect can be skin grafted. Although this flap maintains sensation in the volar surface of the thumb, it does require cortical reorientation, and this may be significantly more difficult in older patients. The donor defect will also lose some protective sensation as the ulnar digital nerve was taken with the pedicle. Consideration should be given to the fact that the donor digit will need to survive on the only remaining vascular pedicle on the opposite aspect, and this may be contraindicated in patients with vascular disease.[11,13,20] This significant donor site morbidity has limited modern use of this flap.

First Dorsal Metacarpal Artery/Kite Flap

Defects that include the volar tip, particularly the ulnar portion, or the middle region of the thumb, are appropriate candidates for the first dorsal metacarpal artery flap, also known as a kite flap. This is a workhorse local flap for thumb coverage, as it keeps sensation while generally providing more robust coverage than the comparable Littler flap, with decreased donor site morbidity. The donor artery pedicle lies on the radial border of the first metacarpal and is accompanied by two venae comitantes. The terminal branches of the radial sensory nerve are present over the dorsal proximal phalanx of the index finger. The flap is elevated to include the pedicle and underlying fascia, off of the paratenon underneath. The donor site is skin grafted (▶ Fig. 11.7).[11,13]

The skin flap can be designed several ways depending on the requirements to fill the defect. The island version is the traditional design. The racquet version allows for better venous outflow through the remaining skin, and does not require tunneling or a skin bridge, but may be less aesthetically pleasing. The bilobed option incorporates the second metacarpal artery and can be designed in either island or racquet fashion—it is used for large defects.

Like the Moberg flap, this reconstruction will provide innervation, but cortical reorientation is necessary. Common complications include mild (< 20 degree) flexion deficits at the index and thumb IP joints, as well as decreased protective sensation at the donor site. There may be more noticeable cosmetic defects with this flap. However, it remains a consistent option for larger thumb defects.[24]

11.6 Nail Plate and Nail Bed (▶ Fig. 11.8)

11.6.1 Anatomy

The nail apparatus is a specialized structure that is useful to hand function by providing counter pressure and rigid

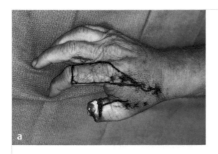
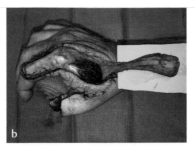
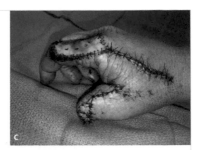
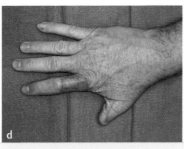
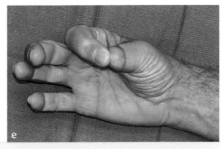

Fig. 11.7 First dorsal metacarpal artery (kite) flap for thumb defect after amputation through the interphalangeal joint with exposed bone. **(a)** Preoperative markings of the dorsal metacarpal artery pedicle and planned skin paddle. **(b)** Elevation of the flap including desired fascia is complete. **(c)** The flap is inset into the distal thumb defect, and the pedicle has been tunneled underneath. The donor site is closed with assistance of a full-thickness skin graft. **(d)** Follow-up demonstrating well-healed flap and donor site. **(e)** Pinch on to the sensate flap at the tip of the thumb.

tactile feedback during pinch and other finger manipulation. Fingers that lack nails have decreased two-point discrimination and more difficulty with manipulation and picking up small items. The nail plate is formed from keratinized cells produced by the germinal matrix. The distal extent of the germinal matrix is visualized just distal to the eponychial fold (the proximal fold of skin superficial to the nail plate). This portion of the germinal matrix is known as the lunula. The germinal matrix extends much further proximally, however, to the midpoint between the eponychial fold and the DIP joint. Distal to the lunula where the nail appears pink is the sterile matrix. This is made up of cells that form a strong adherence to the nail plate until the hyponychium (the distal fingertip area under the nail plate where the nail no longer adheres). Although the germinal matrix is responsible for the vast majority of nail plate production, there are contributions to the plate from the sterile matrix and the dorsal roof (the underside of the eponychial fold). The sterile matrix contributions assist with adherence of the plate to the sterile matrix, and the dorsal roof contributions cause the shine on the nail. Nails that grow in the absence of the dorsal roof appear dull. The sterile matrix covers a dense network of capillaries. Deep to the sterile matrix is the periosteum of the distal phalanx. The axial folds of skin on either side of the nail plate are known as paronychium, and contribute to lateral finger pinch grip and nail matrix protection.

The vascular supply to the nail apparatus originates from the common volar digital arteries. There are several arcades of anastomosis that arc through the dorsal tissue prior to anastomosing to the other common volar digital artery. There are arterial arcades reliably at the base of the nail fold and at the level of the lunula. Venous outflow coalesces and drains just deep to the dorsal skin, enlarging from distal to proximal. The innervation of the nail apparatus is supplied by the common volar digital nerves, branches of which occur at the DIP joint and travel dorsally. Innervation of the dorsal finger originates from the volar nerves to the level of around the PIP joint when dorsal nerves take over. Therefore, the nail apparatuses of the thumb, index, middle, and radial half of ring fingers are supplied by the median nerve, while the ulnar halves of the ring and small fingernail apparatuses are supplied by the ulnar nerve.

Fingernail growth occurs at a rate of 0.1 mm per day, four times more rapid than toenail growth. The rate of nail growth from germinal matrix to hyponychium is ~100 days and there is a delay of 3 weeks after an injury as the nail thickens prior to distal growth.

11.6.2 Reconstruction

Nail Bed

Removal of the nail plate is a necessary step in many Mohs procedures, and varying degrees of sterile and germinal matrix may need to be resected. Reconstruction of the nail bed depends on both how much of the germinal matrix is left and how strongly the patient feels about

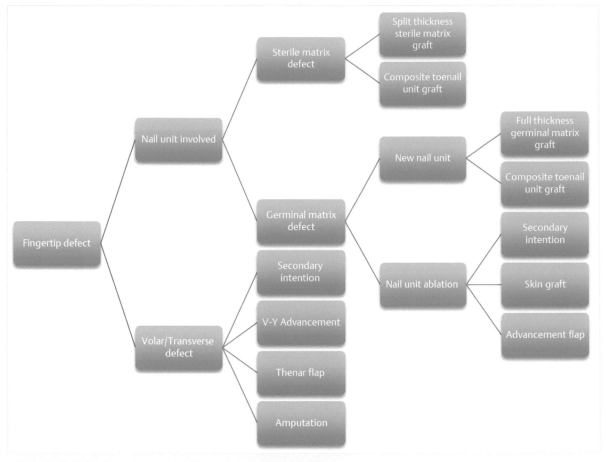

Fig. 11.8 Algorithm for reconstruction of fingertip and nail unit defects.

having a nail unit in the future. If the entire germinal matrix is maintained, but sterile matrix has been lost, the nail bed soft tissue can be restored by several methods including secondary intention,[25] skin grafting,[26] local advancement flaps,[25] or grafting from a toe donor nail bed.[27] If additional pulp is required for soft-tissue bulk, this can be taken as a free tissue transfer from the great toe or the medial second toe. As long as the germinal matrix is intact, the nail plate can be expected to regrow, but the sterile matrix must be replaced by a sterile matrix graft in order for the nail to stick down to the bed properly.

In many cases, all or some of the sterile matrix is resected. If a significant portion of sterile matrix remains intact, a split-thickness sterile matrix graft can be performed from the remaining healthy tissue to the region where it was resected. If most or all of the nail bed and sterile matrix are gone, however, and the patient wants a nail on this digit, a composite toenail bed graft is the other available option. This is typically raised by marking out the size of the matrix defect on the donor toe (usually the great toe) and harvesting a split-thickness graft with a razor blade. Careful inset with correct orientation is critical for nail growth. Although this technique does have

reported success, the nail is not always aesthetically normal in appearance and, when possible, a split-thickness graft from the same bed may be the preferred option.[28]

When the entire nail unit, including the germinal matrix, has been destroyed, the nail plate will not grow back. Another source of germinal matrix is required, usually from a toe donor. The second toe is usually considered to be a more acceptable cosmetic donor than the great toe. A full-thickness germinal matrix graft can be harvested.[20] A composite nail unit graft can also be attempted. This can be harvested and transplanted as a composite graft and secured in much the same way that a skin graft would be.[29] Alternatively, microsurgical techniques can be used to transfer the entire composite nail unit with vascular anastomoses in a free toe wraparound flap.[30]

Discussion of patient preferences is important, because not all patients will be motivated to pursue reconstructive techniques to obtain a new nail plate, and may prefer nail ablation and soft-tissue closure instead. Nail ablation, or matricectomy, can be performed in several ways. Surgical excision may naturally be performed as part of the Mohs procedure or after the procedure. Sharp excision with a blade and electrocautery excision are common

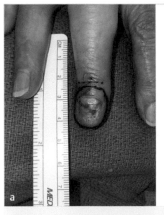
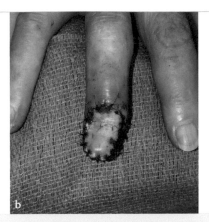
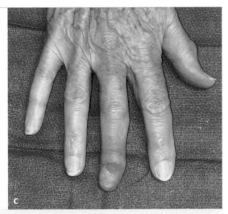

Fig. 11.9 Resection of nail unit for squamous cell carcinoma. **(a)** Preoperative markings for intended resection of the entire nail unit, including nail bed, all paronychium, and the germinal matrix. **(b)** Inset of a full-thickness skin graft for coverage of the entire defect. **(c)** Follow-up demonstrating well-healed graft with reasonable cosmetic result.

methods—the physician must ensure that all of the germinal matrix has been excised to prevent aberrant nail growth later. Chemical matricectomy is also accepted as standard, either with phenol solution or 10% sodium hydroxide. After matricectomy, the wound may be allowed to heal by secondary intention. Alternatively, soft-tissue reconstruction may be performed with skin grafts (▶ Fig. 11.9) or advancement flaps over the no-longer covered nail bed as indicated.[31]

Secondary Intention

Healing by secondary intention is successful in many fingertip defects, especially volar finger pad injuries. Candidate defects are still preferably less than 1 cm² without exposed tendon or bone in the wound bed. Healing by secondary intention is a particularly useful option in fingertip injuries, as it may give the best opportunity for restoration of protective sensation.[25,32] However, in the cases where this fails or where patients lack both the padding and sensation normally present on the finger pad, a free pulp graft may be taken from the either the great toe or the medial second toe.

V-Y Advancement Flaps

Transverse or obliquely resected finger tips can often be repaired with advancement flaps. Volar defects are suitable for bilateral V-Y advancement (Kutler) flaps that are elevated from the axial borders of the digit and advanced toward the distal end. Fascial attachments may need to be released, and care should be taken not to damage the neurovascular bundles during dissection. If the injury is more dorsally oriented, a volar advancement (Atasoy–Kleinert) flap may be appropriate. The flap should be designed so that the apex of the V is located at the DIP joint. Up to 1 cm of advancement can usually be obtained while still achieving primary closure of the donor site.[11,13,17,33]

Thenar Flap

The thenar flap can provide versatile coverage for a wide variety of distal phalanx defects. Although initially described to replace the volar glabrous skin of the fingertip, it can also be designed to replace transverse or dorsal nail bed defects. It is more often utilized in younger patients who are at lower risk of stiffness and joint contractures. The flap should be designed to be about 1.5 times the diameter of the fingertip with the defect, and it should be designed at about the level of the MCP skin crease (▶ Fig. 11.10a). This will be a full-thickness flap raised on the thenar muscle fascia. The radial digital nerve of the thumb can run through this area and care should be taken to avoid injuring it. Beasley notes that the MCP joint of the recipient finger should be fully flexed to limit flexion of the PIP.[34] The thumb should be in full palmar abduction. The pedicle can be divided after about 2 weeks. After this, the donor site can usually be closed primarily, but skin grafts can be used if this is not the case (▶ Fig. 11.10b–d).[11,17,20,35]

Amputation

There are certainly patients who may be best served by a revision amputation. Factors taken into consideration should be the current defect and anticipated course of healing, balanced with the patient's comorbidities as well as their functional needs. Patients who are particularly motivated to return to work may do so faster if a revision amputation is performed at the time of the procedure. This should be an individualized and informed discussion with the patient.

11.7 Conclusion

The dermatologic surgeon will inevitably encounter cutaneous malignancies of the hand throughout their career,

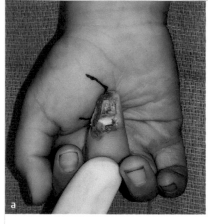
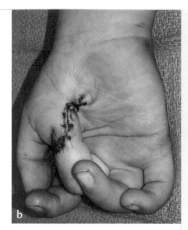
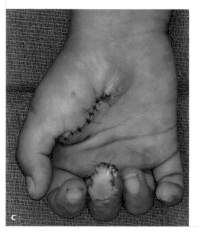
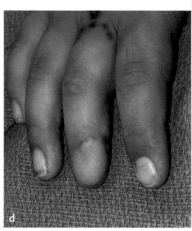

Fig. 11.10 Thenar flap for distal finger defect. **(a)** Design of thenar flap paddle for dorsal coverage of distal finger defect. The flap is designed just proximal to the MCP crease. **(b)** Inset of the thenar flap. **(c)** Immediately after division of the flap, demonstrating good flap take with primary closure of the donor site. **(d)** Follow-up after the flap is totally healed, demonstrating a skin fingertip with no nail unit.

and should be familiar with the unique considerations to maximize function and cosmesis in these cases. Care should be taken to customize the reconstruction to the defect, drawing from the many reconstructive techniques discussed earlier. Plastic and reconstructive surgeons, and in particular hand surgeons, should be considered partners in the care of these patients and can offer guidance and assistance as needed to provide the best possible outcomes in patient care.

References

[1] Trost LB, Bailin PL. History of Mohs surgery. Dermatol Clin. 2011; 29 (2):135–139, vii

[2] Society TAC. Key Statistics for Basal and Squamous Cell Cancers. Vol. 2020. The Atlanta, GA: The American Cancer Society; 2020

[3] Loh TY, Rubin AG, Brian Jiang SI. Basal cell carcinoma of the dorsal hand: an update and comprehensive review of the literature. Dermatol Surg. 2016; 42(4):464–470

[4] Forman SB, Ferringer TC, Garrett AB. Basal cell carcinoma of the nail unit. J Am Acad Dermatol. 2007; 56(5):811–814

[5] Dijksterhuis A, Friedeman E, van der Heijden B. Squamous cell carcinoma of the nail unit: review of the literature. J Hand Surg Am. 2018; 43(4):374–379.e2

[6] Martin DE, English JC, III, Goitz RJ. Squamous cell carcinoma of the hand. J Hand Surg Am. 2011; 36(8):1377–1381, quiz 1382

[7] Husain Z, Allawh RM, Hendi A. Mohs micrographic surgery for digital melanoma and nonmelanoma skin cancers. Cutis. 2018; 101 (5):346–352

[8] Turner JB, Rinker B. Melanoma of the hand: current practice and new frontiers. Healthcare (Basel). 2014; 2(1):125–138

[9] Terushkin V, Brodland DG, Sharon DJ, Zitelli JA. Digit-sparing Mohs surgery for melanoma. Dermatol Surg. 2016; 42(1):83–93

[10] Bosley R, Leithauser L, Turner M, Gloster HM, Jr. The efficacy of second-intention healing in the management of defects on the dorsal surface of the hands and fingers after Mohs micrographic surgery. Dermatol Surg. 2012; 38(4):647–653

[11] Hansen S, Lang P, Sbitany H. Soft tissue reconstruction of the upper extremity. In: Thorne C, ed. Grabb and Smith's Plastic Surgery. 7th ed. Philadelphia, PA: Lippincott Williams & Wilkins; 2014:737–749

[12] Rehim SA, Chung KC. Local flaps of the hand. Hand Clin. 2014; 30(2):137–151, v

[13] Biswas D, Wysocki RW, Fernandez JJ, Cohen MS. Local and regional flaps for hand coverage. J Hand Surg Am. 2014; 39(5):992–1004

[14] Jakubietz RG, Bernuth S, Schmidt K, Meffert RH, Jakubietz MG. The fascia-only reverse posterior interosseous artery flap. J Hand Surg Am. 2019; 44(3):249.e1–249.e5

[15] Cavadas PC, Thione A, Rubí C. The simplified posterior interosseous flap. J Hand Surg Am. 2016; 41(9):e303–e307

[16] Al-Qattan MM, Al-Qattan AM. Defining the indications of pedicled groin and abdominal flaps in hand reconstruction in the current microsurgery era. J Hand Surg Am. 2016; 41(9):917–927

[17] Wink JD, Gandhi RA, Ashley B, Levin LS. Flap reconstruction of the hand. Plast Reconstr Surg. 2020; 145(1):172e–183e

[18] Parrett BM, Bou-Merhi JS, Buntic RF, Safa B, Buncke GM, Brooks D. Refining outcomes in dorsal hand coverage: consideration of aesthetics and donor-site morbidity. Plast Reconstr Surg. 2010; 126 (5):1630–1638

[19] Huang YC, Liu Y, Chen TH. Use of homodigital reverse island flaps for distal digital reconstruction. J Trauma. 2010; 68(2):429–433

[20] Mailey B, Neumeister MW. The finger tip, nail plate, and nail bed: anatomy, repair, and reconstruction. In: Chang J, Neligan P, eds. Plastic Surgery. Vol. 6. Hand and Upper Extremity. 4th ed. Philadelphia, PA: Elsevier; 2017:122–145

[21] Atasoy E. The reverse cross finger flap. J Hand Surg Am. 2016; 41(1):122–128

[22] Balan JR, Mathew S, Kumar P, et al. The reverse dorsal metacarpal artery flap in finger reconstruction: a reliable choice. Indian J Plast Surg. 2018; 51(1):54–59

[23] Gregory H, Heitmann C, Germann G. The evolution and refinements of the distally based dorsal metacarpal artery (DMCA) flaps. J Plast Reconstr Aesthet Surg. 2007; 60(7):731–739

[24] Couceiro J, de Prado M, Menendez G, Manteiga Z. The first dorsal metacarpal artery flap family: a review. Surg J (NY). 2018; 4(4):e215–e219

[25] O'Neill PJ, Litts C. Hand and forearm reconstruction after skin cancer ablation. Clin Plast Surg. 2004; 31(1):113–119

[26] Lazar A, Abimelec P, Dumontier C. Full thickness skin graft for nail unit reconstruction. J Hand Surg [Br]. 2005; 30(2):194–198

[27] Saito H, Suzuki Y, Fujino K, Tajima T. Free nail bed graft for treatment of nail bed injuries of the hand. J Hand Surg Am. 1983; 8(2):171–178

[28] Koh SH, You Y, Kim YW, et al. Long-term outcomes of nail bed reconstruction. Arch Plast Surg. 2019; 46(6):580–588

[29] Das SK. Nail unit matrix transplantation: a plastic surgeon's approach. Dermatol Surg. 2001; 27(3):242–245

[30] Shibata M, Seki T, Yoshizu T, Saito H, Tajima T. Microsurgical toenail transfer to the hand. Plast Reconstr Surg. 1991; 88(1):102–109, discussion 110

[31] Baran R, Haneke E. Matricectomy and nail ablation. Hand Clin. 2002; 18(4):693–696, viii, discussion 697

[32] Magliano J, Rossi V, Turra N, Bazzano C. Secondary-intention healing following Mohs micrographic surgery for squamous cell carcinoma of a finger. Int Wound J. 2019; 16(3):860–861

[33] Lim JX, Chung KCVY. VY advancement, thenar flap, and cross-finger flaps. Hand Clin. 2020; 36(1):19–32

[34] Melone CP Jr, Beasley RW, Carstens JH Jr. The thenar flap: an analysis of its use in 150 cases. J Hand Surg Am. 1982;7(3):291–297

[35] Rinker B. Fingertip reconstruction with the laterally based thenar flap: indications and long-term functional results. Hand (N Y). 2006; 1(1):2–8

159

12 Reconstruction of the Genital

Jenny C. Hu and Richard G. Bennett

Summary

To minimize injury to crucial underlying structures and to achieve an optimal reconstructive result, genital area reconstruction requires understanding the anatomy of the male and female external genitalia. The usual types of genital wounds managed by dermatologists are those subsequent to extirpations of tumors such as squamous cell carcinoma or extramammary Paget's disease. This chapter discusses the reconstructive options by superficial external genitalia subunit, but does not discuss repair of deeply invasive and extensive surgical defects that would not be typically encountered in dermatologic surgery. The following information provides a foundation for managing superficial surgical external genital wounds and setting expectations of their functional and cosmetic outcomes. It should also be emphasized that unlike most other specialties, dermatologists often allow genital wounds to heal by second intention. Oftentimes, this results in an excellent cosmetic and functional result. Genital skin in particular is often loosely attached to underlying fascia, allowing greater mobility during contraction or repair. Thus, contractures or excess scarring are rare in this area.

Keywords: genital, reconstruction, dermatologic surgery, dermatology, Mohs micrographic surgery, primary closure, skin flap, skin graft, second intention

12.1 Anatomy

12.1.1 Anatomy of the Male External Genitalia

The male external genitalia are comprised of the penis, urethra, and scrotum (▶ Fig. 12.1). The penis is further divided into the penile shaft and glans penis. Within the penile shaft, there are three columns of erectile tissue that run longitudinally—one corpus spongiosum and two corpora cavernosa. The corpus spongiosum is ventral and surrounds the urethra; it widens distally to become the glans penis. The two corpora cavernosa run along the dorsal side of the penis. The corpora cavernosa is surrounded by a white fibrous envelope known as the tunica albuginea; it helps trap blood during erection. More dorsal to the corpora cavernosa are a central deep dorsal vein, a dorsal artery on either side of the dorsal vein, and a dorsal nerve adjacent to each dorsal artery. All of these structures are then enveloped by a deep penile fascia of the penis known as Buck's fascia. Superficial to Buck's fascia are a central superficial dorsal vein and two lateral superficial veins. These superficial veins are encompassed by the superficial fascia of the penis known as the dartos fascia and then finally the skin.[1] During reconstruction, it is important to undermine carefully in the plane above the dartos fascia when possible, particularly on the dorsal side of the penile shaft to avoid laceration of the superficial dorsal vein or lateral superficial veins. However, skin cancers may require resection through the dartos fascia; if so, one tries to undermine superficially to Buck's fascia. Laceration to the superficial dorsal vein, beneath the dartos fascia, or to the deep dorsal vein of the penis, beneath Buck's fascia, can lead to a large hematoma that mimic's penis fracture—an acute penis in which there is a tear in the corpus spongiosum or a corpora cavernosa.[2,3] A superficial dorsal vein injury causes ecchymosis and swelling through the subcutaneous tissue of the genitalia including the scrotum and perineum, whereas a deep dorsal vein injury causes ecchymosis and swelling only within the penile shaft due to the confinement of space beneath Buck's fascia.[2,3] Ligation of a tear in either of the veins is crucial to prevent other adverse outcomes, such as infection and necrotizing fasciitis from an unevacuated hematoma.[3]

The scrotum is a thin external sac of skin that is divided into two compartments, with each compartment containing a testis and epididymis. The layers of tissue beneath the scrotal skin, from superficial to deep, that protect these internal structures are the superficial fascia of the scrotum known as the dartos fascia, external spermatic fascia, cremaster muscle and fascia, internal spermatic fascia, parietal layer of the tunica vaginalis, and finally the visceral layer of the tunica vaginalis directly covering the testis.[1] Undermining in the plane above the dartos fascia is recommended.

12.1.2 Anatomy of the Female External Genitalia

The female external genitalia are composed of the central and superior mons pubis, labia majora, labia minora, clitoris, vestibule of the vagina (an inner cleft surrounded by the labia minora), greater vestibular (Bartholin's) glands, and urethral meatus. These structures are collectively known as the vulva or pudendum, and they surround the opening to the vagina. The labia majora are covered with skin-bearing hair (after puberty) on the outer sides and smooth, hairless skin on the inner sides. They are composed mostly of adipose tissue, but deep to this subcutaneous fat is the superficial perineal (Colles') fascia, then another thin layer of fat, followed by the deep perineal (investing or Gallaudet's) fascia covering the underlying muscle.[1,4] During reconstruction in dermatologic surgery, it is important to undermine superficially in the subcutaneous fat plane above Colles' fascia. The labia minora lie medial to the labia majora and are small thin folds of skin and connective tissue that lack adipose tissue.[1,4]

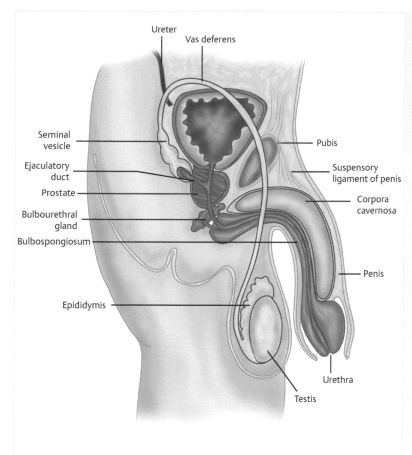

Fig. 12.1 Anatomy of the male external genitalia: penis and scrotum. (Reproduced from Genital Anatomy. In: Agrawal K, Mahajan R, Gupta M, ed. Textbook of Plastic, Reconstructive, and Aesthetic Surgery: Volume IV Reconstruction of Trunk, Genitalia, Lower limb, and Maxillofacial Traumae. 1st Edition. Delhi, India: Thieme; 2019.)

12.1.3 Anatomy of the Perineum

Clinically, the perineum is the region between the scrotum or posterior vaginal introitus and the anus in the male and female, respectively. Anatomically, it is a diamond-shaped region bordered by the pubic symphysis, pubic arches, ischial tuberosities, and coccyx. An arbitrary line between the ischial tuberosities further divides the perineum into an anterior urogenital triangle and posterior ischioanal triangle. Beneath the skin of the perineum is subcutaneous fat, followed by the superficial perineal (Colles') fascia, then deeper fat, followed by the deep perineal (investing or Gallaudet's) fascia that covers the underlying muscle.[1,5] It is recommended to undermine in the plane of the subcutaneous fat above Colles' fascia.

12.2 Anesthesia

The skin (epidermis and dermis) is relatively thin in both the male and female genitalia. This thinness allows topical anesthetics to penetrate and provide complete anesthesia for small biopsies. Also, prior to local anesthetic infiltration, use of topical anesthesia prevents needle stick pain in the genitalia.

Most of the penis can be anesthetized with a nerve block of the dorsal nerve of the penis. A branch of the pudendal nerve, the dorsal nerve of the penis runs dorsally along the penis and gives off numerous branches laterally that eventually innervate the urethra both ventrally and laterally. As the main dorsal nerve of the penis enters the glans penis, it has fine fibers that distribute three dimensionally within the glans penis.[6] There are various ways of performing a penile nerve block; one method is a ring block subcutaneously at the penile base that avoids damaging vessels within the penis that could lead to complications such as extensive hematoma.[7] However, additional local anesthesia may be required in the area of the ventral glans or periurethral area of the glans.

We have found that nerve block anesthesia is best performed with 2% Xylocaine without epinephrine. The 2% anesthetic solution allows local anesthetic to pass down a concentration gradient into the nerve. Nerve blocks take time to become complete, usually about 15 minutes. The addition of epinephrine is unnecessary to achieve an adequate nerve block.

The addition of epinephrine to local anesthesia for infiltration of the penis is often discouraged in the literature. However, because of the rich vascular supply in this area, we do not believe epinephrine is contraindicated, and we know of no instances where its use led to any problems such as necrosis.

12.3 Reconstruction

12.3.1 Reconstruction of the Male External Genitalia

When possible, reconstruction of male external genitalia surgical defects should be confined within the following individual anatomic subunits when possible: glans penis, penile shaft, scrotum, and perineum. If the surgical defect involves more than one anatomic subunit, then the reconstruction may be more appropriately further divided into separate reconstructions of individual subunits.

When possible, isolated surgical defects of the glans penis are repaired with a primary linear closure.[8] Reconstruction of larger surgical defects of the glans can be achieved with either a split-thickness skin graft or full-thickness skin graft harvested from the medial, anterior, or posterolateral thigh, preferably with non-hair-bearing skin[8,9,10,11] (► Fig. 12.2). One word of caution when operating on the glans penis is that the tissue is very vascular, resulting in excessive bleeding. If the foreskin is still present, it can be utilized as a flap to cover large defects on the glans penis (► Fig. 12.3).

When considering the use of skin grafts or flaps, it is important to note that tobacco users have a higher risk of skin graft and flap necrosis due to reduced peripheral perfusion, leading to poor wound healing and surgical outcomes. Similarly, electronic cigarettes have been shown to be as toxic as tobacco cigarettes with respect to surgical outcomes.[12]

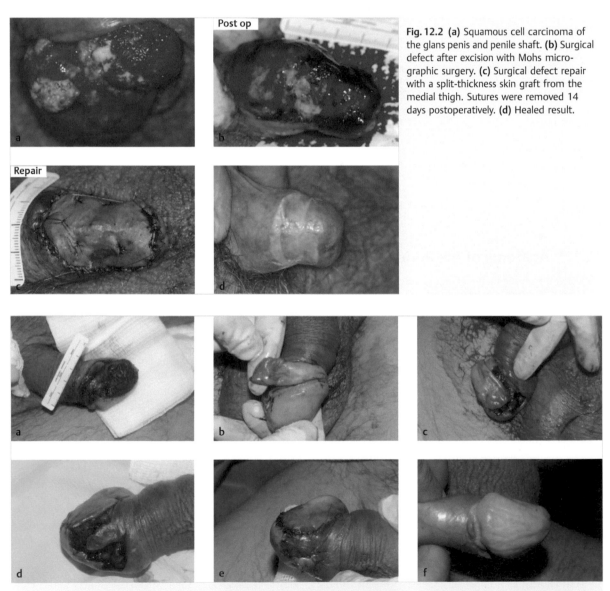

Fig. 12.2 (a) Squamous cell carcinoma of the glans penis and penile shaft. **(b)** Surgical defect after excision with Mohs micrographic surgery. **(c)** Surgical defect repair with a split-thickness skin graft from the medial thigh. Sutures were removed 14 days postoperatively. **(d)** Healed result.

Fig. 12.3 (a) Large surgical defect of the glans penis after Mohs micrographic surgery for a superficial Bowen's disease-type squamous cell carcinoma. **(b,c)** Using foreskin to repair most of the wound. **(d)** A single-lobe transposition flap used to complete the closure. **(e)** Sutured closure. **(f)** Healed result at 1 year.

Alternatively, healing by secondary intention can also be considered for surgical defects of the glans penis. If the wound is small and superficial, the cosmetic result is usually excellent. However, for a deeper wound in the glans, a smooth depressed scar with steep edges can result, which is cosmetically undesirable. In such a case, a skin graft gives a more pleasing result than granulation.[13] One word of caution is that granulation of surgical defects in the glans also involving the urethral meatus can result in meatal stenosis, consequently requiring referral to urology for further management and possible surgical correction.[13] This complication can be avoided by catheterization and placement of a skin graft.

If small, a surgical defect of the penile shaft can be repaired primarily with a linear closure directed horizontally when possible (► Fig. 12.4). A large surgical defect of the penile shaft can be repaired with split-thickness skin graft, especially those in which the wounds run circumferentially around the penis.[11] Use of a thick split-thickness skin results in minimal scar formation and contraction.[14] On the other hand, large full-thickness skin grafts in this area may have suboptimal survival as these grafts have higher metabolic needs and, thus, require a well-vascularized recipient bed and more optimal conditions for graft perfusion and survival.[14,15] In cases of large surgical defects that may have a high risk of poor skin graft take with consequent penile contracture and scarring, such as in diabetic patients or tobacco users, reconstruction with a scrotal skin flap can be considered.[14] The use of scrotal skin is suitable, since it possesses similar properties as penile skin in that it is loose, elastic, and expandable.[14] An alternative option for surgical defects in this area is healing by secondary intention, with excellent results demonstrated even with large noncircumferential surgical defects with no ensuing penile contracture at long-term follow-up.[13,16]

Many scrotal surgical defects can be repaired primarily. Due to the vascularity, redundancy, and elasticity of scrotal skin, surgical defects of up to 50% scrotal skin loss can be repaired primarily.[14,17] Other reconstructive considerations include skin grafts or local skin flaps.[14] When considering scrotal reconstruction options, it is important to also consider the age and fertility status of the patient, as the type of reconstruction may disrupt the thermoregulation of the testicles, thereby affecting testicular function and spermatogenesis.[14,17,18] A study in rats showed that the use of skin grafts resulted in diminished testicular function, whereas the use of skin flaps exhibited testicular function comparable to a control group that did not undergo surgery.[18] However, diminished testicular function has also been exhibited with thick skin flaps.[19]

An alternative for repair of the scrotum is second intention. Because of the looseness of scrotal tissue, when even large wounds granulate, the cosmetic and functional results are equivalent to primary closure (► Fig. 12.5). The

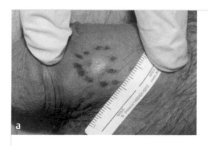
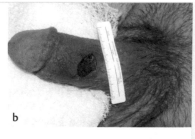
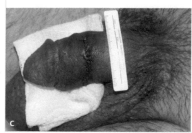
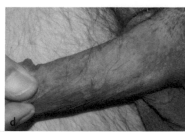

Fig. 12.4 (a) Bowen's disease carcinoma positive for human papillomavirus 16. **(b)** Surgical defect after excision by Mohs micrographic surgery. **(c)** Linear closure using buried dermal–subdermal and percutaneous sutures. **(d)** Healed result at 8 months.

Fig. 12.5 (a) Surgical defect of the scrotum after removal of extramammary Paget's disease by Mohs micrographic surgery. **(b)** Result after healing by second intention.

major difference is that wounds that are allowed to heal by granulation take on average 6 weeks to completely heal, whereas if a wound is sutured primarily, it will be completely healed in 2 weeks.

We recommend that all patients when healing by granulation in the genitalia soak in a sitz bath once a day. The gentle water action helps keep the wound clean.

12.3.2 Reconstruction of the Female External Genitalia

As in male genitalia reconstruction, reconstruction of the female external genitalia should follow the anatomic subunit principles. In females, the anatomic subunits of the external genitalia most likely involved in dermatologic surgery would include the mons pubis, labia majora, and labia minora.

Surgical defects of the mons pubis can be closed primarily as a linear closure or, for larger defects, with a local skin flap. With either of these repairs, caution must be taken to ensure that the closure tension vector should be directed so as to avoid opening of the labia majora, thereby exposing the clitoris to external friction. Full-thickness skin grafts can also be considered for larger surgical defects, although the graft will be devoid of hair in this hair-bearing area.

For labia majora surgical defects, primary closure is preferred if reasonable. As in the mons pubis, it is essential to consider orienting the closure tension vector in the labia majora to prevent opening of the labia majora that would result in drying of the introitus and friction to the clitoris and urethral meatus.[14] Local skin flaps and skin grafts are also reconstructive options for small defects.[20] For large and more extensive defects, variations of a V-Y advancement flap from the medial thigh pedicled on the medial circumflex femoral artery perforator have been described.[20,21,22]

Reconstruction options of the labia minora are limited, mostly achieved with primary linear closure or

healing by secondary intention. Reconstruction of this area should be considered, if possible, in order to maintain the protection of the underlying urethral meatus and vaginal introitus.

Our experience with the female genitalia is that wounds, large or small, do very well with second intention healing (▶ Fig. 12.6). Because of the rich vascular supply and loose tissue, wounds will granulate with an imperceptible scar and good functional result. Although this can result in asymmetry of the labia, this does not seem to be a problem for patients, particularly in the elderly. One problem we have seen is that if a wound is large and circumferential around the introitus, it could result in stricture. As long as there is no impedance of urinary flow, stricture is not usually problematic.

12.3.3 Reconstruction of the Perineum

With surgical defects of the perineum, repair with primary closure is the preferred reconstructive method.[14,17] If closure is difficult because of excess tension, then reconstruction with a local skin flap is recommended over skin grafts.[14] Skin graft survival is suboptimal due to the shearing forces and bacterial colonization of the area.[14] Furthermore, a graft in the perineum may result in an unstable scar prone to epidermal breakdown due to the external pressure exerted on this area with certain positions such as sitting.[14] A reconstructive approach that does not shorten the perineum is most favorable.[14] In the sitting position, the majority of the external pressure is directed on the perineum and the ischial tubercles. With a shortened perineum, the point of highest pressure is subsequently shifted to the anus, leading to chronic hygiene issues, soiling, and possible skin ulcerations.[14]

Healing by granulation is possible in the perineum. With granulation, the surgical defect is allowed to contract from all sides, often leading to less overall perineal shortening than with suturing a wound (▶ Fig. 12.7).

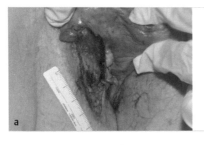
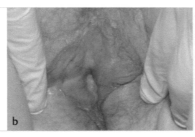
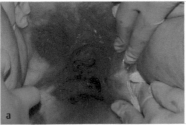
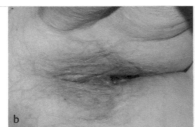

Fig. 12.6 (a) Surgical defect of the labia majora after excision of extramammary Paget's disease by Mohs micrographic surgery. **(b)** Result after healing by secondary intention.

Fig. 12.7 (a) Surgical defect of the perineum, labia minora and labia majora after removal of extramammary Paget's disease by Mohs micrographic surgery. **(b)** Result after healing by secondary intention.

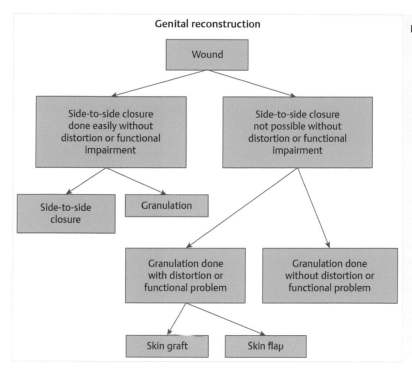

Fig. 12.8 Genital reconstruction algorithm.

12.4 Conclusion

Reconstruction of the genitalia, whether in men or women, can be challenging due to the complex anatomy and the importance of preserving normal function. Both the rich vasculature and ample loose tissue in this area help provide excellent cosmetic and functional scars that are often minimal (► Fig. 12.8).

References

[1] Netter FH. Atlas of Human Anatomy. 2nd ed. Teterboro, NJ: MediMedia USA, Inc.; 2001

[2] Sharma GR. Rupture of the superficial dorsal vein of the penis. Int J Urol. 2005; 12(12):1071–1073

[3] Truong H, Ferenczi B, Cleary R, Healy KA. Superficial dorsal venous rupture of the penis: false penile fracture that needs to be treated as a true urologic emergency. Urology. 2016; 97:e21–e22

[4] Yavagal S, de Farias TF, Medina CA, Takacs P. Normal vulvovaginal, perineal, and pelvic anatomy with reconstructive considerations. Semin Plast Surg. 2011; 25(2):121–129

[5] Morton DA. Gross Anatomy: The Big Picture. New York City, NY: McGraw-Hill Professional Publishing; 2011

[6] Kozacioglu Z, Kiray A, Ergur I, Zeybek G, Degirmenci T, Gunlusoy B. Anatomy of the dorsal nerve of the penis, clinical implications. Urology. 2014; 83(1):121–124

[7] Soh CR, Ng SB, Lim SL. Dorsal penile nerve block. Paediatr Anaesth. 2003; 13(4):329–333

[8] Ralph DJ, Garaffa G, García MA. Reconstructive surgery of the penis. Curr Opin Urol. 2006; 16(6):396–400

[9] Parnham AS, Albersen M, Sahdev V, et al. Glansectomy and split-thickness skin graft for penile cancer. Eur Urol. 2018; 73(2):284–289

[10] Morelli G, Pagni R, Mariani C, et al. Glansectomy with split-thickness skin graft for the treatment of penile carcinoma. Int J Impot Res. 2009; 21(5):311–314

[11] Xu XY, Shao N, Qiao D, et al. Reconstruction of defects in 11 patients with penile Paget's diseases with split-thickness skin graft. Int Urol Nephrol. 2013; 45(2):413–420

[12] Rau AS, Reinikovaite V, Schmidt EP, Taraseviciene-Stewart L, Deleyiannis FW. Electronic cigarettes are as toxic to skin flap survival as tobacco cigarettes. Ann Plast Surg. 2017; 79(1):86–91

[13] Machan M, Brodland D, Zitelli J. Penile squamous cell carcinoma: Penis-preserving treatment with Mohs micrographic surgery. Dermatol Surg. 2016; 42(8):936–944

[14] Kolehmainen M, Suominen S, Tukiainen E. Pelvic, perineal and genital reconstructions. Scand J Surg. 2013; 102(1):25–31

[15] Thornton JF. Skin grafts and skin substitutes. Selected Readings in Plastic Surgery. 2004; 10(1):1–23

[16] Nguyen H, Saadat P, Bennett RG. Penile basal cell carcinoma: two cases treated with Mohs micrographic surgery and remarks on pathogenesis. Dermatol Surg. 2006; 32(1):135–144

[17] Bickell M, Beilan J, Wallen J, Wiegand L, Carrion R. Advances in surgical reconstructive techniques in the management of penile, urethral, and scrotal cancer. Urol Clin North Am. 2016; 43(4):545–559

[18] Demir Y, Aktepe F, Kandal S, Sancaktar N, Turhan-Haktanir N. The effect of scrotal reconstruction with skin flaps and skin grafts on testicular function. Ann Plast Surg. 2012; 68(3):308–313

[19] Wang D, Zheng H, Deng F. Spermatogenesis after scrotal reconstruction. Br J Plast Surg. 2003; 56(5):484–488

[20] Tan BK, Kang GC, Tay EH, Por YC. Subunit principle of vulvar reconstruction: algorithm and outcomes. Arch Plast Surg. 2014; 41(4):379–386

[21] Gentileschi S, Servillo M, Garganese G, et al. Surgical therapy of vulvar cancer: how to choose the correct reconstruction? J Gynecol Oncol. 2016; 27(6):e60

[22] Lee JH, Shin JW, Kim SW, et al. Modified gluteal fold V-Y advancement flap for vulvovaginal reconstruction. Ann Plast Surg. 2013; 71(5):571–574

13 Reconstruction of Lower Legs

Kira Minkis, Thomas S. Bander, and Kristina Navrazhina

Summary

Reconstruction of surgical defects on the lower legs is challenging. Increased venous hydrostatic pressure and congestion lead to edema and slow wound healing. Common comorbidities also contribute to less reliable vascular supply and increased skin fragility. Wound tension is often high due to lack of tissue laxity and desire for postoperative ambulation. Ultimately, these complicating factors can lead to higher risk of infection, prolonged wound-healing time, increased risk of wound dehiscence, and even chronic wounds. Reconstructive approaches for lower extremity wounds include primary linear closure, secondary intention healing with or without the use of tissue substitutes and dressings, grafts, and flaps. In this chapter, we present an evidence-based approach to lower extremity reconstruction. We discuss how clinicians can incorporate patient lifestyle, comorbidities, and preferences while selecting an approach that will deliver optimal functional and cosmetic outcomes.

Keywords: graft, flap, lower extremity reconstruction, dermatologic surgery, Unna boot, keystone flap

13.1 Introduction

Approximately 5 to 10% of skin cancers arise on the lower extremities, with a higher proportion of squamous cell carcinoma (SCC) compared to other sites. Lower extremity SCC and melanoma occur more commonly in women, likely due to clothing habits resulting in increased sun exposure.[1,2]

Small keratinocyte carcinomas on the lower legs are low risk and may be treated with destructive methods in selected patients. For melanoma and higher-risk keratinocyte carcinomas, surgery remains the standard of care. Keratinocyte carcinomas with high-risk features or location on the pretibial lower leg and foot are best treated with Mohs micrographic surgery (MMS), which offers complete marginal assessment. Approaches to tumor extirpation are beyond the scope of this text; however, a thorough understanding of tumor biology should guide margin assessment and surgical approach. Complex reconstruction should only be considered once clear margins have been achieved.

Reconstruction of surgical defects on the lower legs is challenging (▶ Fig. 13.1). Gravity increases venous hydrostatic pressure in the lower legs compared to other locations, and venous congestion through valve incompetence or partial obstruction may result in edema and delayed wound healing. Common comorbidities such as venous insufficiency, peripheral arterial disease, lymphedema, diabetic microangiopathy, and neuropathy also contribute to less reliable vascular supply and increased skin fragility. There are few reservoirs of skin laxity on the lower legs to alleviate wound tension, and postoperative

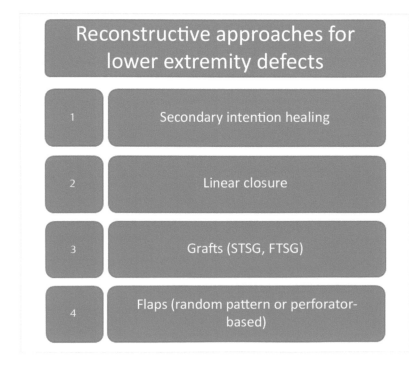

Fig. 13.1 Overview of reconstructive approaches for lower extremity defects. FTSG, full-thickness skin grafts; STSG, split-thickness skin grafts.

mobility adds further strain on surgical wounds. Anterior legs are also frequent sites of trauma, which can increase risk of dehiscence. Ultimately, these complicating factors can lead to higher risk of infection, poor and delayed wound healing, dehiscence, and even chronic wounds (▶ Fig. 13.2).

As in other locations of the body, our approach to reconstruction of the lower extremities starts with preservation of function. Surgical repair on the lower legs must prioritize joint and limb mobility. We also aim to decrease the risk of chronic wounds by closing wounds primarily, minimizing wound tension, and rigorously avoiding wound contamination with preoperative antiseptic use, intraoperative sterile technique, and robust postoperative dressings. Cosmesis is commonly less of a concern on the legs than on the head and neck but remains a consideration after preservation of function and shortening of postoperative recovery time.

In this chapter, we will discuss reconstructive options for the lower legs and our preferred approach. The repair options apply to all areas of the lower leg, though the plantar foot is outside the scope of this chapter. We will also emphasize our pre- and postoperative interventions to optimize wound healing and minimize infection.

13.2 Anatomy of Lower Extremity

13.2.1 Arterial Supply

A review of lower extremity vasculature is key to understanding reconstructive options. The large vessels of the leg course deep and send perforating vessels through the musculature to supply the skin. The abdominal aorta branches into right and left common iliac arteries that supply their respective legs. The common iliac arteries divide into the internal iliac, which supplies the pelvic, gluteal, and thigh regions, and the external iliac, which proceeds to supply the distal leg as the common femoral artery after passing under the inguinal ligament. The common femoral artery gives off a deep femoral branch that divides into the medial and lateral circumflex arteries and terminates in perforating arteries that extend through the adductor magnus muscle to supply the muscles and skin of the thigh.

The external iliac continues as the superficial femoral artery (SFA) through the adductor canal, where it dives through the adductor hiatus at the medial knee to the posterior compartment of the lower leg and becomes the popliteal artery. The popliteal artery gives off genicular branches to the knee joint and anterior and posterior tibial branches.

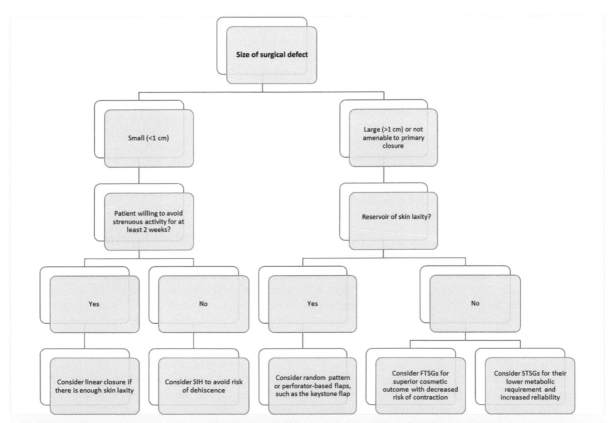

Fig. 13.2 Approach to reconstruction of surgical defects on the lower extremity. Abbreviations: FTSGs, full-thickness skin grafts; SIH, secondary intention healing; STSGs, split-thickness skin grafts.

The posterior tibial artery gives off the fibular (also called peroneal) artery to supply the lateral compartment of the lower leg, and then runs along the superficial surface of the gastrocnemius muscle before entering the foot via the tarsal tunnel. The posterior tibial artery pulse can be palpated posterior to the medial malleolus before it divides into the lateral and medial plantar arteries that anastomose with branches of the anterior tibial artery.

The anterior tibial artery supplies the anterior compartment of the lower leg, running through the interosseous membrane between the tibia and fibula and becoming the dorsalis pedis artery as it enters the dorsal foot. The deep plantar artery between the first and second metatarsal phalangeal joints then anastomoses with the lateral plantar artery from the posterior tibial branch to form the deep plantar arch of the foot.

Although there are significant anastomoses in the foot composed of branches from the anterior and posterior tibial arteries, the remaining blood supply of the lower extremity is dependent on relatively few large and deep vessels, especially compared to the rich network of anastomoses of the head and neck. Whereas random pattern flaps that utilize the subdermal plexus can be effective in selected patients, we frequently turn to flaps that draw from the subcutaneous, fascial, and muscular perforators, such as the keystone advancement flap. The more robust vascular supply helps overcome the limitations imposed by comorbidities that compromise blood flow.

13.2.2 Venous Drainage

Deep venous drainage of the lower leg mirrors its arterial supply and is located deep to the muscle fascia. Branches of the dorsal venous arch drain into the anterior tibial vein, and the medial and lateral plantar veins converge as the posterior tibial vein just posterior to the medial malleolus. The anterior tibial, posterior tibial, and fibular veins course along the lower leg to form the popliteal vein, which travels with the popliteal artery. Above the knee and through the adductor canal, the popliteal vein becomes the femoral vein and travels under the inguinal ligament as the external iliac vein. There are also perforating veins through the thigh muscles that drain into the deep femoral vein.

Superficial venous drainage is achieved through the great and small saphenous veins, which lie superficial to the muscular fascia. The lateral aspect of the dorsal venous arch of the foot drains to the small saphenous vein, which then travels along the posterior lateral malleolus, up the posterior lower leg, and into the popliteal vein. The great saphenous vein drains the medial aspect of the dorsal foot and passes anterior to the medial malleolus, up the medial lower leg, and posteriorly to the medial condyle of the knee. Numerous superficial veins drain into the great saphenous vein until it ends in the femoral vein at the inguinal ligament. There are extensive perforator branches between the superficial and deep venous systems to encourage venous return to the heart.

Normal venous outflow depends on lower extremity muscles to pump deoxygenated blood against the flow of gravity. A system of one-way valves prevents backflow when the muscles are not activated. Prolonged hydrostatic pressure may overwhelm this system, resulting in valvular incompetence. Increased intraluminal pressures dilate vessels and increase permeability to blood cells and plasma, which travel into the interstitial space and cause the signs and symptoms of venous stasis, including edema, venous varicosities, brown pigmentation from hemosiderin deposition, and chronic inflammation that impairs wound healing. With chronic inflammation and poor oxygenation, the skin may become sclerotic and indurated, termed lipodermatosclerosis. Risk factors for venous insufficiency include deep venous outflow obstruction (via thrombosis or trauma), obesity, leg immobility, family history, pregnancy, advanced age, and prolonged standing. External application of graded compression, either via stockings or wraps, has been demonstrated to improve lower extremity swelling, pain, dyspigmentation, and varicosities, hasten healing and minimize recurrence of venous ulcerations.[3]

13.2.3 Cutaneous Innervation

Cutaneous innervation of the lower extremity follows a dermatomal distribution derived from the lumbosacral plexus at spinal levels L1 through S5. In general, the anterior leg and medial foot are innervated from nerve roots at L1–L5, while the posterior leg and lateral foot are innervated by roots S1–S5. Named nerves carry sensory information from the skin. Whereas small sensory nerves may be damaged during skin surgery, the resulting numbness or tingling is generally minimal. Lower extremity motor nerves run deep to the musculature and are rarely encountered by the dermatologic surgeon.

13.3 Reconstructive Approaches for Lower Extremity Defects

13.3.1 Preoperative Consultation

Before any reconstruction, it is important to discuss risks and benefits of the selected approach, alternatives, and expected postoperative course. Setting expectations early is crucial, especially when optimal healing requires a significant change in activity level and extensive postoperative care. Some patients approach surgery on the legs with less concern than more visible locations, but it is important to prepare them for at least 2 to 3 weeks of reduced activity postoperatively if reconstruction is pursued. Patient activity levels vary drastically at baseline, so we inquire about their habits before surgery to provide specific instructions about which activities to avoid and to select the reconstructive plan that best fits their lifestyle.

It is also important to assess the patient's support network. Wound care can be complicated and intimidating, so it is wise for caregivers to attend the surgical visit to receive specific instructions. Knowledge of the patient's home situation aids in wound care planning. Are the patient and caregiver capable of twice daily dressing changes? Would it be reasonable for the patient to present to the office for weekly dressing changes? Or would a visiting nurse be the best fit? Furthermore, some patients may require more assistance with their activities of daily living in the postoperative period. They may plan to have a family member on call in case issues arise. Since compression and wound care are particularly important for lower extremity reconstruction, we provide recommendations for compression stockings and recommend that patients wear them for 1 to 2 weeks before surgery. A preoperative consultation, either by phone or in person, facilitates this important coordination of postoperative care.

13.3.2 Overview of Reconstructive Approaches

Approaches to lower extremity reconstruction include secondary intention healing (SIH), primary linear closure, split-thickness skin grafts (STSGs), full-thickness skin grafts (FTSGs), and local flaps. Although primary linear closure is often preferred for its speed and reliability, there is no consensus on the optimal method of reconstruction of larger wounds or wounds that are not amenable to primary closure.[4] We will discuss the advantages and disadvantages of each repair option and the considerations that inform our eventual selection. Along with our clinical experience and preferences, we include evidence-based recommendations when possible.

13.3.3 Secondary Intention Healing

SIH is a low-cost and straightforward option for superficial defects on the lower legs, especially when there is minimal local skin laxity.[5,6] In carefully selected patients, small superficial surgical defects, abrasions, lacerations, and wounds following cryosurgery and electrodessication can heal well by SIH with minimal downtime (▶ Fig. 13.3a). Postoperative wound management after SIH is relatively simple, requiring only topical petrolatum or antibacterial ointment and an occlusive or semi-occlusive dressing. Complications with SIH are uncommon but include bleeding, prolonged wound healing with possible secondary infection, scar contracture and depression, and dyspigmentation.[6] Patients should be counseled to expect longer healing times of 4 to 12 weeks compared to other body sites.[7]

Active and otherwise healthy patients may prefer SIH because there is no risk of dehiscence, allowing them to return to normal activities earlier than with sutured

defects (generally after 48 hours). On the other hand, patients with limited mobility may struggle to reach healing wounds on the lower legs, and poor wound care and comorbid conditions may lead to prolonged healing times with increased risk of infections (▶ Fig. 13.3b). Some patients may require a visiting health care provider to assist with dressing changes.[8]

In appropriately selected cases, SIH can result in good functional and cosmetic outcomes. A prospective, randomized, evaluator-blinded clinical trial evaluated outcomes following SIH or complete purse-string closure for circular or oval postoperative wounds larger than 8 mm on the trunk and extremities. There were no significant differences in cosmetic outcomes, ratio of scar to defect area, pain level at 1-week follow-up, and postprocedural complications between the SIH and purse-string groups.[9] A retrospective study compared defects on the plantar foot repaired with FTSGs to those left to heal by secondary intention.[10] Whereas FTSGs had faster healing times (8 weeks compared to 12 weeks), cosmesis was better in the SIH group, based on blinded evaluation of scar topography, color match, edge contour, and pigmentation.

SIH should be part of the dermatologic surgeon's armamentarium for selected patients with superficial lower extremity defects.

13.3.4 Linear Repair

Primary linear repair is an excellent option for deeper wounds that are small enough to close with minimal tension. This approach is fast, reliable, and hastens wound-healing time compared to SIH (▶ Fig. 13.4). The main disadvantages are higher risk of dehiscence due to lack of adjacent tissue laxity and depressed scars that alter normal leg contour. Primary linear repair is our first choice for deeper wounds under minimal tension.

13.3.5 Skin Grafts

Skin grafting is another approach for reconstruction of lower extremity defects. STSGs include the epidermis and a variable thickness of dermis, whereas FTSGs involve the entire epidermis and dermis.[11] To optimize cosmetic outcomes, the donor site should be selected to match the recipient site in thickness, texture, color, and density of adnexal structures. In general, FTSGs are thicker and more resistant to trauma, contract less as they heal, and have superior cosmetic outcomes compared to STSGs. Despite these advantages, there are situations where STSGs remain useful.

STSGs are frequently used in reconstruction of burn wounds and diabetic foot and leg wounds.[8,12,13] They heal more rapidly than SIH and can be meshed to reliably cover a large surface area.[14] Their low metabolic requirement is desirable on lower extremities, where vascular supply may be compromised. Scar quality may be similar to SIH

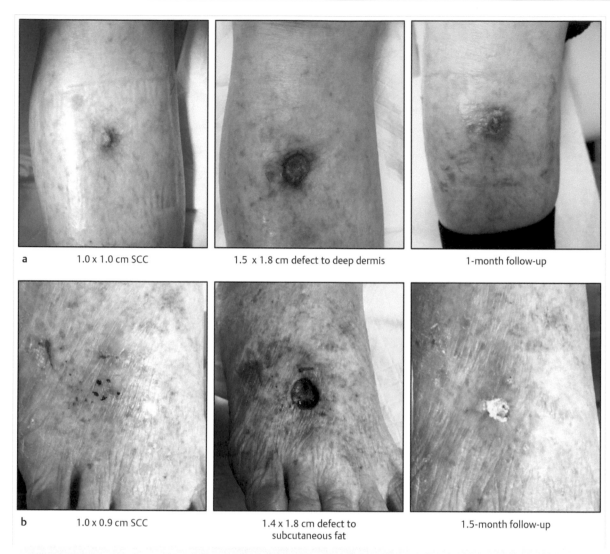

a   1.0 x 1.0 cm SCC   1.5 x 1.8 cm defect to deep dermis   1-month follow-up

b   1.0 x 0.9 cm SCC   1.4 x 1.8 cm defect to   1.5-month follow-up
                                      subcutaneous fat

Fig. 13.3 Examples of secondary intention healing. **(a)** An 81-year-old woman with squamous cell carcinoma (SCC) on the right shin treated with Mohs micrographic surgery (MMS) and allowed to heal by secondary intention. At 1-month follow-up, the wound was granulating well with peripheral re-epithelialization. **(b)** A 71-year-old woman with SCC on the dorsal foot treated with MMS. The patient opted for secondary intention healing (SIH). The surgical site was still healing with a fibrinous center at 2 months and completely healed at 4 months. Patients should be counseled on the prolonged healing time with secondary intention.

at the recipient site, but persistent erythema (in certain cases for over a year) and poor cosmesis of both the donor and recipient sites are major disadvantages.[5]

FTSGs have superior cosmetic outcomes with better tissue match than STSGs and less contraction than STSGs or SIH.[5] They are also less painful and more durable, which is important on trauma-prone areas of the lower legs.[15] The higher metabolic demand of FTSGs has traditionally been thought to impair graft survival; however, several studies have shown comparable graft take between FTSGs and STSGs on the lower limb.[14,16] Similarly, several retrospective studies have demonstrated good graft take, cosmesis, and functionality of FTSGs on the lower legs.[4,5,8,14,17,18] In studies with longer follow-up, all

patients healed without further surgical intervention, indicating that even in cases of partial graft loss, the resulting biological bandage supports SIH.[5,8,15]

Lower limb skin grafts have higher rates of graft failure compared to other regions of the body, with one study reporting a third of lower extremity grafts failing at the 6-week follow-up.[14] A different study compared FTSGs with STSGs in 89 patients following sentinel lymph node biopsies on the trunk and extremities and found that 65% of FTSGs had complete take compared to only 32% of STSGs.[16] This outcome was likely affected by selection bias, as the surgeons avoided FTSGs in larger areas or in cases with high risk of nodal metastasis. The STSG cohort had significantly higher rates of complications (56%)

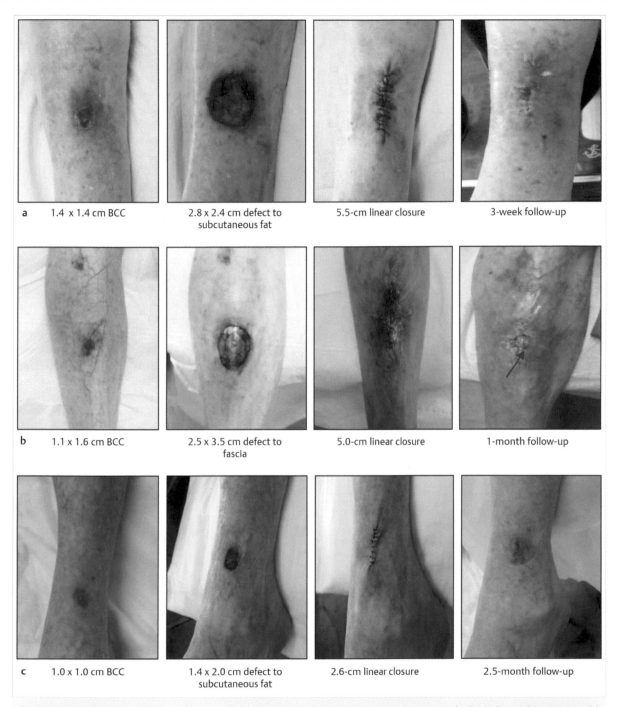

a   1.4 x 1.4 cm BCC   2.8 x 2.4 cm defect to subcutaneous fat   5.5-cm linear closure   3-week follow-up

b   1.1 x 1.6 cm BCC   2.5 x 3.5 cm defect to fascia   5.0-cm linear closure   1-month follow-up

c   1.0 x 1.0 cm BCC   1.4 x 2.0 cm defect to subcutaneous fat   2.6-cm linear closure   2.5-month follow-up

Fig. 13.4 Examples of primary linear closure and possible complications that are more common on the lower legs. **(a)** An 88-year-old woman with basal cell carcinoma (BCC) on the lower leg treated with Mohs micrographic surgery (MMS) and repaired with a linear closure without complications. **(b)** A 98-year-old woman with pretibial BCC treated with MMS and repaired with a linear closure. Central dehiscence (*red arrow*) developed 2 weeks postoperatively and had fully healed by 7 months. Risk of dehiscence is higher for larger defects in this location and should be considered when selecting this reconstructive method. **(c)** A 75-year-old woman with BCC on the ankle treated with MMS and repaired with linear closure. A culture-positive wound infection developed 1.5 months following surgery, and the patient was successfully treated with cephalexin. After 2.5 months, there was a well-healed scar with minimal central thin crust.

compared to the FTSG group (24%). The most common complications were minor seroma or edema. The authors also reported superior cosmetic outcomes in the FTSG cohort at 4 to 8 weeks of follow-up.

Graft failure is correlated with higher body mass index (BMI), peripheral vascular disease, and immunosuppression, possibly due to decreased microperfusion and tissue oxygenation.[14,19] Other causes of graft failure include infection, poor graft–recipient contact, poor recipient site vascularity, and significant tension on the graft. Anticoagulant use and graft size were not associated with worse graft take in a retrospective study of 50 lower extremity FTSGs.[8] There was no difference in graft failure rates between patients on bed rest and those allowed to ambulate on the day of surgery.[14]

Modifications in technique, such as delayed grafting, postoperative immobilization, or quilting the graft to the wound bed, may increase graft take. The resulting base of granulation tissue that forms when grafting is delayed may make the wound bed more receptive to graft placement and decrease the contour irregularity of the final wound; however, small retrospective studies have shown similar rates of graft take with delayed and same-day grafting.[5,17] The authors generally reserve delayed grafts for situations where the recipient bed is not likely to provide adequate blood flow to the graft (as with deep wounds extending to periosteum) or when it is more convenient for the patient to return on a different day. As long as the partially granulated wound is freshened with a curette or a blade before delayed grafting, we do not notice a difference in graft take between immediate and delayed grafting.

It has been suggested that postoperative immobilization of up to 5 days can increase graft uptake, particularly for FTSGs on the lower limb.[20] A retrospective review of 70 lower leg defects repaired with lower extremity FTSGs and immobilized for 5 days had greater than 90% graft take in 91.4% of patients.[20] The most common complications included hematoma formation, infection, and venous thrombosis. Nevertheless, postoperative immobilization carries significant risks that limit its practicality, which will be addressed in a later section.

Quilted or meshed skin grafts may also increase graft uptake. Quilted FTSGs that are fixed to the recipient bed with basting sutures may decrease risk of hematoma and damaging shearing forces during the critical stages of graft imbibition and inosculation. A cohort of 92 lower extremity defects repaired with quilted FTSGs demonstrated 100% graft take in 89.4% of patients at 2-week follow-up.[15] The grafts were quilted to the deep fascia with nylon sutures and tied loosely, thus immobilizing the graft without adding additional tension (▶ Fig. 13.5). This study did not directly compare quilted FTSG to traditional FTSG, but it is our standard approach to place basting sutures through the graft and into the recipient bed, though we rarely place these sutures as deep as the fascia. Another study demonstrated that patients with meshed lower extremity grafts had less graft loss than those without meshing, reinforcing the importance of minimizing graft tension and risk of seroma and hematoma.[21]

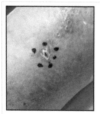

Lesion measuring 0.5 x 0.5 cm

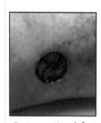

Postoperative defect measuring 2.0 x 2.0 cm

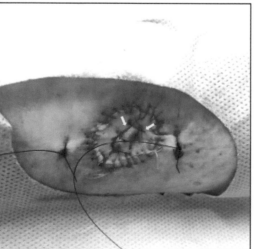

FTSG quilted to the recipient bed

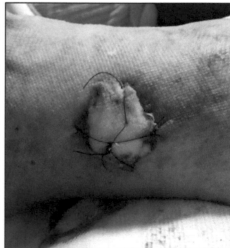

Bolster secured with tie-over sutures

Fig. 13.5 Example of quilted full-thickness skin graft (FTSG) on the shin. An 89-year-old man with a significantly atypical melanocytic proliferation on the shin treated with staged excision and repaired with an FTSG from the inner upper arm. The defect was debrided to freshen the wound edges and the FTSG was tacked down inferiorly and superiorly. The graft was quilted to the recipient bed with basting sutures (*yellow arrows*) and tied loosely, immobilizing the graft while reducing tension. A bolster consisting of petrolatum gauze was secured into place with tie-over sutures secured into surrounding unaffected skin. Zinc oxide compression bandage (Unna boot) was applied.

Even in the best of circumstances, the cosmetic drawbacks of skin grafts are substantial. Graft recipient sites have significant textural, contour, and pigmentary demarcation from surrounding skin. Furthermore, grafts require two surgical wounds to repair one defect, increasing the risk of complications in patients with comorbidities that impair wound healing. On the lower extremity, the authors reserve grafts for cases where function would be impaired with other types of repairs. When we use grafts, they are frequently taken from the Burow's triangle of the adjacent repair to ensure optimal tissue match and reduce morbidity from a second surgical wound.[22,23]

13.3.6 Random Pattern Flaps

Random pattern flaps derive their nutrient supply from subdermal vascular plexus and are dependent on the capillary perfusion pressure of their pedicle. These flaps have a high rate of survival on areas of skin with a rich vascular supply but should be approached more cautiously on the lower extremity, especially in patients with any comorbidity that impedes wound healing. Furthermore, we find that the limited reservoirs of tissue laxity on the lower extremity reduce the opportunity to utilize random pattern flaps because significant tension reduces their viability. We prefer perforator flaps that have a robust blood supply able to withstand high tension and less reliable vasculature.

13.3.7 Perforator Flaps

Perforator flaps utilize a deep pedicle supplied by larger arteries perpendicular to the skin.[24,25] There are many applications of V-Y advancement flaps on the lower extremities, including modifications, such as the cone flap, which combines a V-Y advancement with rotation, and the horn flap, which is an arced V-Y flap.[26,27,28,29,30,31,32]

The keystone perforator island flap, or the keystone flap, was first described by Felix Behan and has emerged as a reliable and effective flap to repair large and deep wounds.[33,34] Named for its resemblance to the central piece of an architectural arch, the keystone flap has a strong vascular supply due to preservation of the musculocutaneous and fasciocutaneous perforator vessels, which pierce through the fascia and feed into the subcutis.[35,36] It has multiple advantages including relative ease of design and execution, robust vascularity of the flap, short operative time, and high reproducibility.[37]

The keystone flap is typically oriented with the long axis along relaxed skin tension lines to minimize tension and optimize cosmesis. This orientation also preserves superficial veins, lymphatics, and cutaneous nerves.[38] The flap requires a local reservoir of tissue laxity; however, in our experience, its robust blood supply allows it to withstand much greater tension than random pattern flaps. Keystone flaps oriented perpendicular to relaxed skin

tension lines generally interrupt lymphatics on the lower legs and carry a risk of swelling, lymphedema, and interruption of future lymphatic mapping should recurrence require it. A perpendicular orientation can be pursued with excellent cosmesis but only if the defect is oriented in that direction or to take advantage of local tissue laxity.

The classic keystone flap is best visualized as two V-Y flaps on opposite sides of the surgical defect.[33] Four variations of the keystone flap were originally described.[33,34] Type I is typically attempted first, but if there is not enough tissue laxity to cover the defect, intraoperative conversion to types II to IV may follow (▶ Fig. 13.6).[39] In the type IIa keystone, the outer arc is incised to the deep fascia to increase lateral mobility, while type IIb utilizes an STSG to cover the secondary defect. The type III keystone flap is used to cover large defects, and is composed of two opposing keystone flaps. Type IV entails undermining up to half of the flap in the subfascial plane to increase advancement.

In addition to the four traditional keystone flap variations, other modifications of the flap have been described in the literature.[40,41] Moncrieff et al introduced an approach where the flap is designed around the original circular defect without first transforming the primary defect into an ellipse. During advancement, a skin bridge opposite the defect is left intact, resulting in fewer suture lines and a shorter scar. Additionally, blunt spreading dissection preserves the subcutaneous vascular and lymphatic structures, offering a more robust vascular pedicle with retained subdermal plexus.[41] The efficacy of this modification was compared to the traditional approach in 176 patients who underwent wide excision for primary melanoma located between the dorsum of the foot and the proximal leg. Of these defects, 65 were reconstructed with the Moncrieff modified keystone flap (also called the Sydney Melanoma Unit modification), 106 with the traditional keystone flap, and 5 with the double-opposing keystone flap. There were significantly fewer complications associated with the modified keystone flap.[41]

In our practice, we often utilize a unilateral modification, also known as the V-Y hemi-keystone advancement flap[42] (▶ Fig. 13.7). Many defects on the lower extremities can be closed with one arm of the keystone, preserving a larger vascular pedicle, saving time, and decreasing scar size (▶ Fig. 13.8). If tension remains high with the unilateral modification, it can easily be converted to the traditional design intraoperatively. We have found that this modification leads to similar rates of complications compared to the traditional keystone flap, while decreasing the total area of surgical manipulation and surgery-associated morbidity.[42] After placement of sufficient deep buried sutures to relieve tension, we frequently utilize surgical staples for epidermal apposition with excellent cosmetic outcomes.

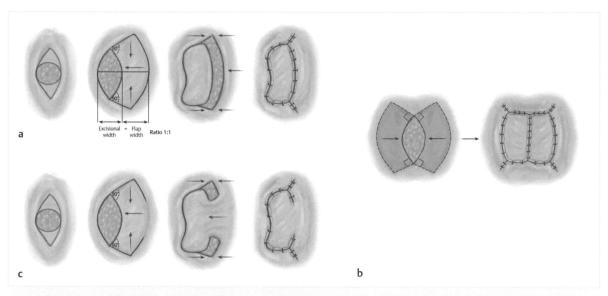

Fig. 13.6 Schematic of the traditional keystone flap and published modifications. **(a)** In the classic type I keystone flap, the flap width is equivalent to the width of the defect, and flap length is determined based on conversion of the circular defect to an ellipse. An incision is made at a 90-degree angle from the apices of the elliptical defect. The arc of the flap is mobilized to the level of the subcutaneous fat and sutured into place, with careful technique to ensure preservation of perforating vessels, nerves, and veins. **(b)** The type III keystone flap utilizes two opposing keystone flaps to cover large defects. **(c)** Unlike the traditional keystone design, the Sydney Melanoma Unit (SMU) modification leaves an intact skin bridge along the greater arc, preserving the subcutaneous vasculature and minimizing the total amount of surgical manipulation.

Several studies have demonstrated the effectiveness of the keystone flap for lower extremity defects.[37,38,39,40,41,43] A systematic review of 9 articles involving 282 keystone flaps on 273 patients found an overall complication rate of 9.6%, including wound dehiscence (5.7%), infection (1.8%), and partial flap loss (1.1%). These complication rates are significantly lower than those reported for free- and perforator-pedicle propeller flaps (19.0 and 21.4%, respectively).[44] In a cohort of over 100 defects, we demonstrated that the keystone flap leads to more rapid healing and superior cosmetic outcomes compared to FTSGs for reconstruction of lower extremity defects (unpublished data). Repairs with concurrent keystone flaps and FTSGs exemplify these observations (▶ Fig. 13.9, ▶ Fig. 13.10). The keystone flap has also been successfully employed following radiation therapy.[45]

Reconstruction of lower extremity defects may be challenging, but SIH, linear repair, skin grafts, and local flaps are excellent options when applied to maximize their inherent advantages.

13.4 Postoperative Care Following Lower Extremity Reconstruction

13.4.1 Dressings

In addition to protecting the postoperative wound from contamination and further trauma, dressings should maintain an optimal healing environment by absorbing wound exudate and preventing excess fluid loss and desiccation. For the lower extremity in particular, compression also speeds healing.[46] Our approach to dressing selection depends on location and wound type.

Occlusive dressings decrease the transmission of fluids or water vapor from the wound to the external environment, thus creating an insulated and moist environment. Patients experience less pain and four to five times faster wound healing with occlusive dressings compared to wounds left exposed to air.[46,47,48,49,50] Occlusive dressings can be both biologic, which include allografts, xenografts, and skin substitutes, and nonbiologic, which include hydrocolloids, hydrogels, alginates, and films.[46]

13.4.2 Unna Boot

Zinc oxide dressings that combine occlusion and compression were first described in 1896 by dermatologist Paul Gerson Unna, and are now commonly referred to as "Unna boots."[51] The Unna boot is a gauze bandage saturated with a moistened paste consisting of zinc oxide, glycerin, and calamine lotion, depending on the formulation.[52] The bandage is wrapped around the leg to be worn continuously and changed weekly (▶ Fig. 13.11). Petrolatum is frequently applied to the skin before Unna boot placement similar to an occlusive dressing.[49] A systematic review demonstrated that an Unna boot was superior to a moist but noncompressive dressing for treatment of venous leg ulcers,[53] suggesting a possible benefit for its use in lower

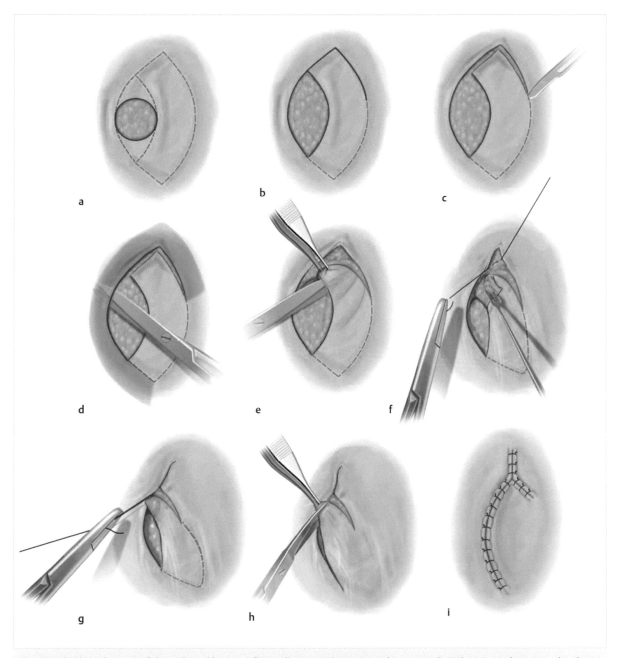

Fig. 13.7 (a–i) A schematic of the unilateral keystone flap. Following Mohs micrographic surgery (MMS) or surgical excision, the classic keystone flap is designed, but only a partial incision is made along the outer arc of the flap. The incision may be extended as necessary, and a larger portion of the flap may be mobilized in order to close the defect. In our experience, this technique alleviates tension while minimizing surgical manipulation to provide excellent cosmetic outcomes and faster operative times.

extremity surgical wounds.[54] The Unna boot provides both compression and an ideal local wound environment while minimizing the burden of postoperative wound care on the patient.

Several animal studies have also demonstrated zinc's potential role in wound healing.[55] Histologically, wounds treated with zinc oxide exhibited advanced re-epithelization with minimal inflammation, whereas those treated with zinc chloride or saline showed incomplete re-epithelization, wound debris, and chronic inflammatory infiltration.[56,57,58,59] Additional studies have demonstrated that zinc oxide has both anti-inflammatory and antibacterial properties, particularly against *Staphylococcus aureus*.[60,61]

In addition to the benefits of compression and zinc oxide, weekly in-office dressing changes may be particularly

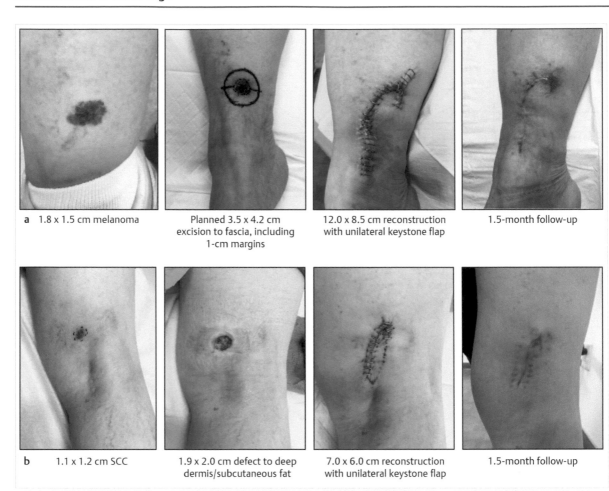

a   1.8 x 1.5 cm melanoma | Planned 3.5 x 4.2 cm excision to fascia, including 1-cm margins | 12.0 x 8.5 cm reconstruction with unilateral keystone flap | 1.5-month follow-up

b   1.1 x 1.2 cm SCC | 1.9 x 2.0 cm defect to deep dermis/subcutaneous fat | 7.0 x 6.0 cm reconstruction with unilateral keystone flap | 1.5-month follow-up

Fig. 13.8 Examples of the unilateral keystone flap demonstrate excellent healing and cosmetic outcomes with fewer incisions. **(a)** An 80-year-old woman with superficial spreading melanoma (Breslow depth of 0.65 mm, Clark level I) on the distal pretibial region treated with staged excision with 1.0-cm margins. Horizontal mattress pulley sutures were placed for tissue expansion. After clear margins were confirmed, the patient returned for reconstruction with a unilateral keystone flap and postoperative Unna boot application. The patient was completely healed at the 3-week suture removal visit. At 1.5-month follow-up, the patient had healed well without complications. **(b)** A 64-year-old woman with squamous cell carcinoma (SCC) on the right posterior thigh treated with Mohs micrographic surgery (MMS) and repaired with a unilateral modification of the keystone flap. The wound healed well without complications.

important for patients unable to perform more frequent and rigorous postoperative wound care on their own. Indeed, patient anxiety may be lessened and satisfaction increased with weekly Unna boot dressing, even when SIH is pursued.[49]

The combination of occlusion, compression, and protection from mechanical trauma also leads to an objective improvement in wound-healing time with fewer complications.[49,54] Thompson et al compared outcomes of standard postoperative wound care consisting of gauze and tape (44 patients) to weekly zinc oxide compression bandages (36 patients) following excision of cutaneous lesions on the lower extremities. At 19 days, 92% of patients with zinc oxide compression bandages were fully healed compared to only 66% in the control group. There were no complications in the zinc oxide compression group compared to a complication rate of 13.6% in patients receiving standard wound care. The most common complications in the standard wound care cohort included infection (9.1%), bleeding (2.3%), dehiscence (4.5%), pain (2.3%), and excessive swelling (2.3%). When adjusted for age, sex, and complexity of surgical closure, patients with zinc oxide compression had better healing times without any postoperative complications.[54] Further studies are needed to compare Unna boots to other compressive dressings on the lower extremities.

Potential disadvantages of the Unna boot are dermatitis, irritation, inability to accommodate significant changes in leg volume, pain if the bandage is applied too tightly, increased application time, and additional office visits. Visiting nursing services are often required for weekly dressing

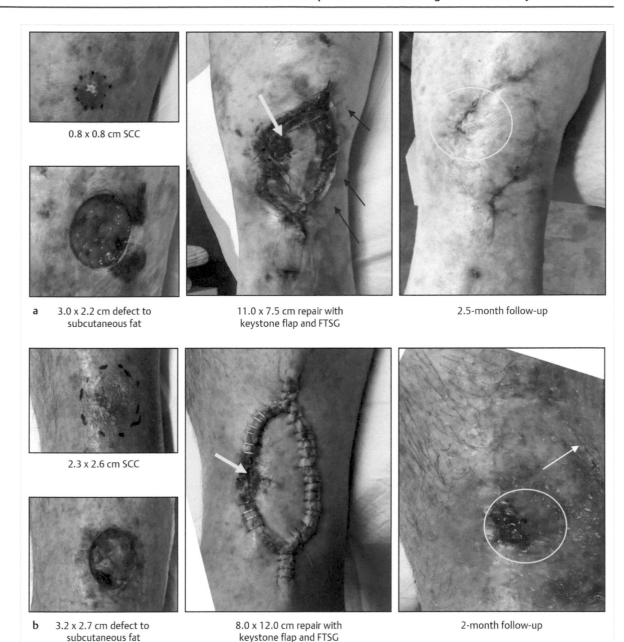

Fig. 13.9 Examples of concurrent keystone advancement flaps and full-thickness skin grafts (FTSGs) in the same location demonstrate faster and more reliable healing with flap reconstruction. **(a)** A 75-year-old woman with squamous cell carcinoma (SCC) on the pretibial region treated with Mohs micrographic surgery (MMS) and repaired with a keystone advancement flap and Burow's FTSG from the standing cones of the elliptical incision (*yellow arrow*). The patient's fragile skin resulted in epidermal tearing and difficulty placing deep buried sutures; therefore, sutures were placed through steri-strips parallel to the wound edge (*blue arrows*). An Unna boot was applied and changed weekly. At 2.5-month follow-up, the keystone flap had healed well, but a small area of granulation tissue remained at the graft site (*yellow circle*). The wound had completely healed at 4.5 months. **(b)** An 82-year-old man with SCC on the pretibial region treated with MMS and repaired with a keystone advancement flap and Burow's FTSG from the standing cones of the elliptical incision (*yellow arrow*). An Unna boot was placed and changed weekly. At the 1- and 2-month follow-ups, the keystone flap had healed well with an inconspicuous scar (*white arrow*), while the graft had not taken and continued to granulate (*yellow circle*).

changes if patients are unable to return to the office.[51,52] These adverse effects are minimal compared to the benefits of more reliable and rapid wound healing, decreased risk of complications, and increased patient satisfaction.

13.4.3 Postoperative Immobilization

Most dermatologic surgery is performed in the outpatient setting, eliminating the cost of postoperative hospitalization

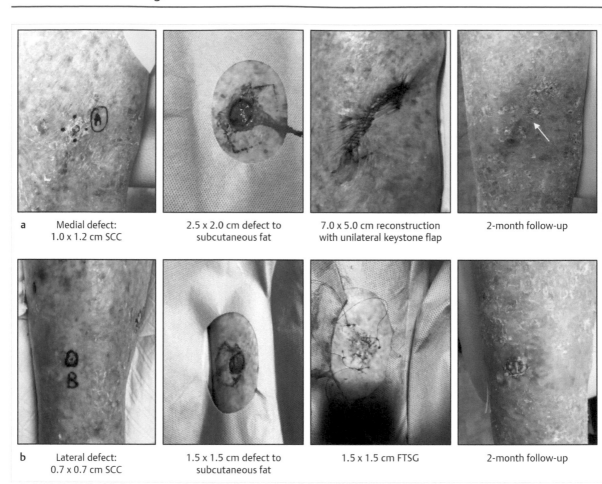

a	Medial defect:	2.5 x 2.0 cm defect to	7.0 x 5.0 cm reconstruction	2-month follow-up
	1.0 x 1.2 cm SCC	subcutaneous fat	with unilateral keystone flap	

b	Lateral defect:	1.5 x 1.5 cm defect to	1.5 x 1.5 cm FTSG	2-month follow-up
	0.7 x 0.7 cm SCC	subcutaneous fat		

Fig. 13.10 Adjacent defects in the same patient demonstrate superior healing and cosmetic outcomes with the keystone flap compared to full-thickness skin graft (FTSG). An 84-year-old man with stasis dermatitis and two squamous cell carcinomas (SCCs) on the right medial and lateral pretibial region, both treated with Mohs micrographic surgery (MMS). The medial defect **(a)** was repaired with a unilateral modification of the keystone flap, and the lateral defect **(b)** was repaired with an FTSG from the Burow's triangle of the adjacent keystone flap. An Unna boot was applied and changed weekly. At the 2-month follow-up, the patient presented with a well-healing keystone flap and a viable FTSG. This direct comparison of flap reconstruction (*white arrow*) and FTSG on the same patient with the same postoperative care demonstrates the superior cosmetic outcome and faster healing time of the keystone flap.

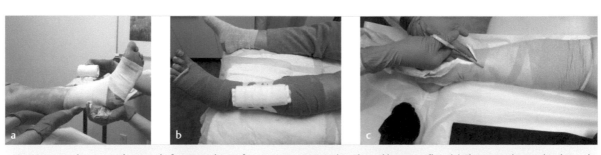

Fig. 13.11 Application and removal of an Unna boot after reconstruction with unilateral keystone flap. **(a)** The surgical wound is dressed with a mixture of mupirocin 2% ointment and petrolatum, and covered with a nonadherent dressing. Petrolatum is also applied to the entire lower leg to prevent irritation and pruritus. Then, gauze impregnated with zinc oxide is carefully wrapped around the lower extremity to provide mild compression without vascular compromise. Toes remain exposed to test capillary refill and ensure the dressing is not applied too tightly. **(b)** The zinc dressing is covered with a layer of dry gauze and then a self-adherent elastic wrap. An additional focal pressure dressing is placed over the surgical site to absorb wound exudate (this can be applied over or under the elastic wrap). **(c)** After 1 week, the Unna boot is removed carefully with scissors to avoid trauma to the underlying skin, either in the office or with a visiting nurse. The Unna boot is then replaced weekly for 2 to 4 weeks depending on patient tolerability and healing.

and the associated risk of nosocomial infections in an already vulnerable elderly population.[17] For larger cases requiring hospitalization, immobilization of the lower limb for up to 5 postoperative days (PODs) has been suggested following reconstruction of the lower extremity, particularly in patients receiving skin grafts.[41,62] Proponents of postoperative immobilization argue that ambulating before revascularization could increase the risk of graft failure.[62] On the other hand, there are significant risks associated with even short periods of immobilization, including physical deconditioning, increased risks of deep vein thrombosis and pulmonary embolism, and the cost and time required to care for an immobilized patient.[63]

Multiple recent studies have shown that immobilization is not necessary following reconstruction of lower extremity defects.[4,8,62,64] A prospective, randomized trial compared early mobilization with inpatient bed rest for an average hospital stay of 12 days following STSG repair of pretibial lacerations in the elderly.[64] At the 1- and 3-week follow-ups, the authors found no statistical difference in percentage of skin graft take. A third of the patients in the delayed ambulation group reported difficulty returning to an independent lifestyle. Another study randomized patients who received skin grafts on the lower extremity to ambulate within 24 hours or to remain on bed rest until POD 5. There was no significant difference in the number of patients who had graft loss between the two groups, and patients who began ambulating early reported less pain in both donor and graft sites.

Immobilization carries inherent risks, especially in elderly patients. Current evidence suggests that immobilization following dermatologic surgery is not necessary. In our center, we instruct patients to eliminate strenuous activity for three postoperative weeks. We also recommend leg elevation when possible but allow patients to slowly and carefully ambulate and pursue normal activities of daily living in the postoperative period.

13.5 Complications

13.5.1 Infection

Infection rates following excisions or MMS for cutaneous malignancies are low, ranging between 1 and 4%.[65,66,67] Below-the-knee surgery carries a higher rate of postoperative infections, with reports ranging between 3.3 and 17.6%.[20,65,68,69,70] Postoperative infections on the lower extremity can lead to wound dehiscence, flap necrosis, delayed healing, and poor cosmetic outcomes in an already technically challenging location.[65]

Dixon et al assessed 448 below-the-knee defects following dermatologic surgery and reported an infection rate of 6.92% in the absence of prophylactic antibiotics.[65] These rates were significantly higher than the 1.47% for other regions of the body. Interestingly, the authors reported that the majority of infections in below-the-knee

wounds progressed to cellulitis or infection necrosis, rather than an abscess. The authors postulated that the relative skin tightness and subsequent lack of dead space contributed to the decreased formation of abscesses. Not surprisingly, surgical site infection (SSI) rates for more complex dermatologic reconstructions are higher, with reports of 2.3 to 8.7% for reconstructive procedures (grafts and flaps) compared to 0.54 to 1.6% for simple excisions.[65,71] Increasing age and BMI, smoking, immunosuppression, and peripheral vascular disease are all factors that increase rates of SSIs.[72]

The medical team and patient must be vigilant with postoperative care to minimize risks of SSIs and intervene early if signs and symptoms of infection arise.

Antisepsis

Preoperative antiseptic treatment of the operative site is an important aspect of preventing SSIs. Careful attention to intraoperative antisepsis is especially important in locations at high risk of infection.

Povidone-iodine (PVI) and chlorhexidine gluconate (CHG) are the two most commonly utilized preoperative antiseptic preparations. Both PVI and CHG are available in aqueous and alcoholic solutions, and are effective against bacteria, fungi, and viruses.[73] A landmark study found that 2% chlorhexidine in 70% isopropyl alcohol was more efficacious than aqueous 10% PVI; however, the study was confounded by the addition of alcohol, itself an antiseptic, to chlorhexidine.[74] In another prospective trial, patients were randomized to either 0.5% CHG in 70% alcohol or 0.5% CHG in aqueous solution prior to minor skin excisions. At 30-day follow-up, there was no statistically significant difference in rates of SSIs between the treatment arms.[75]

In our practice, patients undergoing lower extremity procedures are instructed to decolonize the skin with daily chlorhexidine application at home for 1 week preoperatively. The skin is rigorously prepared from knee to foot with chlorhexidine before incision and an Unna boot applied after the operation is complete.

Prophylactic Antibiotics

Large-scale randomized trials have demonstrated that prophylactic topical antibiotics are not effective in preventing SSIs following dermatological surgery[76,77,78]; however, the evidence for prophylactic oral antibiotics is less certain for surgical sites on the lower extremities. Since wounds on the lower limb have higher rates of SSIs compared to other regions of the body, a 2008 advisory statement suggested consideration of cephalexin 2 g for prophylaxis prior to procedures in the groin and below the knee but noted a lack of high-quality data.[79,80] Several small studies have demonstrated possible decrease in SSI incidence with a single perioperative dose of cephalexin 2 g.[20,81]

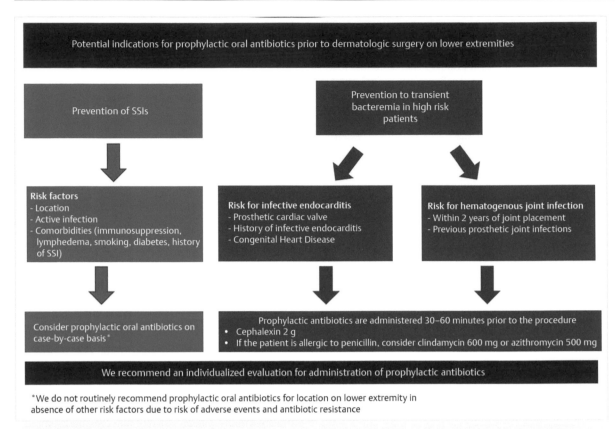

Fig. 13.12 Algorithm for antibiotic prophylaxis for patients undergoing reconstruction of lower extremity defects. Abbreviation: SSI, surgical site infection. (Recommendations are based on Wright et al,[79] Mourad et al,[82] and Lee and Paver.[83])

Other studies, however, have demonstrated no difference in infection rates with prophylactic oral antibiotics. A retrospective review of 271 cases of MMS or wide local excision (WLE) for below-the-knee cutaneous malignancies demonstrated no statistically significant difference in SSI frequency with prophylactic antibiotics.[80] The overall rates of SSI at 2 weeks were 2.3% in the MMS cohort and 8.3% in the WLE cohort. A recent meta-analysis including 839 patients randomized to receive either oral antibiotic prophylaxis or placebo prior to MMS on the ear and nose demonstrated no statistically significant reduction in SSIs with antibiotic prophylaxis.[82] Additionally, overuse of antibiotics exposes patients to potential adverse drug reactions and antibiotic resistance.

Our approach is to evaluate each patient's risk of postoperative infection individually, factoring in surgical location and other comorbidities such as immunosuppression, lymphedema, smoking, diabetes, and history of SSI. We do not routinely recommend prophylaxis based on lower leg location alone. In those at high risk, we typically administer cephalexin 2 g 30 to 60 minutes before incision. For patients with penicillin allergy, we consider clindamycin 600 mg or azithromycin 500 mg[79,83] (▶ Fig. 13.12). Further study is needed to better delineate the risks and benefits

of antibiotics in this population to prevent overuse and reduce bacterial resistance.

As in other surgical locations, prophylactic oral antibiotics are recommended in contaminated, dirty, or infected wounds, or in patients with high risk of infective endocarditis or hematogenous joint infection (generally within the first 2 years of joint replacement).

13.5.2 Dehiscence

Wound dehiscence is multifactorial, resulting from high tension at the surgical site, poor postoperative care, or atrophic and fragile skin quality often seen in elderly patients. Typically, wound dehiscence occurs within the first 7 PODs. A study of STSGs and primary closures on the lower extremity found the incidence of surgical site failure (graft failure or primary closure dehiscence) to be as high as 53.4%. STSGs, advanced age, SSI, and hematoma formation were significantly correlated with the risk of surgical site failure in patients undergoing ambulatory dermatologic surgery on the lower limb.[84] Postoperative edema following lower extremity reconstruction may also contribute to delayed healing and dehiscence.[85]

Wound dehiscence may also result from other wound complications, and these should be managed appropriately. This includes drainage of seroma or hematoma and management of any infections. Debridement of any necrotic or nonviable tissue followed by repeat wound closure is an option; however, the authors generally prefer conservative management and SIH for any dehisced areas. Delayed revision could be considered if the patient desires. As with any other surgical complication, patients should be closely followed to ensure eventual improvement.

13.5.3 Contact and Stasis Dermatitis

Each step of cutaneous surgery may expose the patient to contact allergens, including PVI, nickel-plated instruments, sutures, surgical glues, dressings, bacitracin, and neomycin.[86,87,88,89,90] Preoperative evaluation should elicit history of allergies or sensitivities. Allergens should be avoided, and dermatitis treated with topical steroids.

As discussed previously, compression therapy is the best option for prevention and management of stasis dermatitis. Increasing age, prolonged immobilization, female gender, obesity, deep venous thrombosis (DVT), and pregnancy are risk factors for stasis dermatitis.[91] Treatment of secondary cutaneous pigmentation due to stasis dermatitis is challenging, with the use of noncoherent intense pulsed light source showing promise.[92] Any laser procedure on the lower extremities should be performed with caution, as complications like dyspigmentation are more common.

13.5.4 Hematoma or Seroma

Development of a hematoma is one of the most common postoperative complications in dermatologic surgery. A prospective study of 1,343 MMS cases found that hematomas make up 32% of all complications.[93] Hematomas and seromas can lead to an increased risk of wound infection, dehiscence, and necrosis.[94]

Preoperative assessment and meticulous surgical technique are critical in predicting and preventing hemorrhagic complications. We do not recommend routine discontinuation of anticoagulants before cutaneous surgery, as the risks are often higher than the risk of postoperative bleeding. Multiple studies have clearly demonstrated that aspirin, warfarin, and nonsteroidal anti-inflammatory agents do not significantly increase the risk of postoperative complications in dermatologic surgery.[95,96] This is particularly true on the lower extremities. Even with larger flap and graft reconstruction, we have not observed an increase in bleeding complications in patients on anticoagulants (unpublished data). Postoperative wound pressure dressings decrease bruising and prevent hematomas and seromas.

Table 13.1 Comparison of reconstructive outcomes for flaps versus grafts on the lower extremity

Outcome	Most effective		Least effective
Reliability	Flap	STSG	FTSG
Tissue match	Flap	FTSG	STSG
Contour match	Flap	FTSG	STSG

Abbreviations: FTSG, full-thickness skin grafts; STSG, split-thickness skin grafts.

13.5.5 Management of Scarring

Scarring is inevitable after cutaneous surgery. Hypertrophic scars can often be managed with noninvasive methods, including silicone gel sheets, pressure or massage therapy, intralesional corticosteroid injections, carbon dioxide and pulsed-dye lasers, or even revision if contractures limit function.[97] Keloid scars are often more difficult to manage. In addition to the above modalities, a combination of surgical excision, radiation therapy, and intralesional 5-fluorouracil and corticosteroids may be used for management of keloids.[98,99,100,101,102] Scars or postoperative edema that limit range of motion often improve with physical therapy.

13.6 Conclusion

Reconstruction of lower extremity surgical defects remains a clinical challenge. Patient comorbidities and lifestyle must be considered when selecting a reconstructive approach. SIH and primary linear closure are frequently utilized for small defects. Large wounds not amenable to a more conservative approach are better repaired with skin grafts and local flaps. In our experience, skin grafts have less reliable healing with variable cosmetic outcomes, leading to our increased use of perforator flaps like the keystone advancement flap (▶ Table 13.1). Clear preoperative counseling, meticulous intraoperative technique, careful postoperative wound care, and early intervention for complications can help overcome the challenges of lower extremity surgery and lead to successful reconstructive outcomes.

References

[1] Gallagher RP, Ma B, McLean DI, et al. Trends in basal cell carcinoma, squamous cell carcinoma, and melanoma of the skin from 1973 through 1987. J Am Acad Dermatol. 1990; 23(3, Pt 1): 413–421

[2] Kim C, Ko CJ, Leffell DJ. Cutaneous squamous cell carcinomas of the lower extremity: a distinct subset of squamous cell carcinomas. J Am Acad Dermatol. 2014; 70(1):70–74

[3] Eberhardt RT, Raffetto JD. Chronic venous insufficiency. Circulation. 2014; 130(4):333–346

[4] Oganesyan G, Jarell AD, Srivastava M, Jiang SI. Efficacy and complication rates of full-thickness skin graft repair of lower extremity wounds after Mohs micrographic surgery. Dermatol Surg. 2013; 39(9):1334–1339

[5] Rao K, Tillo O, Dalal M. Full thickness skin graft cover for lower limb defects following excision of cutaneous lesions. Dermatol Online J. 2008; 14(2):4

[6] Zitelli JA. Secondary intention healing: an alternative to surgical repair. Clin Dermatol. 1984; 2(3):92–106

[7] Perper M, Eber A, Lindsey SF, Nouri K. Blinded, randomized, controlled trial evaluating the effects of light-emitting diode photomodulation on lower extremity wounds left to heal by secondary intention. Dermatol Surg. 2020; 46(5):605–611

[8] Audrain H, Bray A, De Berker D. Full-thickness skin grafts for lower leg defects: an effective repair option. Dermatol Surg. 2015; 41(4):493–498

[9] Joo J, Custis T, Armstrong AW, et al. Purse-string suture vs second intention healing: results of a randomized, blind clinical trial. JAMA Dermatol. 2015; 151(3):265–270

[10] Jung JY, Roh HJ, Lee SH, Nam K, Chung KY. Comparison of secondary intention healing and full-thickness skin graft after excision of acral lentiginous melanoma on foot. Dermatol Surg. 2011; 37(9):1245–1251

[11] Adams DC, Ramsey ML. Grafts in dermatologic surgery: review and update on full- and split-thickness skin grafts, free cartilage grafts, and composite grafts. Dermatol Surg. 2005; 31(8, Pt 2):1055–1067

[12] Anderson JJ, Wallin KJ, Spencer L. Split thickness skin grafts for the treatment of non-healing foot and leg ulcers in patients with diabetes: a retrospective review. Diabet Foot Ankle. 2012; 3(3):1024–1030

[13] Kirsner RS, Falanga V. Techniques of split-thickness skin grafting for lower extremity ulcerations. J Dermatol Surg Oncol. 1993; 19(8):779–783

[14] Reddy S, El-Haddawi F, Fancourt M, et al. The incidence and risk factors for lower limb skin graft failure. Dermatol Res Pract. 2014; 2014:582080

[15] Harvey I, Smith S, Patterson I. The use of quilted full thickness skin grafts in the lower limb: reliable results with early mobilization. J Plast Reconstr Aesthet Surg. 2009; 62(7):969–972

[16] Lewis JM, Zager JS, Yu D, et al. Full-thickness grafts procured from skin overlying the sentinel lymph node basin; reconstruction of primary cutaneous malignancy excision defects. Ann Surg Oncol. 2008; 15(6):1733–1740

[17] Coldiron BM, Rivera E. Delayed full-thickness grafting of lower leg defects following removal of skin malignancies. Dermatol Surg. 1996; 22(1):23–26

[18] Ochoa SA. Nonfacial reconstructive techniques. Dermatol Surg. 2015; 41 Suppl 10:S229–S238

[19] Wilson JA, Clark JJ. Obesity: impediment to postsurgical wound healing. Adv Skin Wound Care. 2004; 17(8):426–435

[20] Struk S, Correia N, Guenane Y, Revol M, Cristofari S. Full-thickness skin grafts for lower leg defects coverage: interest of postoperative immobilization. Ann Chir Plast Esthet. 2018; 63(3):229–233

[21] Sharpe DT, Cardoso E, Baheti V. The immediate mobilisation of patients with lower limb skin grafts: a clinical report. Br J Plast Surg. 1983; 36(1):105–108

[22] Quatrano NA, Samie FH. Modification of Burow's advancement flap: avoiding the secondary triangle. JAMA Facial Plast Surg. 2014; 16(5):364–366

[23] Metz BJ, Katta R. Burow's advancement flap closure of adjacent defects. Dermatol Online J. 2005; 11(1):11

[24] Khouri JS, Egeland BM, Daily SD, et al. The keystone island flap: use in large defects of the trunk and extremities in soft-tissue reconstruction. Plast Reconstr Surg. 2011; 127(3):1212–1221

[25] Huang J, Yu N, Long X, Wang X. A systematic review of the keystone design perforator island flap in lower extremity defects. Medicine (Baltimore). 2017; 96(21):e6842

[26] Dini M, Innocenti A, Russo GL, Agostini V. The use of the V-Y fasciocutaneous island advancement flap in reconstructing postsurgical defects of the leg. Dermatol Surg. 2001; 27(1):44–46

[27] Georgeu GA, El-Muttardi N. The horn shaped fascio-cutaneous flap usage in cutaneous malignancy of the leg. Br J Plast Surg. 2004; 57(1):66–76

[28] Penington AJ, Mallucci P. Closure of elective skin defects in the leg with a fasciocutaneous V-Y island flap. Br J Plast Surg. 1999; 52(6):458–461

[29] Behan FC, Terrill PJ, Breidahl A, et al. Island flaps including the Bezier type in the treatment of malignant melanoma. Aust N Z J Surg. 1995; 65(12):870–880

[30] Niranjan NS, Price RD, Govilkar P. Fascial feeder and perforator-based V-Y advancement flaps in the reconstruction of lower limb defects. Br J Plast Surg. 2000; 53(8):679–689

[31] Venkataramakrishnan V, Mohan D, Villafane O. Perforator based V-Y advancement flaps in the leg. Br J Plast Surg. 1998; 51(6):431–435

[32] Calderón W, Andrades P, Leniz P, et al. The cone flap: a new and versatile fasciocutaneous flap. Plast Reconstr Surg. 2004; 114(6):1539–1542

[33] Behan F, Findlay M, Lo CH. The Keystone Perforator Island Flap Concept. 1st ed. Sydney: Churchill Livingstone; 2012

[34] Behan FC. The keystone design perforator island flap in reconstructive surgery. ANZ J Surg. 2003; 73(3):112–120

[35] Martinez JC, Cook JL, Otley C. The keystone fasciocutaneous flap in the reconstruction of lower extremity wounds. Dermatol Surg. 2012; 38(3):484–489

[36] Hessam S, Sand M, Bechara FG. The keystone flap: expanding the dermatologic surgeon's armamentarium. J Dtsch Dermatol Ges. 2015; 13(1):70–72

[37] Rao AL, Janna RK. Keystone flap: versatile flap for reconstruction of limb defects. J Clin Diagn Res. 2015; 9(3):PC05–PC07

[38] Hu M, Bordeaux JS. The keystone flap for lower extremity defects. Dermatol Surg. 2012; 38(3):490–493

[39] Magliano J, Falco S, Agorio C, Bazzano C. Modified keystone flap for extremity defects after Mohs surgery. Int J Dermatol. 2016; 55(12):1391–1395

[40] Stone JP, Webb C, McKinnon JG, Dawes JC, McKenzie CD, Temple-Oberle CF. Avoiding skin grafts: the keystone flap in cutaneous defects. Plast Reconstr Surg. 2015; 136(2):404–408

[41] Moncrieff MD, Bowen F, Thompson JF, et al. Keystone flap reconstruction of primary melanoma excision defects of the leg-the end of the skin graft? Ann Surg Oncol. 2008; 15(10):2867–2873

[42] Petukhova TA, Navrazhina K, Minkis K. V-Y hemi-keystone advancement flap: a novel and simplified reconstructive modification. Plast Reconstr Surg Glob Open. 2020; 8(2):e2654

[43] Yoon CS, Kim SI, Kim H, Kim KN. Keystone-designed perforator island flaps for the coverage of traumatic pretibial defects in patients with comorbidities. Int J Low Extrem Wounds. 2017; 16(4):302–309

[44] Bekara F, Herlin C, Somda S, de Runz A, Grolleau JL, Chaput B. Free versus perforator-pedicled propeller flaps in lower extremity reconstruction: what is the safest coverage? A meta-analysis. Microsurgery. 2018; 38(1):109–119

[45] Behan F, Sizeland A, Porcedu S, Somia N, Wilson J. Keystone island flap: an alternative reconstructive option to free flaps in irradiated tissue. ANZ J Surg. 2006; 76(5):407–413

[46] Lionelli GT, Lawrence WT. Wound dressings. Surg Clin North Am. 2003; 83(3):617–638

[47] Helfman T, Ovington L, Falanga V. Occlusive dressings and wound healing. Clin Dermatol. 1994; 12(1):121–127

[48] Eaglstein WH, Mertz PM. New methods for assessing epidermal wound healing: the effects of triamcinolone acetonide and polyethelene film occlusion. J Invest Dermatol. 1978; 71(6):382–384

[49] Stebbins WG, Hanke CW, Petersen J. Enhanced healing of surgical wounds of the lower leg using weekly zinc oxide compression dressings. Dermatol Surg. 2011; 37(2):158–165

[50] Nemeth AJ, Eaglstein WH, Taylor JR, Peerson LJ, Falanga V. Faster healing and less pain in skin biopsy sites treated with an occlusive dressing. Arch Dermatol. 1991; 127(11):1679–1683

[51] Kikta MJ, Schuler JJ, Meyer JP, et al. A prospective, randomized trial of Unna's boots versus hydroactive dressing in the treatment of venous stasis ulcers. J Vasc Surg. 1988; 7(3):478–483

[52] Koksal C, Bozkurt AK. Combination of hydrocolloid dressing and medical compression stockings versus Unna's boot for the treatment of venous leg ulcers. Swiss Med Wkly. 2003; 133(25–26):364–368

[53] Fletcher A, Cullum N, Sheldon TA. A systematic review of compression treatment for venous leg ulcers. BMJ. 1997; 315(7108): 576–580

[54] Thompson CB, Wiemken TL, Brown TS. Effect of postoperative dressing on excisions performed on the leg: a comparison between zinc oxide compression dressings versus standard wound care. Dermatol Surg. 2017; 43(11):1379–1384

[55] Lansdown AB, Mirastschijski U, Stubbs N, Scanlon E, Agren MS. Zinc in wound healing: theoretical, experimental, and clinical aspects. Wound Repair Regen. 2007; 15(1):2–16

[56] Lansdown AB. Influence of zinc oxide in the closure of open skin wounds. Int J Cosmet Sci. 1993; 15(2):83–85

[57] Arslan K, Karahan O, Okuş A, et al. Comparison of topical zinc oxide and silver sulfadiazine in burn wounds: an experimental study. Ulus Travma Acil Cerrahi Derg. 2012; 18(5):376–383

[58] Agren MS. Zinc in wound repair. Arch Dermatol. 1999; 135(10): 1273–1274

[59] Agren MS, Chvapil M, Franzén L. Enhancement of re-epithelialization with topical zinc oxide in porcine partial-thickness wounds. J Surg Res. 1991; 50(2):101–105

[60] Akiyama H, Yamasaki O, Kanzaki H, Tada J, Arata J. Effects of zinc oxide on the attachment of Staphylococcus aureus strains. J Dermatol Sci. 1998; 17(1):67–74

[61] Sunzel B, Lasek J, Söderberg T, Elmros T, Hallmans G, Holm S. The effect of zinc oxide on Staphylococcus aureus and polymorphonuclear cells in a tissue cage model. Scand J Plast Reconstr Surg Hand Surg. 1990; 24(1):31–35

[62] Lorello DJ, Peck M, Albrecht M, Richey KJ, Pressman MA. Results of a prospective randomized controlled trial of early ambulation for patients with lower extremity autografts. J Burn Care Res. 2014; 35 (5):431–436

[63] Gawaziuk JP, Peters B, Logsetty S. Early ambulation after-grafting of lower extremity burns. Burns. 2018; 44(1):183–187

[64] Budny PG, Lavelle J, Regan PJ, Roberts AH. Pretibial injuries in the elderly: a prospective trial of early mobilisation versus bed rest following surgical treatment. Br J Plast Surg. 1993; 46(7):594–598

[65] Dixon AJ, Dixon MP, Askew DA, Wilkinson D. Prospective study of wound infections in dermatologic surgery in the absence of prophylactic antibiotics. Dermatol Surg. 2006; 32(6):819–826, discussion 826–827

[66] Whitaker DC, Grande DJ, Johnson SS. Wound infection rate in dermatologic surgery. J Dermatol Surg Oncol. 1988; 14(5):525–528

[67] Rabb DC, Lesher JL, Jr. Antibiotic prophylaxis in cutaneous surgery. Dermatol Surg. 1995; 21(6):550–554

[68] Garland R, Frizelle FA, Dobbs BR, Singh H. A retrospective audit of long-term lower limb complications following leg vein harvesting for coronary artery bypass grafting. Eur J Cardiothorac Surg. 2003; 23(6):950–955

[69] Bordeaux JS, Martires KJ, Goldberg D, Pattee SF, Fu P, Maloney ME. Prospective evaluation of dermatologic surgery complications including patients on multiple antiplatelet and anticoagulant medications. J Am Acad Dermatol. 2011; 65(3):576–583

[70] Penington A. Ulceration and antihypertensive use are risk factors for infection after skin lesion excision. ANZ J Surg. 2010; 80(9):642–645

[71] Rogues AM, Lasheras A, Amici JM, et al. Infection control practices and infectious complications in dermatological surgery. J Hosp Infect. 2007; 65(3):258–263

[72] Maragh SL, Otley CC, Roenigk RK, Phillips PK, Division of Dermatologic Surgery, Mayo Clinic, Rochester, MN. Antibiotic prophylaxis in dermatologic surgery: updated guidelines. Dermatol Surg. 2005; 31(1):83–91

[73] Heal CF, Charles D, Hardy A, et al. Protocol for a randomised controlled trial comparing aqueous with alcoholic chlorhexidine antisepsis for the prevention of superficial surgical site infection after minor surgery in general practice: the AVALANCHE trial. BMJ Open. 2016; 6(7):e011604

[74] Darouiche RO, Wall MJ, Jr, Itani KM, et al. Chlorhexidine-alcohol versus povidone-iodine for surgical-site antisepsis. N Engl J Med. 2010; 362(1):18–26

[75] Charles D, Heal CF, Delpachitra M, et al. Alcoholic versus aqueous chlorhexidine for skin antisepsis: the AVALANCHE trial. CMAJ. 2017; 189(31):E1008–E1016

[76] Saco M, Howe N, Nathoo R, Cherpelis B. Topical antibiotic prophylaxis for prevention of surgical wound infections from dermatologic procedures: a systematic review and meta-analysis. J Dermatolog Treat. 2015; 26(2):151–158

[77] Smack DP, Harrington AC, Dunn C, et al. Infection and allergy incidence in ambulatory surgery patients using white petrolatum vs bacitracin ointment. A randomized controlled trial. JAMA. 1996; 276(12):972–977

[78] Dixon AJ, Dixon MP, Dixon JB. Randomized clinical trial of the effect of applying ointment to surgical wounds before occlusive dressing. Br J Surg. 2006; 93(8):937–943

[79] Wright TI, Baddour LM, Berbari EF, et al. Antibiotic prophylaxis in dermatologic surgery: advisory statement 2008. J Am Acad Dermatol. 2008; 59(3):464–473

[80] Bari O, Eilers RE, Jr, Rubin AG, Jiang SIB. Clinical characteristics of lower extremity surgical site infections in dermatologic surgery based upon 24-month retrospective review. J Drugs Dermatol. 2018; 17(7):766–771

[81] Smith SC, Heal CF, Buttner PG. Prevention of surgical site infection in lower limb skin lesion excisions with single dose oral antibiotic prophylaxis: a prospective randomised placebo-controlled double-blind trial. BMJ Open. 2014; 4(7):e005270

[82] Mourad A, Gniadecki R, Taher M. Oral and intraincisional antibiotic prophylaxis in Mohs surgery: a systematic review and meta-analysis. Dermatol Surg. 2020; 46(4):558–560

[83] Lee MR, Paver R. Prophylactic antibiotics in dermatological surgery. Australas J Dermatol. 2016; 57(2):83–91

[84] Stankiewicz M, Coyer F, Webster J, Osborne S. Incidence and predictors of lower limb split-skin graft failure and primary closure dehiscence in day-case surgical patients. Dermatol Surg. 2015; 41 (7):775–783

[85] Unal C, Gercek H. Use of custom-made stockings to control postoperative leg and foot edema following free tissue transfer and external fixation of fractures. J Foot Ankle Surg. 2012; 51(2):246–248

[86] Jacob SE, James WD. From road rash to top allergen in a flash: bacitracin. Dermatol Surg. 2004; 30(4, Pt 1):521–524

[87] Cohen DE, Kaufmann JM. Hypersensitivity reactions to products and devices in plastic surgery. Facial Plast Surg Clin North Am. 2003; 11 (2):253–265

[88] Bitterman A, Sandhu K. Allergic contact dermatitis to 2-octyl cyanoacrylate after surgical repair: humidity as a potential factor. JAAD Case Rep. 2017; 3(6):480–481

[89] Jacob SE, Amado A, Cohen DE. Dermatologic surgical implications of allergic contact dermatitis. Dermatol Surg. 2005; 31(9, Pt 1):1116–1123

[90] Sánchez-Morillas L, Reaño Martos M, Rodríguez Mosquera M, Iglesias Cadarso A, Pérez Pimiento A, Domínguez Lázaro AR. Delayed sensitivity to Prolene. Contact Dermat. 2003; 48(6):338–339

[91] Sundaresan S, Migden MR, Silapunt S. Stasis dermatitis: pathophysiology, evaluation, and management. Am J Clin Dermatol. 2017; 18(3):383–390

[92] Pimentel CL, Rodriguez-Salido MJ. Pigmentation due to stasis dermatitis treated successfully with a noncoherent intense pulsed light source. Dermatol Surg. 2008; 34(7):950–951

[93] Cook JL, Perone JB. A prospective evaluation of the incidence of complications associated with Mohs micrographic surgery. Arch Dermatol. 2003; 139(2):143–152

[94] Bunick CG, Aasi SZ. Hemorrhagic complications in dermatologic surgery. Dermatol Ther (Heidelb). 2011; 24(6):537–550

[95] Billingsley EM, Maloney ME. Intraoperative and postoperative bleeding problems in patients taking warfarin, aspirin, and nonsteroidal antiinflammatory agents. A prospective study. Dermatol Surg. 1997; 23(5):381–383, discussion 384–385

[96] Otley CC, Fewkes JL, Frank W, Olbricht SM. Complications of cutaneous surgery in patients who are taking warfarin, aspirin, or nonsteroidal anti-inflammatory drugs. Arch Dermatol. 1996; 132 (2):161–166

[97] Alster TS. Improvement of erythematous and hypertrophic scars by the 585-nm flashlamp-pumped pulsed dye laser. Ann Plast Surg. 1994; 32(2):186–190

[98] Jones K, Fuller CD, Luh JY, et al. Case report and summary of literature: giant perineal keloids treated with post-excisional radiotherapy. BMC Dermatol. 2006; 6:7

[99] Norris JE. Superficial X-ray therapy in keloid management: a retrospective study of 24 cases and literature review. Plast Reconstr Surg. 1995; 95(6):1051–1055

[100] Klumpar DI, Murray JC, Anscher M. Keloids treated with excision followed by radiation therapy. J Am Acad Dermatol. 1994; 31(2, Pt 1):225–231

[101] Akita S, Akino K, Yakabe A, et al. Combined surgical excision and radiation therapy for keloid treatment. J Craniofac Surg. 2007; 18 (5):1164–1169

[102] Shah VV, Aldahan AS, Mlacker S, Alsaidan M, Samarkandy S, Nouri K. 5-fluorouracil in the treatment of keloids and hypertrophic scars: a comprehensive review of the literature. Dermatol Ther (Heidelb). 2016; 6(2):169–183

14 Reconstruction of Scars

Jill Waibel, Chloe Gianatasio, and Rebecca Lissette Quinonez

Summary

Scarring is a complex cutaneous phenomenon with many different profiles, presentations, and prognoses. Some scars, such as typical surgical scars, fade in time until ultimately blending seamlessly into the rest of the skin, while some, such as keloid scars, continue to grow and develop worsening symptomatology for many years after injury. Variations in physical characteristics are dependent on the source of the scarring, the timing and measures taken for prevention, and the healing capabilities of the individual. However, certain factors remain consistent across scar profiles:

- Cutaneous insults deeper than 0.56 ± 0.03 mm will form a human scar (with the exception of keloids, which can result from even a superficial injury).[1]
- Lack of appropriate scar treatment can cause physical and psychosocial consequences of long-term, if not permanent, duration.

Keywords: scar, fractional ablative-non-ablative laser, CO_2 laser, hypertrophicr, keloidr, atrophic scar, hypopigmented scar, Z plasty, W plasty

14.1 Introduction: Why Do We Scar?

Any insult to the skin initiates a wound-healing response. At sufficient depths of dermal injury, the complexity of the wound exceeds the body's ability to restore normal skin structure. A major component of cutaneous strength and flexibility is in the collagen, which has three subtypes: types I, II, and III. Collagen acts as a scaffold in connective tissue and plays a major role in multiple important wound-healing processes such as protein synthesis of the extracellular matrix (ECM), cytokine and growth factor synthesis and release, and regulation/interaction of other key players in the global wound-healing process such as matrix metalloproteinases (MMPs) and tissue inhibitors. It also undergoes substantial remodeling following injury. Human skin is composed primarily of type III collagen, which dominates fetal wound healing, the predominant model of scarless healing. In normal early adult wounds, type III collagen is the first to be laid down.[2] Type I collagen (mature collagen) dominates scar tissue and the proportion compared to type III collagen increases with the degree of scar formation.[3] Excess proliferation of this primarily type I collagen outcompetes the normally coordinated other components of the ECM by healing not only in excess but also without coordination.[4] This imbalance is an unsuccessful attempt to rapidly restore skin strength, the primary responsibility of type I collagen, but it instead causes rigidity and limits recovery to a maximum of 70% of its prior strength.[5] Recently, an additional theory has emerged to help explain this differential wound healing, which

involves the importance of papillary fibroblasts. Papillary dermal fibroblasts have been associated with improved keratinocyte viability and ECM development compared to reticular dermal fibroblasts.[6] In vitro models have revealed more stratified and differentiated epidermis development from young papillary fibroblasts than both reticular fibroblasts and even old papillary fibroblasts. As such, dysregulation of fibroblast production may also play a critical role in the development of scar tissue.

14.2 Types of Scars

The basic underlying mechanism of scar formation as outline above is consistent in any wound of sufficient depth. However, variations in the cutaneous recovery process result in categorization into specific scar subtypes based on their morphologies: atrophic, hypertrophic, keloid, and contracture.

14.2.1 Atrophic

One of the most common causes of atrophic scarring is acne. The presentation of acne scars is largely location dependent with bodily acne scars commonly resulting in hypertrophy and facial scars resulting in atrophy. The primary contributor to this scarring is inflammation, the root of acne lesions, helping explain why such a large percentage of atrophic scarring is acne related. The longer and slower the inflammatory reaction, the worse the resultant scarring. Whether the collagen deposition is over- or underactive is influenced by the communication of extracellular MMPs and their tissue inhibitors. MMPs degrade the ECM in the wound-healing process to allow for remodeling. However, overactive MMPs degrade faster than the remodeling can occur, leading to the formation of atrophic scarring.[7] Atrophic acne scars present in three different forms: "ice pick" (approximately 2-mm punctiform, deep scars), boxcar (shallow and sharp edged), and rolling (wider and untapered) scars.[8] Atrophic scarring can also occur from inflammatory diseases such as chicken pox or from trauma (▶ Fig. 14.1). Once scarring has occurred, these scars undergo minimal to no change.

14.2.2 Hypertrophic

Hypertrophic scarring also occurs from prolonged inflammation and imbalanced anabolic versus catabolic mechanisms, but in the opposite direction from atrophic scarring (▶ Fig. 14.2). In hypertrophic scarring, deposition reigns accompanied by overproduction of fibroblasts, proteoglycans, vasculature, and other ECM components. Hypertrophy does not occur immediately, but begins at approximately 4 to 7 months following burn injury. Hypertrophy in surgical scars can begin as soon as 1 month following insult,

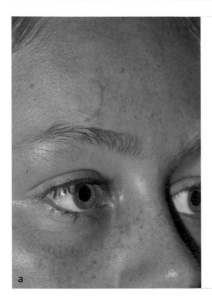
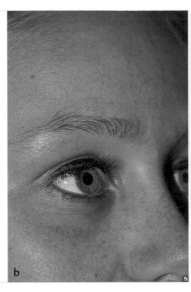

Fig. 14.1 A 22-year-old Caucasian woman who received a scar from a chemistry experiment causing scar to be atrophic before (a) and after (b) one treatment of fractional ablative laser along with laser-assisted delivery of poly-L-lactic acid. (Reprinted from Facial Plastic Surgery Clinics of North America. 25(1). Jill S Waibel and Ashley Rudnick. Laser-assisted delivery to treat facial scars. Copyright [2017] with permission from Elsevier.)

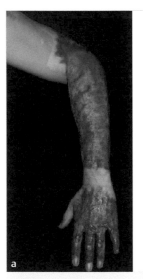
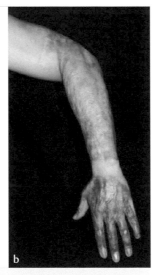

Fig. 14.2 A 30-year-old male Fitzpatrick skin type (FST)-III plane crash survivor before (a) and after (b) undergoing a series of seven treatments of combined IPL, 1927-nm Thulium, AFL erbium, and Kenalog 10.

particularly in areas of high tension. Some hypertrophic scars can spontaneously regress, improving with time, but rarely resolve completely. Hypertrophic scarring also does not surpass the lateral confines of the original wound, but it can continue to build vertically for months to several years.[9]

14.2.3 Keloid

Keloids possess much of the features of hypertrophic scars, with excess deposition of collagen and overactivity of extracellular protein/fibroblast proliferation. But keloids also have unique characteristics that require highly specialized treatment considerations. Keloids have

a strong genetic component[10] and occur often in areas of high tension such as the shoulders and chest. However, genetics vary; some are prone to forming keloids with any minor assault, including acne, on any part of the body surface. Others develop keloids specifically of the ears with completely normal scarring from bodily trauma. Keloids can continue to grow substantially longer than hypertrophic scars and spread beyond the confines of the initial injury margins. They are also rare in their ability, and seeming eagerness, to recur.

14.2.4 Contracture

Formation of contractures is generally limited to burn and trauma injury with severity correlating with depth of burn. Deep dermal or full-thickness burns cause destruction of deep epidermal structures, leading to inhibition of adequate re-epithelialization.[11] Contractures are a dense, excessive thickening and tightening of mature scar tissue that limits range of motion, often exacerbated by factors such as skin grafting, which limit the body's production of new tissue and lead to irregular closure of the wounds around the additional tissue. One study found that more than a third of major burn injuries developed a contracture upon hospital discharge.[12] The mechanism is poorly understood but suspected to be largely mediated by myofibroblasts, which are responsible for the contraction of skin in normal wound healing.[13]

14.3 Scar Prevention

14.3.1 Early Intervention

Evidence is increasingly mounting to support that the best treatment of scarring is to prevent it from occurring.[14,15] If proper action is taken during the healing process, the risk of pathological scarring can be reduced or the results

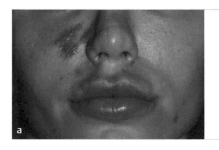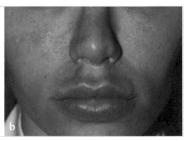

Fig. 14.3 A 30-year-old female Fitzpatrick skin type (FST)-III before (a) and after (b) undergoing two treatment sessions with PDL, 1927-nm and AFL on the right cheek after a dog bite. Image (a) was taken 1 month after her surgical revision.

minimized. Depending on the source of scarring, there are several different prevention mechanisms (▶ Fig. 14.3).

14.3.2 Passive and Active Therapies

Passive: Silicone and Sun Protection

There are certain features of scar formation that are essentially universal in humans. One such feature is epithelial disruption and resultant water loss in wounded tissue. Skin injury upsets sodium channel homeostasis in keratinocytes, causing sodium influx and activation of proinflammatory cytokines that induce fibroblast activation through the cyclooxygenase-2 (COX-2)/prostaglandin E2 (PGE2) pathway.[16] Inflammation is a well-studied contributor to scar exacerbation,[17] and, as such, prolonging this phenomenon promotes the scar-inducing cascade. Passive therapies are available to help mitigate this risk through superficial moisturization. One of the primarily used and most effective mechanisms in this arena is silicone both in gel and sheet form. Silicone products locally retain moisture to help reduce underlying dehydration and calm the inflammatory cycle. The use of sheeting adds the additional beneficial component of pressure, helping mitigate fibroblast proliferation, which will be further addressed in active therapies.

In addition to inflammation, sun exposure has been widely purported to worsen the appearance of scarring, particularly in darker skinned patients. In some cases, this is simply due to the darkening of pigmentation or the increase in discrepancy between a scar and the surrounding skin. In others, the sun is expected to have a negative impact on the process of wound healing itself. One study in murine models examined the impact of ultraviolet B (UVB) on wound healing and epidermal keratinocyte motility and found that wound closure was delayed significantly compared to normal mice. Keratinocyte motility was also inhibited substantially through alteration of focal adhesion turnover and cytoskeletal dynamics. Healing of full thickness wounds was accordingly delayed.[18] Delayed wound healing suggests prolonged inflammation, which, again, exacerbates scar formation. Studies in humans have suggested that a healing time of over 21 days greatly increases the risk of hypertrophic scarring.[19] Impedance of cellular adhesion and migration also likely interferes with the ability of the new skin structure to

form normally or adequately. Regardless of the mechanism at play and the type of scar, sun protection is a beneficial passive therapy. This can be achieved through physical sunscreens (zinc oxide or titanium dioxide base) or full coverage of the healing area. The growing popularity of passive scar treatments has also produced recent products that provide both silicone hydration and physical sunscreen in the same product, allowing easy maximization of home remedies to mitigate scar risk. For simple scars such as many surgical scars, these passive measures may be enough to prevent or minimize scarring on their own. As injuries become deeper and more complex, more extensive measures must be taken to avoid pathological scarring.

Active: Physical Therapy (Stretching, Massage), Compression/Pressure Garments

In more severe injuries such as burn and trauma wounds, scar prevention is more complicated than hydration and sun protection. Although these passive measures will still provide some benefit, they are far less likely to be sufficient on their own. As mentioned, large surface area and/or full-thickness wounds are at high contracture risk. Once a wound has settled into a contracture, the result is often restrictive, painful, pruritic, and psychologically devastating. Active measures aim to redirect healing and reduce the ability of the scarring process to progress. One such method is compression. Compression is an effective treatment both stand-alone and in conjunction with other treatments such as laser or surgery. Wounds treated with approximately 15 to 25 mm Hg of compression have been shown to soften, reduce in thickness, and improve in overall clinical appearance.[20,21] The suspected mechanism is the reduction of capillary flow, limiting oxygen and nutrients that would promote collagen production and fibroblast proliferation. Although collagen is important for skin strength, this helps prevent the excess proliferation. Not only does it limit production but it also limits the capacity to build vertically from mechanical restriction. When this pressure is provided through silicone gel sheeting, a combination product of silicone gel and compression, it provides the added benefits of hydration of the stratum corneum through reduction of transepidermal water loss.[22] Coverage also aids in sun protection and, when kept clean, preventative infection control.

Though less extensively studied, massage and strategic stretching have also shown beneficial effects on scar quality and progression. It is important to note for these strategies, however, that full healing must be complete, which was not the case for sun avoidance, silicone gels, or compression. Stretching skin during the proliferative and remodeling phases, particularly on suture lines, may increase tension, a common cause of hypertrophic and keloid scarring. While the skin is healing, stretching should be avoided. However, hypertrophic scars may benefit from massage and physical therapy stretching to help break up scar fibers and increase pliability, assisting particularly in range-of-motion deficits.[23]

14.3.3 To Skin Graft or not to Skin Graft

Burn rehabilitation is complex with wide variability in patient response and success. Understandably, the primary concern of the burn unit has been focused on saving the patient's life by reestablishing skin integrity. This is done largely through skin grafting, both autologous and allogenic. Although not widely studied at this point, there is increasing discussion about whether skin grafting should be used as widely as is current practice. Skin grafting increases scarring through multiple mechanisms. First, it typically leaves an obvious skin mismatch (complete with waffling, hair growth, color gradients, and thickness discrepancies) due to the donor site often being from a completely different part of the body that has different cutaneous characteristics. Additionally, there can be a large scar formed at the donor site, which, in rare cases, can even be worse than that of the area being grafted. The combination of several cumbersome visible scars can be psychologically detrimental.

Of course, the decision of whether or not to skin graft is more complicated than just the desire to avoid scarring. The burn surgeon has to make this challenging decision based on the size of the injury, whether or not the blood vessels are viable to allow healing, the patient's pain level, and other situational factors. If the wound is partial thickness, the skin may be able to heal without grafting, but it may take several weeks that are painful and require meticulous wound care to avoid infection. This also raises the question of which is worse, the scarring from the skin graft or the scarring from the known association between extended wound healing/inflammation and the severity of scarring. For full-thickness burns, lack of skin grafting may result in wound healing that takes years or lack of wound healing all together. Studies have also shown that delayed grafting worsens scar hypertrophy, so a burn injury that is grafted is likely better off being grafted early in the wound-healing process to mitigate extended inflammation.[24]

14.4 Scar Revision

If scars are insufficiently prevented, they can develop several different characteristics. As discussed, they can be categorized into atrophic, hypertrophic (e.g., after a burn or tension subjected injury), keloid (e.g., after an ear piercing), and contracture (e.g., after large area burn/trauma injury) scars. They can also be further subcategorized by clinical features including flat (e.g., after abrasions), linear (e.g., after laceration), punctate (e.g., after acne), patterned (e.g., after meshed skin grafting), hyperpigmented, hypopigmented, erythematous, edematous, hard, soft, etc. For best outcomes, multimodal approaches that combine specifically targeted approaches for each feature simultaneously provide the fastest and most impactful results.

14.4.1 Discoloration

Scars from minor traumas and surgery are frequently highly manageable. Surgical scars typically heal well on their own without any intervention at all.[25] As such, minimal, if any, scar revision is necessary. Although early intervention is the new hallmark paradigm for scar treatment, surgical scars are the exception that can be left to resolve on their own. However, depending on skin type, surgical technique, sun exposure, location, and genetics, scarring can still form. Minor assaults such as abrasion, cryotherapy, shave removal of nevi, etc., can leave impressions that, while lacking in substantial collagen alteration, become pigmented or erythematous due to hemosiderin staining or increased vascularity. A highly effective way to treat such scars is through nonablative vascular and pigment-targeting lasers. Minor scars often can be resolved by these tactics alone. For surgical scars under tension or in highly cosmetic areas, laser treatment can be done as soon as the sutures are removed or as soon as the scar begins to hypertrophy to help ensure that more extensive treatment is not needed. More substantial hypertrophic or atrophic scarring, however, often possesses additional discoloration that would benefit from these tactics as well.

14.4.2 Laser Treatment of Erythema

Erythema can be treated by vascular lasers that selectively target small blood vessels for destruction. The most common of these is the pulsed-dye laser (PDL), which operates on a millisecond domain at 585 or 595 nm.[26] The operating principle of such lasers is the theory of selective photothermolysis, discovered in 1983 by Anderson and Parrish,[27] which encompasses the process of selective heating of target chromophores based on wavelength. For erythema, the chromophore is oxyhemoglobin. Effective treatment occurs when the wavelength of the treatment device is paired as closely as possible to the absorption spectrum of the target. In practice, the most effective wavelengths for vasculature have been 585- or

595-nm wavelengths[28] against the spectrum of oxyhemoglobin, which has peaks at 418, 542, and 577 nm (the *blue*, *green*, and *yellow* portions of the visible range, respectively). Optimization of the match between laser wavelength and laser target allows selective heating of the target without heating the surrounding tissue. Heating leads to endothelial damage and blood coagulation for overall destruction. The body then eliminates the damaged tissue through macrophages and normal waste elimination mechanisms. It is now well established that thermal relaxation time should also be proportional to the square of the target diameter,[27] which drastically affects the choice of pulse duration. Lower wavelengths limit the depth into the skin that can be reached, causing the longer wavelengths to be more favorable. Years of research support utilization of a range of 0.4 to 20 milliseconds for pulse duration, particularly for inflamed, erythematous scars with pruritus and/or pain.[29] Shorter pulse durations can better target the microcirculatory system without excess heat that could bulk heat the superficial skin. Lower fluences of 4 to 7 J/cm^2 have also been found to be more effective than higher fluences[30] though this is recently being challenged following the invention of optical coherence tomography (OCT) and its ability to image vasculature.[31] The combination of short pulse duration and low fluence induces local damage to the vascular endothelium, hemorrhage, and platelet-mediated adherence of thrombi, whereas high fluences and long pulse durations typically cause immediate intravascular coagulation, denaturation, and resulting cessation of blood flow with less mechanical vessel damage.[32,33] Intense pulsed light (IPL) can also be used to treat scar vasculature due to its broad spectrum of wavelengths and its positive impact on pigmentation and collagen stimulation. However, it is less targeted and therefore, for intense erythema, less impactful on its own.

Removal of the vascular component of the scar not only eliminates the red coloring associated with blood vessels but also can help eliminate the excess vasculature that may be a culprit in hypertrophic scar formation. However, while it can be helpful, it is less effective at removing scars that are already hypertrophic. It is also not impactful in treatment of mature, hypopigmented, or strictly pigmented scars.

14.4.3 Laser Treatment of Pigmentation

Scars come in a wide variety of different color profiles. Dark brown pigmentation occurs typically from hemosiderin staining due to leaky blood vessels or postinflammatory hyperpigmentation from inflammatory injury into melanocytes. Treatment of pigmentation relies on the same basic principle of treating vascularity: selective photothermolysis. In this case, the target chromophore is melanin. Melanin is different than oxyhemoglobin in that it has no real peaks. Many different wavelengths can target pigment as can be seen by the wide variety of pigment-targeting devices available. The key then becomes the depth of the pigment and the isolation of wavelengths that do not preferentially target something else. This feature of melanin is also what makes dark skin so difficult to treat. Because of the propensity of these devices to target pigment, regular skin pigment is vulnerable as well, making most devices unsafe to use outside of Fitzpatrick skin types I, II, and III (▶ Fig. 14.4). However, there are now pigment-oriented lasers that are safe in all skin types such as the 1,927-nm thulium. As the absorption of melanin decreases with increasing wavelength, these high-wavelength devices are generally less effective overall at removing pigment and may require several treatments. However, they also allow for a much greater depth of treatment than other lasers, making them very useful for deeper dermal pigment. Though not originally indicated for pigment, ablative fractional lasers, which are safe in all skin types, have been shown to help pigmentation as well.

The approach to pigmentation of scars can be different than that for other pigmented lesions such as nevi or lentigines because scar pigmentation is often varied and multimodal. Depending on the scar, pigment-targeting lasers alone are often not the best treatment option. The use of devices such as the 1,927-nm thulium rolling laser and the IPL can provide increased efficacy in the treatment of scars due to their ability to treat globally by rolling technique and large footprint/wavelength spectrum,

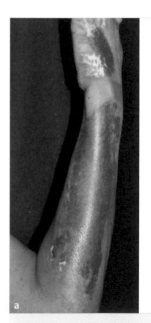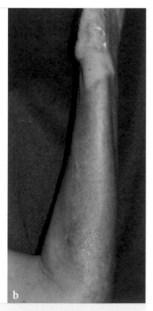

Fig. 14.4 A 55-year-old female Fitzpatrick skin type (FST)-V patient before **(a)** and after **(b)** a total of five treatments with a combination of 1927-nm Thulium and Ultra Pulse Laser.

respectively. Additionally, it is rare that a scar has color abnormality without any textural abnormality. Both the thulium laser and IPL impact texture through stimulation of collagen production that can help smooth out scars with added mild textural components.

14.4.4 Discoloration in Hypertrophic and Keloid Scars

Although some scarring consists of primarily discoloration, hypertrophic and keloid scarring also experience substantial discoloration in addition to textural change (▶ Fig. 14.5). They are typically red in color, but they can also be accompanied by sections of brown from hemosiderin staining and/or areas of hypopigmentation. Regardless of scar severity, these components should be targeted individually using selective and fractional photothermolysis as discussed previously. What changes the treatment approach for these scar types is the variation in depth compared to flat scars. The heterogeneous organization of tissue also coincides with a heterogenous size and organization of blood vessels as well as dermal/epidermal location of hemosiderin deposition. Traditionally, this is managed through trial and error in alteration of laser settings. More recently, technologies such as OCT have been developed to aid in noninvasive detection of scar qualities prior to treatment. OCT allows imaging beneath the skin for overall depth of scar and vessels as well as vessel diameter.[29] Once these variables are known, color-targeting laser settings can be adjusted accordingly.

14.4.5 Textural Irregularities

Most scars leave a visible alteration in skin coloration, but many also result in textural irregularities. These stem from the aforementioned disruption between anabolic and catabolic processes that throw deposition of collagen and other ECM components out of balance. Although lasers targeting pigmentation and erythema can help with any added discoloration, they are often insufficient to treat the underlying skin architecture that causes the major features of the resulting tissue.

14.4.6 Atrophic and Hypopigmented Scars

Hypopigmented and atrophic scars are put into the same category partially because they frequently occur together but also because hypopigmentation cannot be treated in the same simple manner as hyperpigmentation. Lasers are very successful at removing pigment, but there is no absorption spectrum for lack of pigment. Similarly, in the case of atrophy, lasers are adept at tissue destruction but not at tissue production. Certain lasers such as fractional ablative lasers stimulate collagen production over time, which may be sufficient in some patients but require supplementation in others (▶ Fig. 14.6). The ultimate goal in treatment is to maximize results with the fewest amount of treatments. As such, treatment strategy must adjust accordingly to each individual scar.

14.4.7 Excision/Punch Biopsies

Due to the challenge involved in the concept of repigmenting or rebuilding skin, one of the oldest methods of treatment of hypopigmentation and atrophy is excision of the tissue or skin grafting of normal tissue onto the affected area.[34] These are effective for the base purpose: eliminating the original hypopigmented or atrophic area. The caveat is that excision of tissue can leave another scar that is either the same or worse, negating the

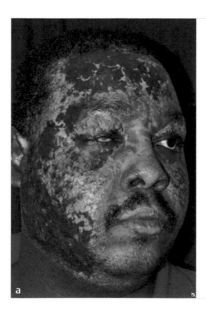
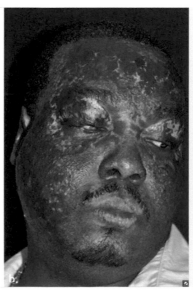

Fig. 14.5 A 41-year-old African American man with hypopigmented scars from a chemical burn before **(a)** and after **(b)** treatment with five fractional ablative laser treatments along with laser-assisted delivery with bimatoprost topical application on chemical burn scars. (Reprinted from Facial Plastic Surgery Clinics of North America. 25(1). Jill S Waibel and Ashley Rudnick. Laser-assisted delivery to treat facial scars. Copyright [2017] with permission from Elsevier.)

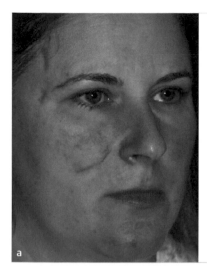
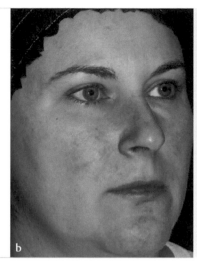

Fig. 14.6 A 43-year-old female Fitzpatrick skin type (FST)-II patient with dog bite trauma to face before **(a)** and after **(b)** being treated a total of six times with a combination of PDL, Fraxel, 1927-nm Thulium, ablative fractional laser CO_2, and poly-L-lactic acid on her right cheek and temple, undergoing a total of 14 and 3 stitches, respectively.

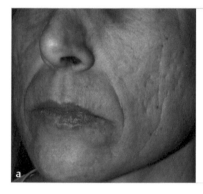
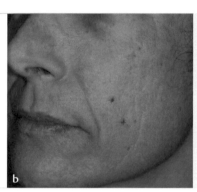

Fig. 14.7 A woman in her 50s with Fitzpatrick skin type (FST)-IV before **(a)** and after **(b)** after treatment for acne scars with punch biopsies, Ultra Pulse Laser, and poly-L-lactic acid.

original treatment. Grafting can not only leave a new scar but also create a mismatch between the treated area and the surrounding skin from lack of continuity. These procedures risk replacing one scar for another, diminishing the efficacy of these types of treatments. However, one type of surgery that has been shown to heal with little to no scarring is a punch biopsy.[35] Punch biopsies of 1 to 3 mm in diameter can heal with no to an imperceptible scar, allowing full removal of hypopigmented and atrophic tissue such as acne scars (which are often both) without negative residual side effects of traditional excision. These are particularly effective for acne scars, which are typically fully encompassed and removed within the area of the punch biopsy (▶ Fig. 14.7). The same applies to other small scars that can be successfully completely removed. However, this can also be done on larger affected areas, particularly of larger-scale hypopigmentation, in pieces until a whole area is removed over time. This is best for areas with sporadic hypopigmentation/atrophy or smaller areas. Larger areas may take many treatments to achieve the desired results. Punch biopsies can also be used in conjunction with laser treatments for a synergistic, highly impactful treatment course.

14.4.8 Laser

Despite the fact that these types of scars cannot be treated sufficiently by traditional nonablative laser techniques, lasers can still be an affective technique for both atrophic and hypopigmented scars. They both respond best to the use of fractional ablative laser treatment. There are a few mechanisms at play. Fractional ablative lasers operate, rather than by selective photothermolysis, by fractional photothermolysis. This involves the creation of an array of microscopic thermal injuries that both vaporize a portion of the tissue away and encourage normal wound healing at a depth insufficient to create resultant scarring.[36] Both atrophy and hypopigmentation benefit from the aspect of tissue destruction because it serves to remove damaged tissue. Additionally, the heat provided by the laser initiates a molecular cascade that stimulates rapid healing and collagen production/remodeling, helping fill in depressed areas of scar. Hypopigmentation has also been reported to repigment from fractional laser, both nonablative and ablative, laser alone, suspected due to repopulation of melanocytes in the hypopigmented areas from surrounding hair follicle stem cells and basal melanocytes.[39] Fractional nonablative lasers can be used as well and, in some cases, have been shown to have better results in repigmentation than fractional ablative lasers.[38] However, results are variable with both treatments due to remaining unknowns in the pathophysiology of hypopigmentation. What has been shown to be even more effective for both types of scarring is the use of fractional ablative laser followed by laser-assisted delivery of topical medications.

14.4.9 Laser-Assisted Delivery

Laser-assisted delivery is growing in popularity for treatment of a variety of cutaneous conditions. It utilizes channels of tunable depths created by fractional ablative lasers as a delivery route for topical medications.[37] The channels provide direct access to the epidermis and dermis, expanding the capability of medications to penetrate and enact their respective effects.

14.4.10 Hypopigmentation

Treatment of hypopigmentation can be aided through laser-assisted delivery of bimatoprost 0.03% topical solution. Originally a medication for glaucoma, bimatoprost was purported to have a negative side effect of periocular hyperpigmentation from increased melanogenesis.[38] This previously negative consequence of treatment was then repurposed as a stimulant of pigmentation to attempt to induce melanogenesis from dormant melanocytes and hopefully repigment areas of hypopigmentation.[39] Though limited in number, studies that evaluate the impact of this technique tend to find over 75% improvement in some patients and over 50% in others.[39,40] There are also often people who show little improvement. Since typically, over half the patients have substantial improvements and some are not very receptive to treatment at all, it suggests that there are multiple factors at play in the mechanism of hypopigmentation, repigmentation, or both. But these results are phenomenal compared to what any previous therapies have been able to achieve at this point, such as surgery that creates more scarring or tattooing, which does not undergo changes with the surrounding skin, making it stand out regardless.

14.4.11 Atrophy

Treatment of atrophy is best aided by the addition of volume. This can be accomplished by using laser-assisted delivery of poly-L-lactic acid, a bioactive filler.[41] Poly-L-lactic acid can be used in the traditional method through needle application to specified areas for volume. This technique is still useful, often in conjunction with subcision, for smaller atrophic scarring such as acne scars. However, the use of laser-assisted delivery for poly-L-lactic acid allows the filler to be distributed broadly and evenly across an area, allowing a very natural spread of the product and optimization of results. This technique provides both immediate results of extra volume from the presence of bulk fluid and long-term results from the bioactivity of the compound stimulating the body's own collagen and fat production. As the fluid and exogenous filler itself degrades over time, the body's production of tissue helps replace it, providing a building effect over time rather than a traditional temporary fill and then subsequent depletion associated with typical fillers. This technique also stands out compared to methods such as excision and fat grafting because it does not require any surgical intervention, which many patients are often hesitant to undergo. There are no stitches, minimal down time, only a few days of wound care, and no additional scar creation. It is also substantially easier and faster than procedures such as fat grafting, which requires additional liposuction. The pros and cons of each procedure may change depending on the size of the scar. If a patient has substantial atrophy over an expansive area, fat grafting may be a beneficial choice.

14.4.12 Fat Grafting

Fat grafting is an old procedure that has found a niche in atrophy. It involves liposuction of bodily area such as the abdomen or the leg, followed by injection of the autologous fat into sites of atrophy. This is hypothesized to utilize the properties of adipose-derived stem cells for induction of epithelial hyperplasia and angiogenesis resultant from growth factor release.[42] There have been positive results seen from microfat injection,[43] and it is a great choice for filling large areas of atrophy that would be very time-consuming and difficult to achieve with laser and filler alone. There can also be a beneficial effect on melanocyte stimulation to encourage pigmentation. However, there are downsides as well. The first is that a portion of the adipose is always reabsorbed into the body and this portion varies from person to person, making results hard to predict reliably. Permanence is also not guaranteed. As an expensive procedure, this can be difficult for patients who need multiple treatments. Patients also may have to undergo multiple rounds of liposuction, which is a cumbersome procedure. This poses an additional challenge for thin patients of low fat content.

14.4.13 Other Techniques (Hyaluronic Acid Filler, Subcision)

There are a few other techniques that can be applied to atrophic scars but will not impact hypopigmented scars. They are also generally adjunct procedures rather than stand-alone techniques. Hyaluronic acid (HA) fillers are a treatment option for atrophy with the acknowledgment that they are temporary. If a patient is worried about taking permanent action or has a remaining amount of HA filler left from another treatment, this may be a good option. Otherwise, previously mentioned treatments are more robust.

Subcision can be a useful technique particularly for acne scars. It involves undermining beneath the surface of scars with a needle tip to help break up dense scar tissue in smaller scars that have adhered to the underlying skin layers to elevate the patient's existing tissue. This is often best combined with bioactive fillers such as poly-L-lactic acid to allow creation of space from separating of the tissue and then population of that space through the filler and subsequent tissue production techniques.

14.4.14 Hypertrophic and Keloid Scars

Hypertrophic scarring can manifest in a variety of ways. They are often combined in treatment strategy with keloid scarring due to the lack of specific and proven keloid treatments available. The underlying principles of treatment are the same: debulking and blending. There are many available tools to achieve this goal that can be tailored to each scar.

14.4.15 Surgery

Basic surgical excision of a scar is not an ideal treatment strategy because it provides scar-prone skin an opportunity for new scar formation. In the case of keloids, this also frequently causes frequent scar recurrence, often more extensive than the initial scar. Depending on the size of the scar, the volume of excised tissues can also lead to excessive pulling of the skin that results in a visually or even functionally suboptimal result. However, there are surgical techniques that allow reorganization of scar tissue that realigns healing vectors in a way that relaxes skin tension and encourages normal wound healing. These techniques include primarily Z-plasty and W-plasty, though punch biopsies can also be utilized in select cases of smaller scars or as an added tool to other treatment types.

14.4.16 Z-Plasty

Hypertrophic scars characteristically disrupt the coordinated lattice of ECM proteins that cause normal, flat, strong skin integrity. The tissue proliferates excessively and lays in dense, linear, irregular formats that are visually and functionally detrimental. Scarring can also lead to contracture formation where the tension is so great that movement is inhibited, particularly around a joint. The Z-plasty aims to reorient the tension vectors and minimize the strain experienced by any one portion of the scar, leading to overall relief and improvement in skin pliability and quality. Z-plasty has many different subtypes, but the basic concept involves making surgical incisions in a Z pattern over a solidified hypertrophic/contracture scar to obtain triangular tissue flaps (▶ Fig. 14.8).[44] These flaps are then rearranged to assume their opposite orientation. This allocates the strain differently and initiates new wound-healing processes on smaller, multidirectional, manageable planes. Instead of having one large wound to bridge haphazardly, the technique creates smaller wounds divided evenly among the surrounding tissue, preventing excessive pulling from any one direction. This surgical technique has been utilized for various applications, including burn scars, for longer than can be reasonably documented (with some reports as early as 1856) but has been included heavily in the literature since the early 1900s.[45,46] It is particularly valuable in range-of-motion impediments as it can release the restriction and subsequently increase mobility. The "zigzag" nature of the result is also less perceptible to the eye than a straight line,[47] allowing for more cosmetically favorable results.

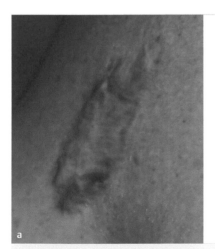
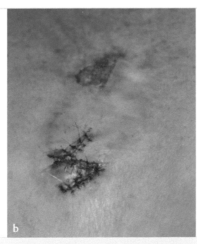
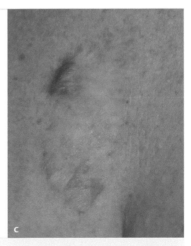

Fig. 14.8 (a–c) A 39-year-old female Fitzpatrick skin type (FST)-II with a chest scar after six treatments of combined PDL, Fraxel, 1927-nm Thulium, AFL, and Z-plasty procedure.

14.4.17 W-Plasty

A W-plasty is similar in concept to a Z-plasty in that it divides scars into triangular flaps. However, it does not reorient the flaps but rather surgically excises some scar tissue and closes in a nonlinear fashion such that the site of excision heals less perceptibly.[48] This also differs from Z-plasty in that Z-plasty does not involve excision of tissue, whereas W-plasty does require some tissue excision. This makes it less desirable for contracture scars as it can increase tension, but it is a viable option for hypertrophic scars that would benefit from tissue excision. W-plasties are best utilized in smaller scar revisions as the repetitive pattern may become discernable if utilized over a large area.

14.4.18 Laser

Laser treatment has emerged at the forefront of treatment for hypertrophic and keloid scars. Although severe contractures may require surgical intervention, the majority of scars can be adequately or better managed with laser treatment because they are outpatient, do not involve general anesthesia, require less downtime, and do not open the possibility of new scar formation in the process. Particularly in keloid scar treatment, surgical intervention often stimulates growth of existing keloids or stimulation of new keloids at the incision site, making laser treatment a safer treatment option. Laser treatment appears to turn off this cytokine storm that promotes recurrence more effectively as well, an emerging theory that is under current investigation.

Treatment of hypertrophic and keloid scars utilizes many of the same tools in laser treatment of atrophic and flat scars as previously discussed. Hypertrophic scars, particularly those caused by burn or trauma, are often broadly heterogenous, requiring several different treatment strategies combined to achieve optimal results. The gold standard is again fractional ablative treatment with low treatment densities. With characteristic aberrant proliferation of tissue, these scars benefit from the vaporization of present tissue and the breakdown of dense, fibrous areas for overall scar softening. The microthermal treatment zones created rewound the tissue in manageable quantities so that wound-healing mechanisms proceed normally rather than stimulating the overactive, disorganized wound-healing response.[49] Countless studies have touted the effects of fractional ablative laser treatment on the color, texture, pliability, vascularity, and symptomatology of hypertrophic scarring.[50,51,52,53,54,55,56] Nonablative fractional lasers can be used effectively as well but do not achieve the same depth as do ablative fractional lasers, making ablative lasers a preferred choice for thick hypertrophic and keloid scars.

14.4.19 Laser-Assisted Delivery

Fractional ablative treatment of hypertrophic scars is an ideal opportunity for laser-assisted delivery of topical medications. Although the laser on its own is an effective treatment, the treatment can be optimized further utilizing agents to further atrophy and combat growth. The most popular current medications for this purpose include corticosteroids and 5-fluorouracil.[57] Corticosteroids break the bonds between collagen fibers and, as a result largely of excess collagen deposition, elevated scars often respond positively. 5-fluorouracil inhibits fibroblast proliferation, delaying cell cycle progression and inducing scar fibroblast apoptosis.[58] For tissue prone to excess proliferation, this helps discourage excess tissue growth or recurrence of scar formation. Both treatments are utilized for the same variety of scars with approximately equal efficacy. However, 5-fluorouracil is associated with fewer side effects although for both treatments, side effects are minimal when delivered in this format (▶ Fig. 14.9). Laser-assisted delivery of these medications as a delivery vehicle is ideal for even distribution of product throughout the scar at tunable depths based on laser settings. This helps avoid inappropriate allocation of medication and consequences such as excessive atrophy.

14.4.20 Adjuvant Therapies
Radiation

The use of radiation has increased in popularity in surgical revision of scars. Following surgical excision, physicians will often apply radiation to prevent reformation or exacerbation of keloid and hypertrophic scars. Keloids are known for extremely high recurrence rates. Although largely in case report form, the literature reports a reduction in recurrence following radiotherapy to anywhere between 8 and 28%.[59] The mechanism is incompletely understood, but it is thought to be a result of its effects on inhibiting fibroblast activity or angiogenesis. Although radiation therapy on its own will not be a stand-alone treatment for hypertrophic and keloid scarring, it is a possible adjuvant to traditional therapies in scars that are historically prone to recur. Radiation must always be used with caution to avoid excess radiation and increased potential for skin malignancy. Excess radiation can also cause scarring in the form of what is known as a "radiation tattoo."

Injections

Before the development of laser-assisted delivery, hypertrophic and keloid scars were historically treated with intralesional corticosteroid injections to achieve the same effect of tissue atrophy. This continues to be done this way for those with limited technology. However, the injection vehicle can be difficult to adequately control and can sometimes result in excess tissue atrophy, leaving an

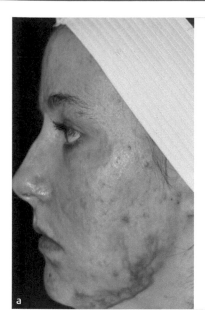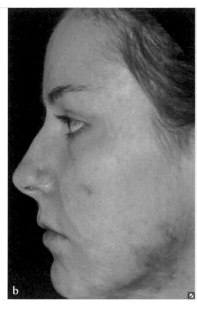

Fig. 14.9 A 22-year-old Caucasian woman with erythematous, hypertrophic burn scars from a bonfire before **(a)** and after **(b)** fractional ablative lasers, nonablative fractional lasers, along with laser-assisted delivery of 5-fluorouracil. (Reprinted from Facial Plastic Surgery Clinics of North America. 25(1). Jill S Waibel and Ashley Rudnick. Laser-assisted delivery to treat facial scars. Copyright [2017] with permission from Elsevier.)

indentation in the treated skin or fat. Small surgical scars can sometimes be treated with Kenalog or 5-flourouracil. In certain circumstances, particularly bulky sections of a scar may benefit from adjuvant injection. However, laser-assisted delivery is typically preferred for optimal scar treatment. Other products have been increasingly utilized in the literature as well such as bleomycin or verapamil with varying results.[60,61]

Compression

Compression has been long utilized in healing scars as an active strategy for scar prevention. However, compression is also an extremely important part of scar therapy. Much like the healing process in the initial wound, healing following laser treatment or surgery can benefit from the moisturization, mechanical pressure, and restricted collagen production of silicone gel sheeting. Silicone gel sheeting can be used as soon as the skin re-epithelializes and continue as much as possible until healing is complete.

14.4.21 Combination Treatment

Scars often vary not only between patients but also within an individual patient. Maximizing treatment technique is typically best done through combination treatment. For example, severe burn and trauma patients may require a baseline Z-plasty to release major range-of-motion restrictions with follow-up treatments of laser and laser-assisted delivery to help blend and normalize the released tissue. Thick scars may benefit from laser treatment with adjuvant steroid injections to particularly thickened sections. Stubborn keloids prone to recurrence may benefit from Z-plasty, followed by laser, and followed up with radiation. Scar treatment should be done

formulaically. Is it a flat surgical scar? Leave it alone. Does it require surgery? If yes, then the surgery should be completed first. Are there color and textural abnormalities? Then laser treatment can be done first by color, then by texture, followed by the appropriate adjuvant. If hypertrophic, each treatment can be accompanied by compression to maximize results.

14.5 Conclusion

In this decade, scar treatment is making astronomical advances with continual improvement in patient outcomes and satisfaction. With the surge in scientific interest and the corresponding creation crescendo of new treatment strategies, options are boundless in choosing a treatment path to follow. In this field, laser has been increasingly at the forefront due to its high efficacy and low downtime nature, but there is no one ultimate treatment that encompasses every scar. Each scar and patient characteristics are unique and, as such, treatment should be customized individually to optimize results.

References

[1] Dunkin CSJ, Pleat JM, Gillespie PH, Tyler MPH, Roberts AHN, McGrouther DA. Scarring occurs at a critical depth of skin injury: precise measurement in a graduated dermal scratch in human volunteers. Plast Reconstr Surg. 2007; 119(6):1722–1732, discussion 1733–1734

[2] Yates CC, Hebda P, Wells A. Skin wound healing and scarring: fetal wounds and regenerative restitution. Birth Defects Res C Embryo Today. 2012; 96(4):325–333

[3] Rangaraj A, Harding K, Leaper D. Role of collagen in wound management. Wounds UK. 2011; 7(2):54–63

[4] Westra I, Verhaegen PDHM, Ibrahim Korkmaz H, et al. Investigating histological aspects of scars in children. J Wound Care. 2017; 26(5): 256–265

[5] Desmoulière A, Redard M, Darby I, Gabbiani G. Apoptosis mediates the decrease in cellularity during the transition between granulation tissue and scar. Am J Pathol. 1995; 146(1):56–66

[6] Rippa AL, Kalabusheva EP, Vorotelyak EA. Regeneration of dermis: scarring and cells involved. Cells. 2019; 8(6):607

[7] Holland DB, Jeremy AH, Roberts SG, Seukeran DC, Layton AM, Cunliffe WJ. Inflammation in acne scarring: a comparison of the responses in lesions from patients prone and not prone to scar. Br J Dermatol. 2004; 150(1):72–81

[8] Jacob CI, Dover JS, Kaminer MS. Acne scarring: a classification system and review of treatment options. J Am Acad Dermatol. 2001; 45(1): 109–117

[9] De Jesus AM, Aghvami M, Sander EA. A combined in vitro imaging and multi-scale modeling system for studying the role of cell matrix interactions in cutaneous wound healing. PLoS One. 2016; 11(2): e0148254

[10] Murray JC. Keloids and hypertrophic scars. Clin Dermatol. 1994; 12 (1):27–37

[11] Wulkan A, Rudnick A, Badiavas E, Waibel JS. Treatment of traumatic hypertrophic scars with 2940-nm fractional ablative erbium-doped yttrium aluminium: a pilot study. Dermatol Surg. 2020; 46(6):789–793

[12] Schneider JC, Holavanahalli R, Helm P, Goldstein R, Kowalske K. Contractures in burn injury: defining the problem. J Burn Care Res. 2006; 27(4):508–514

[13] Hinz B. The role of myofibroblasts in wound healing. Curr Res Transl Med. 2016; 64(4):171–177

[14] Karmisholt KE, Haerskjold A, Karlsmark T, Waibel J, Paasch U, Haedersdal M. Early laser intervention to reduce scar formation: a systematic review. J Eur Acad Dermatol Venereol. 2018; 32(7):1099–1110

[15] Waibel J, Gianatasio C, Rudnick A. Randomized, controlled early intervention of dynamic mode fractional ablative CO_2 laser on acute burn injuries for prevention of pathological scarring. Lasers Surg Med. 2020; 52(2):117–124

[16] Xu W, Hong SJ, Zeitchek M, et al. Hydration status regulates sodium flux and inflammatory pathways through epithelial sodium channel (ENaC) in the skin. J Invest Dermatol. 2015; 135(3):796–806

[17] Ogawa R. Keloid and hypertrophic scars are the result of chronic inflammation in the reticular dermis. Int J Mol Sci. 2017; 18(3):606

[18] Liu H, Yue J, Lei Q, et al. Ultraviolet B inhibits skin wound healing by affecting focal adhesion dynamics. Photochem Photobiol. 2015; 91 (4):909–916

[19] Lonie S, Baker P, Teixeira RP. Healing time and incidence of hypertrophic scarring in paediatric scalds. Burns. 2017; 43(3):509–513

[20] Atiyeh BS, El Khatib AM, Dibo SA. Pressure garment therapy (PGT) of burn scars: evidence-based efficacy. Ann Burns Fire Disasters. 2013; 26(4):205–212

[21] Macintyre L, Baird M. Pressure garments for use in the treatment of hypertrophic scars: a review of the problems associated with their use. Burns. 2006; 32(1):10–15

[22] Mustoe TA. Evolution of silicone therapy and mechanism of action in scar management. Aesthetic Plast Surg. 2008; 32(1):82–92

[23] Cho YS, Jeon JH, Hong A, et al. The effect of burn rehabilitation massage therapy on hypertrophic scar after burn: a randomized controlled trial. Burns. 2014; 40(8):1513–1520

[24] Chan QE, Harvey JG, Graf NS, Godfrey C, Holland AJ. The correlation between time to skin grafting and hypertrophic scarring following an acute contact burn in a porcine model. J Burn Care Res. 2012; 33(2): e43–e48

[25] Gauglitz GG, Pötschke J, Clementoni MT. Therapy of scars with lasers. Hautarzt. 2018; 69(1):17–26

[26] Khetarpal S, Kaw U, Dover JS, Arndt KA. Laser advances in the treatment of burn and traumatic scars. Semin Cutan Med Surg. 2017; 36(4):185–191

[27] Anderson RR, Parrish JA. Selective photothermolysis: precise microsurgery by selective absorption of pulsed radiation. Science. 1983; 220(4596):524–527

[28] Alster TS, Williams CM. Treatment of keloid sternotomy scars with 585 nm flashlamp-pumped pulsed-dye laser. Lancet. 1995; 345 (8959):1198–1200

[29] Waibel JS, Rudnick AC, Wulkan AJ, Holmes JD. The diagnostic role of optical coherence tomography (OCT) in measuring the depth of burn and traumatic scars for more accurate laser dosimetry: pilot study. J Drugs Dermatol. 2016; 15(11):1375–1380

[30] Manuskiatti W, Wanitphakdeedecha R, Fitzpatrick RE. Effect of pulse width of a 595-nm flashlamp-pumped pulsed dye laser on the treatment response of keloidal and hypertrophic sternotomy scars. Dermatol Surg. 2007; 33(2):152–161

[31] Waibel JS, Holmes J, Rudnick A, Woods D, Kelly KM. Angiographic optical coherence tomography imaging of hemangiomas and port wine birthmarks. Lasers Surg Med. 2018; 50(7):718–726

[32] Ma J, Chen B, Zhang Y, Li D, Xing ZL. Multiple laser pulses in conjunction with an optical clearing agent to improve the curative effect of cutaneous vascular lesions. Lasers Med Sci. 2017; 32(6): 1321–1335

[33] Garden JM, Tan OT, Kerschmann R, et al. Effect of dye laser pulse duration on selective cutaneous vascular injury. J Invest Dermatol. 1986; 87(5):653–657

[34] Alster T, Zaulyanov L. Laser scar revision: a review. Dermatol Surg. 2007; 33(2):131–140

[35] Boen M, Jacob C. A review and update of treatment options using the acne scar classification system. Dermatol Surg. 2019; 45(3):411–422

[36] Manstein D, Herron GS, Sink RK, Tanner H, Anderson RR. Fractional photothermolysis: a new concept for cutaneous remodeling using microscopic patterns of thermal injury. Lasers Surg Med. 2004; 34 (5):426–438

[37] Hantash BM, Bedi VP, Kapadia B, et al. In vivo histological evaluation of a novel ablative fractional resurfacing device. Lasers Surg Med. 2007; 39(2):96–107

[38] Kapur R, Osmanovic S, Toyran S, Edward DP. Bimatoprost-induced periocular skin hyperpigmentation: histopathological study. Arch Ophthalmol. 2005; 123(11):1541–1546

[39] Massaki AB, Fabi SG, Fitzpatrick R. Repigmentation of hypopigmented scars using an erbium-doped 1,550-nm fractionated laser and topical bimatoprost. Dermatol Surg. 2012; 38(7, Pt 1):995–1001

[40] Waibel J, Rudnick A, Nagrani N, Gonzalez A. Re-pigmentation of hypopigmentation: fractional laser versus laser assisted delivery of bimatoprost versus novel epidermal melanocyte harvesting system. J Drugs Dermatol. 2019; 18(11):1090–1096

[41] Waibel JS, Rudnick A. Laser-assisted delivery to treat facial scars. Facial Plast Surg Clin North Am. 2017; 25(1):105–117

[42] Riyat H, Touil LL, Briggs M, Shokrollahi K. Autologous fat grafting for scars, healing and pain: a review. Scars Burn Heal. 2017; 3: 2059513117728200

[43] Gu Z, Li Y, Li H. Use of condensed nanofat combined with fat grafts to treat atrophic scars. JAMA Facial Plast Surg. 2018; 20(2):128–135

[44] Borges AF, Gibson T. The original Z-plasty. Br J Plast Surg. 1973; 26 (3):237–246

[45] McCurdy SL. Z-plastic surgery. Surg Gynecol Obstet. 1913; 16:209

[46] Mccurdy SL. Correction of burn scar deformity by the Z-plastic method. J. Bone and Joint Surg. 1924; 6(3):683–688

[47] Rohrer T, Cooke J, Kaufman A. Flaps and Grafts in Dermatologic Surgery. 2nd ed. Philadelphia, PA: Elsevier; 2018

[48] Morais P, Santos P. "W-plasty: the role in the camouflage of an unaesthetic postsurgical facial scar. Surg Cosmet Dermatol. 2016; 8 (3):262–265

[49] Anderson RR, Donelan MB, Hivnor C, et al. Laser treatment of traumatic scars with an emphasis on ablative fractional laser resurfacing: consensus report. JAMA Dermatol. 2014; 150(2):187–193

[50] Kim DW, Hwang NH, Yoon ES, Dhong ES, Park SH. Outcomes of ablative fractional laser scar treatment. J Plast Surg Hand Surg. 2015; 49(2):88–94

[51] Patel SP, Nguyen HV, Mannschreck D, Redett RJ, Puttgen KB, Stewart FD. Fractional CO_2 laser treatment outcomes for pediatric hypertrophic burn scars. J Burn Care Res. 2019; 40(4):386–391

[52] Daoud AA, Gianatasio C, Rudnick A, Michael M, Waibel J. Efficacy of combined intense pulsed light (IPL) with fractional CO_2: laser ablation in the treatment of large hypertrophic scars—a prospective, randomized control trial. Lasers Surg Med. 2019; 51(8):678–685

[53] Waibel JS, Wulkan AJ, Rudnick A, Daoud A. Treatment of hypertrophic scars using laser-assisted corticosteroid versus laser-assisted 5-fluorouracil delivery. Dermatol Surg. 2019; 45(3):423–430

[54] Datz E, Schönberger C, Zeman F, et al. Fractional carbon dioxide laser resurfacing of skin grafts: long-term results of a prospective, randomized, split-scar, evaluator-blinded study. Lasers Surg Med. 2018; 50(10):1010–1016

[55] Rodriguez-Menocal L, Davis SS, Becerra S, et al. Assessment of ablative fractional CO_2 laser and Er:YAG laser to treat hypertrophic scars in a red duroc pig model. J Burn Care Res. 2018; 39(6):954–962

[56] Issler-Fisher AC, Waibel J, Donelan M. Laser modulation of hypertrophic scars. Clin Plast Surg. 2017; 44:757–766

[57] Waibel JS, Wulkan AJ, Rudnick A, Daoud A. Treatment of hypertrophic scars using laser-assisted corticosteroid versus laser-assisted 5-fluorouracil delivery. Dermatol Surg. 2019; 45(3):423–430

[58] Huang L, Wong YP, Cai YJ, Lung I, Leung CS, Burd A. Low-dose 5-fluorouracil induces cell cycle G2 arrest and apoptosis in keloid fibroblasts. Br J Dermatol. 2010; 163(6):1181–1185

[59] Keeling BH, Whitsitt J, Liu A, Dunnick CA. Keloid removal by shave excision with adjuvant external beam radiation therapy. Derm Surg. 2015; 41(8):989–992

[60] Abedini R, Sasani P, Mahmoudi HR, Nasimi M, Teymourpour A, Shadlou Z. Comparison of intralesional verapamil versus intralesional corticosteroids in treatment of keloids and hypertrophic scars: a randomized controlled trial. Burns. 2018; 44(6):1482–1488

[61] Payapvipapong K, Niumpradit N, Piriyanand C, Buranaphalin S, Nakakes A. The treatment of keloids and hypertrophic scars with intralesional bleomycin in skin of color. J Cosmet Dermatol. 2015; 14(1):83–90

15 Mohs and Melanoma

John A. Zitelli

Summary

This chapter discusses the use of Mohs surgery and other techniques to enable histologic evaluation of the entire peripheral margin of a melanoma. Advantages of Mohs surgery include tissue conservation, complete histologic margin assessment, repair in a guaranteed tumor-free plane, same-day repair, and cure rates around 99%. Recurrence rates for standard excision of melanoma range between 8 and 20% versus 1 and 2% with Mohs surgery.

Keywords: melanoma, melanoma in situ, lentigo maligna, lentigo maligna melanoma, Mohs micrographic surgery, staged excision, slow Mohs, melanoma treatment, guidelines

15.1 Melanoma In Situ and Malignant Melanoma

Melanoma is a malignant tumor that arises from the melanocytes. It is most commonly of cutaneous origin but can also arise on the mucosal, uveal, and leptomeningeal surfaces. It is the fifth most common type of skin cancer in men and sixth in women with over 90,000 cases diagnosed in 2018 in the United States alone. Incident rates have been rising for greater than three decades, while the mortality rates have stabilized since the 1990s. Invasive melanomas represent only 1% of skin cancers but result in the most deaths.[1]

Current therapies for primary melanomas are too often inadequate. Standard excisions can result in high recurrence rates up to 20%.[2,3,4] Melanomas in situ (MIS) and invasive melanomas frequently have amelanotic extensions that cannot be seen by visual inspection. Only histologic examination will detect these extensions. Even wide margins of 1 to 2 cm may not completely remove these extensions. Not only can these wide margins be noncurative but they may also lead to unnecessary tissue removal where melanoma extensions are not present. There is a preponderance of evidence demonstrating high recurrence rates of melanomas on the head and neck and inadequately excised tumors on the trunk (Zitelli, unpublished data). The failure of these treatment methods is the incomplete margin examination that is necessary for the complete tumor removal. Most physicians, even dermatologists, are not aware that less than 0.1% of the surgical margins are examined with standard excision pathology.

15.2 Treatment

According to the American Academy of Dermatology Melanoma Guidelines, surgical excision with histologically negative margins is the recommended first-line treatment for cutaneous melanoma.[5] Complete surgical removal can be completed with wide local excision, Mohs micrographic surgery (MMS), or staged excisions. Standard excisions with wide local margins remove the primary visible tumor and the prescribed margin of "normal-appearing" skin. This requires practitioners to have adequate experience and training in identifying the abnormal and normal skin with which to base their initial tumor dimensions. Some dermatologists utilize a Wood's lamp and a dermatoscope to help identify the primary tumor's size and location. The safety margin of "normal skin" is removed to ideally capture any subclinical extensions of melanoma that are not visible to the eye. The excised tissue is then submitted for paraffin-embedded permanent sections for standard "bread loaf" sectioning, which are then examined by the pathologist at minimum 24 hours later. The entire cross section of the specimen is not viewed. In contrast to the other techniques, there is only a small percentage of the actual excised margin that is examined (likely < 1% of the margin). The actual extent of margin examined depends on the interval of sectioning, which may be standardized within a given laboratory, but it is not universally standardized and is highly variable. The interval will determine the likelihood that involved margins will be identified.[6] For example, with standard processing of these specimens of 5 mm between each vertical section, only 12 to 20% of positive margin excisions would be detected. This may explain why melanoma has the tendency to recur 8 to 20% of the time with standard excisions even when the standard pathology reports clear margins.[2,3,4]

Unlike standard excision, MMS and slow Mohs with enface histologic processing examine 100% of the margin and allows for detection of melanoma that is not visible to the eye. It affords complete tumor removal with clear microscopic margins. Clear microscopic margins are essential to reduce local recurrences and thus the need for more surgeries. The processes of "slow mohs" and other staged excisions will be discussed later in this chapter.

Alternative therapies including nonsurgical options are considered second line for the treatment of primary cutaneous melanoma. They should only be considered in a limited patient population who are unable to undergo surgical resection. Topical imiquimod 5% cream has been used as a second-line treatment of MIS, lentigo maligna (LM) type, in these circumstances and has also been used in the adjuvant setting. Hidden histologic disease can persist in at least 25% of cases, and the development of invasive disease with satellite metastasis has been reported.[7,8] Additional alternative treatments including cryosurgery, electrodesiccation and curettage, laser ablation, radiation, azelaic acid, intralesional 5-fluorouracil, and topical tazarotene have been reported.[9] The use of superficial brachytherapy is not recommended for the treatment of melanoma.[5] Careful discussion of the risks, benefits, and uncertainties should take place with the patient and his or her family prior to any nonsurgical treatment.

15.3 Indications for MMS

All melanoma tumors have the potential to have amelanotic or invisible extensions. the wide margins needed to treat melanomas of the head and neck are well described in the literature; however, even well-defined melanomas on the trunk and extremities can have amelanotic extensions.[10] These tumors with would benefit from MMS's ability to detect any microscopic tumor that is not visible to the eye. Additionally, melanoma excisional defects that may require a flap or graft would benefit from complete margin assessment to histologically confirm clearance of the tumor prior to reconstruction. This reduces the likelihood of reoperation and further morbidity. The American Academy of Dermatology, American College of Mohs Surgery, American Society for Dermatologic Surgery Association, and the American Society for Mohs Surgery regarded MMS to be appropriate for primary LM and MIS on the head, neck, hands, feet, genitalia, and pretibial leg and recurrent LM or MIS in any location. Although no consensus has been reached on the use of MMS for invasive melanomas, the likelihood of subclinical extensions or repair with a flap or graft does not differ between MIS and invasive melanoma (▸ Table 15.1).[11]

15.4 Mohs Micrographic Surgery: Procedure

15.4.1 Technique

Unlike standard excision, MMS examines 100% of the peripheral and deep tissue margins. First, the visible tumor (including the biopsy scar) is excised to the adipose tissue. If the diagnostic biopsy reveals a positive deep margin or if there is clinical evidence of a remaining lesion, the central debulk is evaluated by routine histologic processing to determine if there is an upgrade to the Breslow depth. This can also be sent for paraffin sections. After the debulking, a single layer is removed to the deep adipose tissue (▸ Fig. 15.1). The margin of each layer is dependent on the location of the tumor. A 1-cm margin can be taken on the trunk and extremities without compromise to the closure in some circumstances, whereas on the head and neck smaller margins may be needed to preserve anatomic units. Wider margins would be taken if necessitated by the microscopic tissue examination of the margin. After the initial layer, the specimen is then sectioned as the following: the peripheral tissue is sectioned into 1- to 2-cm strips and the center is sectioned appropriately to fit the slide similar to a routine Mohs layer with hematoxylin and eosin (H&E). Stains are utilized on these sections to facilitate localization of the tumor (▸ Fig. 15.2). The peripheral strips are then processed with H&E and melanoma antigen recognized by T-cells 1 (MART-1) immunostains. Any remaining tumor is marked on a map as depicted in ▸ Fig. 15.3 and an additional 3-mm margin is excised and examined. The process is repeated until the tumor is completely removed.

Some centers utilize other immunostains for the evaluation of melanoma. Melanocyte-inducing transcription factor (MITF) is a nuclear stain and is highly specific for melanocytes. MART-1 is a cytoplasmic stain that can highlight keratinocytes and pseudonests. Although MITF is more specific, it stains melanocytes faintly with tiny dots. MART-1 is sensitive and creates a bright stain. Human melanoma black-45 (HMB-45) has also been

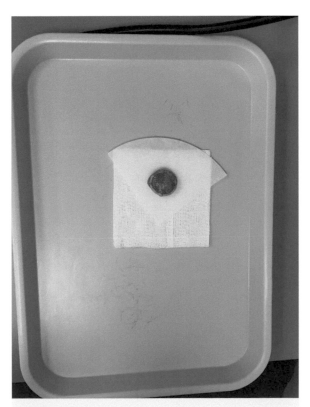

Fig. 15.1 Image of initial layer of melanoma excision prior to sectioning.

Table 15.1 Indications for Mohs micrographic surgery

Primary melanoma on the head and neck, sacral sites, genitalia, and pretibial legs
Locally recurrent melanoma in any location
Locations that may require repair with a flap or a graft

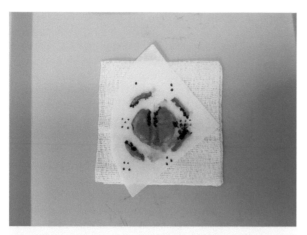

Fig. 15.2 Sectioning of the initial layer including 1- to 2-cm strips of peripheral tissue sectioned and inked. *Dots on filter paper* indicate the numbering of the sections.

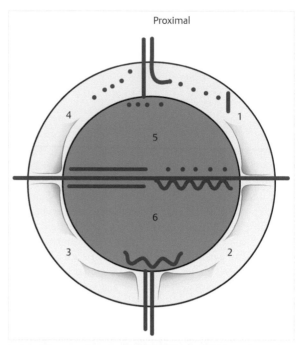

Fig. 15.3 Mohs maps of the excised tissue in ▶ Fig. 15.1 and ▶ Fig. 15.2.

utilized in the past, but it has fallen out of favor due to its lower sensitivity and poorer staining quality in comparison to MART-1.[12]

15.4.2 Positive Margins

Evaluating the margin of a melanoma can seem to be difficult to the untrained professional; however, a set of well-established guidelines for positive margins includes the following: (1) nests of at least three atypical melanocytes, (2) melanocytes above the dermoepidermal junction, and (3) nonuniform crowding of cells along the basement membrane. ▶ Fig. 15.4 depicts a negative margin. ▶ Fig. 15.5 demonstrates a positive margin utilizing MART-1 immunostaining on a frozen section. Other signs of atypical melanocytic proliferations include (1) extension of atypical, crowded melanocytes deep to the follicular infundibulum, (2) nonuniform distribution of pigment, (3) excessive number of melanophages, and (4) brisk inflammatory response. As many melanomas occur on chronically sun-damaged skin, the Mohs surgeon must have a high level of understanding of melanocytes in this type of skin. Hendi et al studied the melanocyte distribution in chronically sun-damaged skin in 149 patients undergoing MMS for a nonmelanoma skin cancer. They found that confluence of up to nine adjacent melanocytes and extension along hair follicles are considered normal in chronically sun-damaged skin, whereas nesting and pagetoid spread are not.[13] When utilizing these criteria, the frozen section interpretation is comparable to that of the paraffin section.[14]

15.5 Slow Mohs and Other Staged Excisions

Staged excision of melanoma is another method of providing complete margin assessment. With this procedure,

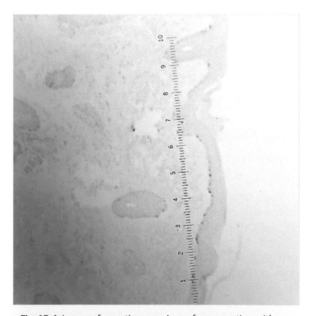

Fig. 15.4 Image of negative margin on frozen section with melanoma-associated antigen recognized by T cells (MART-1) immunostain.

the central tumor is excised to the deep adipose. The perimeter of skin is then removed and inked/marked. A map of the excised tissue is created and often sent with the tissue to the lab. The central debulk is processed with vertical sections to detect any upgrade to Breslow's depth.

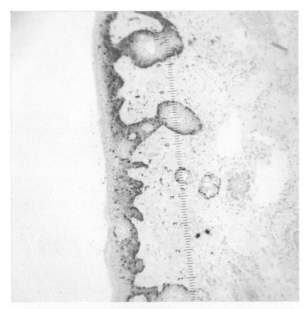

Fig. 15.5 Melanoma-associated antigen recognized by T cells (MART-1) staining of a melanoma on frozen section.

The peripheral tissue is processed en face to allow complete examination of the margin. The resulting wound is bandaged and the patient is sent home that day. This procedure is often called "slow Mohs" as the excised tissue is sent for paraffin sections in formalin-fixed tissue. The tissue is sent to the lab for "rush" permanent Mohs sections, which are then reviewed by the dermatopathologist, not the Mohs surgeon. This may take 2 to 3 days to obtain a result between each layer, hence the name "slow Mohs." When the results are available, the patient returns to have additional layers taken if necessary. This process is then repeated until a tumor-free place is reached. After the tumor is completely excised, the patient returns for reconstruction.

With any form of staged excision, it is imperative that good communication exist between the Mohs surgeon and the dermatopathologist. In order to ensure the entire peripheral margin is being examined, the peripheral tissue should be embedded en face. Other staged excisions utilizing radial sections, vertical, or bread loaf sections do not examine 100% of the peripheral margin and may result in higher recurrence rates by lack of full-margin examination.

15.6 Local Recurrence after MMS

When melanomas recur, 23% recur at the margin with an invasive component. These invasive components recur with a mean Breslow depth of 0.9 mm.[14] Recurrent tumors can track along scars and be multifocal, lowering cure rates even with complete margin assessment. There

is an invasive growth potential of not only inadequately excised primary malignant melanomas but also MIS. It is not uncommon to find an invasive melanoma when examining the margins of an MIS. Incomplete and inaccurate removal of all melanomas at the time of the initial diagnosis and treatment can lead to larger salvage procedures and ultimately morbidity.[15] Complete and exhaustive margin assessment through MMS or slow Mohs affords the smallest possible margins and identifies outliers with wide extensions of disease.

Recurrence rates for the treatment of melanoma with MMS are highly operator dependent. Like any procedure, if the surgeon and/or the technology supporting the surgeon are faulty, then the results can be less than optimal. With high-quality sections and experience, very low recurrence rates are possible.

15.7 Reconstruction after Clear MMS Margins

Mohs surgery provides a unique opportunity for real-time evaluation of the surgical margins completed within the same day, unlike all other excision techniques as described earlier. After the histologic confirmation of a tumor-free field has been obtained, immediate reconstruction is available. Approximately 50% of patients undergoing MMS for facial melanomas require reconstruction with a flap or a graft.[11] When reconstruction is complex, patients certainly benefit from same-day tumor excision, marginal histologic assessment, and reconstruction on the same day. If the patient needs an additional procedure such as a sentinel lymph node biopsy (SLNBx), this can be completed at any time prior to MMS, after clearance of the tumor prior to reconstruction, or after reconstruction. Some may argue that excision may alter the results of the SLNBx; however, that has yet to be proven. In fact, there are five studies that demonstrate wide local excision does not impact the results of SLNBx results.[16,17,18,19,20]

15.8 Controversies

There is no doubt that controversies exist regarding the use of frozen sections for melanoma. Frozen sections are believed to be inferior to permanent paraffin-embedded sections for the examination of atypical melanocytes. Several authors have claimed that the interpretation of H&E-stained frozen sections is unreliable.[21,22] For example, several authors believe that actinic keratoses may stain with MART-1, but with experience, it is easy to read that an actinic keratosis does not stain as darkly as a melanocyte. It has been demonstrated time and again that high-quality H&E-stained slides can be reliable.[23,24]

With the addition of rapid frozen section immunostains, Mohs surgery for melanoma is more accessible and reliable. Many Mohs surgeons have reported high local cure rates for the treatment of melanoma aided by the use of frozen section immunostains.[25,26,27,28,29] With the use of high-quality, reliably thin frozen sections from an experienced histotechnician, low recurrence rates can be achieved. Without these thin sections, the MART-1 stain will appear positive and may lead to overcalling. More stages would be necessary, leading to larger defects. The fact that most melanomas can be excised in one to two stages with recurrence rates between 0 and 2% supports that frozen sections are valid.

Randomized data do not exist and may never be available to support the use of Mohs for melanoma on the head and neck. A truly randomized study may be impossible, as most tumors in this location cannot be excised with 1-cm margins. A study completed by the Mayo clinic reported similar recurrence rates between MMS and WLE; however, these two treatment arms were not randomized. Larger lesions, recurrent tumors, and those on the head and neck were referred for Mohs surgery.[30]

The controversy of the utility of SLNBx is often debated. Although the utility of SLNBx in melanoma is being reevaluated, there are some circumstances when it is utilized.[31,32] It is argued that SLNBx cannot be performed if the patient has Mohs surgery; however, the SLNBx can be performed at any time prior to Mohs surgery, after Mohs surgery prior to reconstruction, or after reconstruction.[16,17,18,19,20] If the use of SLNBx remains a concern to the treating physician or team, then the frozen sections of the debulking specimen can be utilized to detect an upgrade to Breslow's depth. If an upgrade of the depth is found that may warrant an SLNBx, it can be then performed prior to reconstruction.[27]

As gene expression profile testing for several solid organ tumors such as breast cancer and uveal melanoma has become standard of care, its implementation into cutaneous melanoma management has been studied. Some authors have found that its clinical utility has not been well established.[33] There are, however, several studies that have further validated its use in the management of patients with invasive melanoma. These studies have shown to add valuable prognostic information to current American Joint Committee on Cancer (AJCC) staging methods by identifying those cutaneous melanomas that have higher risk factors for metastases.[34,35,36]

Cost is often considered when comparing WLE to MMS. As Mohs surgery frequently results in smaller defects, repairs also tend to be smaller and simpler. The cost of MMS and subsequent repair is often less than that of WLE and repair, especially when this occurs in the operating room. In addition, the cost of recurrent tumor treatment from WLE should be considered when comparing the cost of Mohs surgery to that of standard excision. Evaluating and confirming a clear margin prior to reconstruction is invaluable to avoiding a complicated reconstruction for an inadequately excised primary tumor.

References

[1] American Cancer Society. Key Statistics for Melanoma Skin Cancer. 2018. Available at: https://www.cancer.org/cancer/melanoma-skin-cancer/about/key-statistics.html. Accessed December 26, 2018

[2] Pitman GH, Kopf AW, Bart RS, Casson PR. Treatment of lentigo maligna and lentigo maligna melanoma. J Dermatol Surg Oncol. 1979; 5(9):727–737

[3] Osborne JE, Hutchinson PE. A follow-up study to investigate the efficacy of initial treatment of lentigo maligna with surgical excision. Br J Plast Surg. 2002; 55(8):611–615

[4] Coleman WP, III, Davis RS, Reed RJ, Krementz ET. Treatment of lentigo maligna and lentigo maligna melanoma. J Dermatol Surg Oncol. 1980; 6(6):476–479

[5] Swetter SM, Tsao H, Bichakjian CK, et al. Guidelines of care for the management of primary cutaneous melanoma. J Am Acad Dermatol. 2019; 80(1):208–250

[6] Kimyai-Asadi A, Katz T, Goldberg LH, et al. Margin involvement after the excision of melanoma in situ: the need for complete en face examination of the surgical margins. Dermatologic Surg. 2007; 33 (12):1434–1439–; discussion 1439–1441

[7] Cotter MA, McKenna JK, Bowen GM. Treatment of lentigo maligna with imiquimod before staged excision. Dermatol Surg. 2008; 34(2): 147–151

[8] Fisher GH, Lang PG. Treatment of melanoma in situ on sun-damaged skin with topical 5% imiquimod cream complicated by the development of invasive disease. Arch Dermatol. 2003; 139(7):945–947

[9] Silapunt S, Goldberg L. Lentigo maligna. In: Mikhail G, Snow S, eds. Mohs Micrographic Surgery. 18th ed. Madison: University of Wisconsin Press; 2004:175–182

[10] Stigall L, Brodland DG, Zitelli JA. The use of Mohs micrographic surgery (MMS) for melanoma in situ (MIS) of the trunk and proximal extremities. J Am Acad Dermatol. 2016; 75(5):1015-1021

[11] Etzkorn JR, Sobanko JF, Shin TM, et al. Correlation between appropriate use criteria and the frequency of subclinical spread or reconstruction with a flap or graft for melanomas treated with Mohs surgery with melanoma antigen recognized by T cells 1 immunostaining. Dermatologic Surg. 2016; 42(4):471–476

[12] Zalla MJ, Lim KK, Dicaudo DJ, Gagnot MM. Mohs micrographic excision of melanoma using immunostains. Dermatol Surg. 2000; 26 (8):771–784

[13] Hendi A, Brodland DG, Zitelli JA. Melanocytes in long-standing sun-exposed skin: quantitative analysis using the MART-1 immunostain. Arch Dermatol. 2006; 142(7):871–876

[14] Zitelli JA. Mohs surgery for lentigo maligna. Arch Dermatol. 1991; 127(11):1729–1730

[15] DeBloom JR, II, Zitelli JA, Brodland DG. The invasive growth potential of residual melanoma and melanoma in situ. Dermatol Surg. 2010; 36(8):1251–1257

[16] Gannon CJ, Rousseau DL, Jr, Ross MI, et al. Accuracy of lymphatic mapping and sentinel lymph node biopsy after previous wide local excision in patients with primary melanoma. Cancer. 2006; 107(11): 2647–2652

[17] Leong WL, Ghazarian DM, McCready DR. Previous wide local excision of primary melanoma is not a contraindication for sentinel lymph node biopsy of the trunk and extremity. J Surg Oncol. 2003; 82(3):143–146

[18] Brys AK, Schneider MM, Selim MA, Mosca PJ. Sentinel lymph node biopsy following a rotational flap. BMJ Case Rep. 2015; 2015: bcr2015210762

[19] Karakousis CP, Grigoropoulos P. Sentinel node biopsy before and after wide excision of the primary melanoma. Ann Surg Oncol. 1999; 6(8): 785–789

[20] McCready DR, Ghazarian DM, Hershkop MS, Walker JA, Ambus U, Quirt IC. Sentinel lymph-node biopsy after previous wide local excision for melanoma. Can J Surg. 2001; 44(6):432–434

[21] Prieto VG, Argenyi ZB, Barnhill RL, et al. Are en face frozen sections accurate for diagnosing margin status in melanocytic lesions? Am J Clin Pathol. 2003; 120(2):203–208

[22] Barlow RJ, White CR, Swanson NA. Mohs' micrographic surgery using frozen sections alone may be unsuitable for detecting single atypical melanocytes at the margins of melanoma in situ. Br J Dermatol. 2002; 146(2):290–294

[23] Zitelli JA, Moy RL, Abell E. The reliability of frozen sections in the evaluation of surgical margins for melanoma. J Am Acad Dermatol. 1991; 24(1):102–106

[24] Bienert TN, Trotter MJ, Arlette JP. Treatment of cutaneous melanoma of the face by Mohs micrographic surgery. J Cutan Med Surg. 2003; 7(1):25–30

[25] Bricca GM, Brodland DG, Ren D, Zitelli JA. Cutaneous head and neck melanoma treated with Mohs micrographic surgery. J Am Acad Dermatol. 2005; 52(1):92–100

[26] Kunishige JH, Brodland DG, Zitelli JA. Surgical margins for melanoma in situ. J Am Acad Dermatol. 2012; 66(3):438–444

[27] Etzkorn JR, Sobanko JF, Elenitsas R, et al. Low recurrence rates for in situ and invasive melanomas using Mohs micrographic surgery with melanoma antigen recognized by T cells 1 (MART-1) immunostaining: tissue processing methodology to optimize pathologic staging and margin assessment. J Am Acad Dermatol. 2015; 72(5):840–850

[28] Newman J, Beal M, Schram SE, Lee PK. Mohs micrographic surgery for lentigo maligna and lentigo maligna melanoma using Mel-5 immunostaining: an update from the University of Minnesota. Dermatol Surg. 2013; 39(12):1794–1799

[29] Bhardwaj SS, Tope WD, Lee PK. Mohs micrographic surgery for lentigo maligna and lentigo maligna melanoma using Mel-5

immunostaining: University of Minnesota experience. Dermatol Surg. 2006; 32(5):690–696, discussion 696–697

[30] Hou JL, Reed KB, Knudson RM, et al. Five-year outcomes of wide excision and Mohs micrographic surgery for primary lentigo maligna in an academic practice cohort. Dermatol Surg. 2015; 41(2):211–218

[31] Stiegel E, Xiong D, Ya J, et al. Prognostic value of sentinel lymph node biopsy according to Breslow thickness for cutaneous melanoma. J Am Acad Dermatol. 2018; 78(5):942–948

[32] Zagarella S, Sladden M, Popescu CM. Time to reconsider the role of sentinel lymph node biopsy in melanoma. J Am Acad Dermatol. 2019; 80(4):1168–1171

[33] Marchetti MA, Bartlett EK, Dusza SW, Bichakjian CK. Use of a prognostic gene expression profile test for T1 cutaneous melanoma: will it help or harm patients? J Am Acad Dermatol. 2019; 80(6):e161–e162

[34] Gastman BR, Gerami P, Kurley SJ, Cook RW, Leachman S, Vetto JT. Identification of patients at risk of metastasis using a prognostic 31-gene expression profile in subpopulations of melanoma patients with favorable outcomes by standard criteria. J Am Acad Dermatol. 2019; 80(1):149–157.e4

[35] Greenhaw BN, Zitelli JA, Brodland DG. Estimation of prognosis in invasive cutaneous melanoma. Dermatologic Surg. 2018; 44(12):1494–1500

[36] Gastman BR, Zager JS, Messina JL, et al. Performance of a 31-gene expression profile test in cutaneous melanomas of the head and neck. 2019; 41(4):871–879

16 Prevention and Repair of Internal Nasal Valve Dysfunction for the Reconstructive Surgeon

Parth Patel, Ethan T. Routt, Ziad M. Alshaalan, and David H. Ciocon

Summary

The internal nasal valve is a complex structure of the lower nose that plays an important function in nasal inspiration. It is prudent that the reconstructive surgeon is aware of this construct and is trained to prevent and/or repair any possible dysfunction that may ensue after tumor extirpation or during reconstruction of defects in the region. As with most surgical issues, prevention of internal nasal valve dysfunction is easier than to treat the ensuing complication. With no well-randomized trial to compare the outcomes of different techniques, and with patients presenting with a heterogeneity of pathologies, there is no single technique for all cases of internal nasal valve dysfunction, and thus each case must be considered uniquely.

Keywords: internal nasal valve, dysfunction, obstruction, suspension suture, cartilage graft

16.1 Introduction

The internal nasal valve (INV) is a three-dimensional construct classically defined by the upper lateral cartilage (ULC) superiorly, nasal septum medially, pyriform aperture inferiorly, and head of the inferior turbinate posteriorly (▶ Fig. 16.1a, b). INV dysfunction is a common cause of functional airway obstruction that leads to difficulty with nasal inspiration and a decreased quality of life.[1] The reconstructive surgeon primarily encounters INV dysfunction after tumor extirpation in Mohs micrographic surgery (MMS) or iatrogenically during reconstruction of perialar defects.[2,3] Although it is unknown what rate of INV dysfunction is caused by MMS, Schlosser and Park[4] have reported that trauma of any sort, both surgical and accidental, accounts for 71% of cases.

INV dysfunction is well described in relation to primary otorhinolaryngological issues, but it is not extensively discussed in relation to MMS. Not only is it important to identify preexisting INV dysfunction, for many medical and legal reasons, but it is also important to identify it as a known complication of tumor extirpation and/or reconstruction, so as to best prevent it from occurring and optimize outcomes should it occur.

There are many techniques to prevent and treat INV dysfunction, each depending on the underlying pathophysiology of the defect, as well as patient and surgeon preferences. The purpose of this chapter is to discuss relevant anatomy, note opportunities to prevent INV dysfunction, and explore treatment options from the perspective of the reconstructive surgeon. Techniques that will not be discussed include those that involve rhinoplasties, septoplasties, or turbinoplasties/turbinectomies,

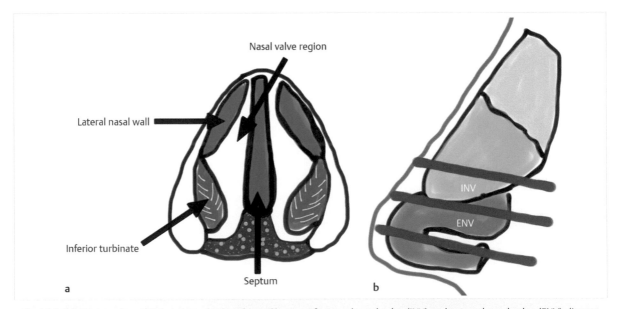

Fig. 16.1 (a) Cross section of internal nasal valve. (b) Profile view of internal nasal valve (INV) and external nasal valve (ENV). (Image courtesy of Dr. Parth Patel.)

or those that require special rhinological instruments or treatment systems not readily available to all reconstructive surgeons.

16.2 Modalities/Treatment Options Available

A multitude of both invasive and noninvasive techniques have been described in the literature to address INV dysfunction, but given the dearth of randomized trials, no single technique stands out as the "gold standard" (▶ Table 16.1). Noninvasive techniques focus on stenting or providing external support to the INV and lateral nasal wall[1]; examples include the use of nasal dilators and clips. Although noninvasive techniques can be successful in select patients, invasive correction is often required for definitive treatment. Invasive techniques focus on widening the nasal valve and/or increasing the rigidity of structures overlying the INV[1,5]; such surgical techniques include the use of suspension sutures,[6,7,8,9,10,11] autologous cartilage grafts,[1,12,13,14] and repositioning and reallocation of scar tissue.[3,15,16]

16.3 Indications and Evaluation of INV Dysfunction

The INV plays an important role in nasal airflow as it is the narrowest portion of the nasal airway, and is the place of maximal resistance, termed the "flow-limiting segment." A standardized preoperative, intraoperative, and postoperative assessment for every surgery involving the INV area should be performed and should include a clinical examination and subjective airflow report by the patient. The symptomatic patient may complain of nasal stuffiness, but in some cases, a history will have to be elicited. In addition, photographs including an anteroposterior, a 45-degree, and a "worm's" view should be taken both before and after surgery.[6]

Table 16.1 Techniques to prevent and treat internal nasal vale dysfunction in Mohs micrographic surgery

Noninvasive techniques	Invasive techniques: intraoperative	Invasive techniques: postoperative
External nasal dilators[17]	Suspension toward local tissue[6,7,10]	Suspension toward the orbital rim[8,9]
Nasal clips[17]	Autologous cartilage graft[12,13,14]	Suspension toward the lateral nasal bone[11]
"Spreader graft injection": calcium hydroxylapatite[18] or hyaluronic acid[19]		Autologous cartilage graft[12,13,14]
		Repositioning and reallocation of scar tissue[15,16]

Examination for INV dysfunction is best done without a speculum, evaluating the outside of the nose for a pinched middle third and evaluating the inside by lightly retracting the ala with a cotton-tip applicator.[20,21,22] The examiner should check closely for dysfunction of the nasal sidewall and narrowing of the septal–lateral cartilage angle.[22,23] The septum should be evaluated for evidence of deviation.[3,22] The limen nasi may be unduly prominent in instances where the critical juncture between the lateral and alar cartilage has been disturbed by prior surgery or inflammation.[3] The mucosa should be evaluated for edema and undue prominence of the anterior edge of the inferior turbinate should be ruled out.[3]

If subjective blockage is noted, in the form of stuffiness or resistance to airflow, Cottle's maneuver should be performed.[21,23] In this maneuver, the cheek is pulled laterally with one to two fingers, during passive inspiration, opening the INV (▶ Fig. 16.2a).[23] A positive result is indicated by the patient reporting improved nasal airflow and indicates that INV dysfunction is contributing to the patient's symptoms.[23] A false-negative result can occur if there is extensive scarring/webbing of the valve or narrowing of the pyriform aperture secondary to congenital malformation or excessive narrowing of the nasal base from prior osteotomy.[23,24] If there is suspicion for a false-negative result, a modified Cottle maneuver can be performed by using a cotton-tip applicator to retract the INV laterally from inside the nare during passive inspiration, which should overcome rigid tissue and improve the patient's nasal airflow (▶ Fig. 16.2b).[24]

INV dysfunction can be categorized as static or dynamic, depending on whether the dysfunction is present at rest or occurs during inspiration, respectively.[25,26] In many cases, static and dynamic INV dysfunction occur together.[25,26]

Static INV dysfunction is defined as a narrowing of the middle third of the nose at rest caused by a relative decrease in the angle between the ULC and nasal septum, which is 10 to 15 degrees in Caucasian patients, and ranges from 22.5 to 52 degrees in non-Caucasians.[21,25] Static dysfunction is often the result of a scarring process or a weakening of support structures caused by elevation of the skin–soft tissue envelope, damage to the nasal dilator muscles, and/or defects in the middle third cartilages.[1,20,25]

Dynamic INV dysfunction is defined as an active narrowing of the ULC and middle third of the nose that only occurs during inspiration, and is typically caused by an inherent weakness in the nasal sidewall.[21,25] Dynamic dysfunction is often the result of a thin, weak, detached, or absent ULC that cannot provide the necessary strength to withstand the negative pressures created by inspiration.[1,20,25]

16.4 Patient Selection/ Considerations

In MMS and reconstruction, nasal valve dysfunction most commonly occurs due to bulky flaps, inappropriate flaps,

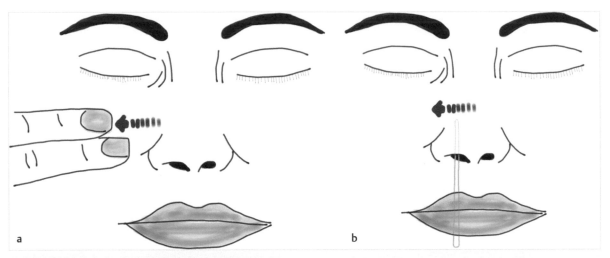

Fig. 16.2 (a) Cottle's maneuver. **(b)** Modified Cottle's maneuver. (Image courtesy of Dr. Parth Patel.)

inadequate structural support, and inappropriate use of healing by secondary intention.[2,3] To preemptively minimize the incidence of INV dysfunction in MMS, the following precautions should be taken. First, bulky flaps should be thinned as the weight of the flap can cause positional impingement on the INV.[3] Second, flaps with significant tension vectors overlying the INV should be avoided as they can cause nasal narrowing with healing.[27] Third, adequate structural support should be provided to the resected areas; in addition to replacing resected native cartilage, it is important to reinforce moderately deep defects of the ala, alar crease, and/or sidewall, even if native cartilage is intact.[27,28,29] Although the dimension of the cutaneous defect is not a direct indicator for the need for structural support, in a retrospective study of 304 cases, Robinson and Burget[2] recommend that wounds be repaired with a cartilage graft if they bridge the alar crease or are located in the ala or lateral sidewall and come within 1 mm of the alar crease with a total diameter of 1.0 cm. Similarly, in a comparative study of 38 patients, Ezzat and Liu[30] suggest that nasal defects greater than 1.2 cm in diameter and involving the alar crease and sidewalls are associated with a lower incidence of postoperative nasal obstruction when either cartilage grafting or suspension suture is used in reconstruction. Additional retrospective studies evaluating various size defects suggest that liberal use of structural reinforcement results in a low overall INV obstruction rate of approximately 3%.[27,28,29] In general, structural reinforcement prevents alar margin elevation and displacement of the alar and lateral cartilages into the nasal vestibule.[2] On a last separate note, it should be highlighted that mucosal defects in the area of the INV should rarely be allowed to heal by secondary intention, because although mucosalization will occur, it will not be before significant contracture and functionally apparent stenotic webbing occur.[3]

16.5 Noninvasive Techniques

For patients who are poor surgical candidates or refuse surgery, external nasal dilators and nasal clips are the best studied potential alternatives to surgical intervention.[17] Less studied but possible alternatives are calcium hydroxylapatite[18] or hyaluronic acid[19] injected submucoperichondrially and/or submucosally along the ULC and nasal dorsum to function as a spreader graft. Importantly, not only do noninvasive techniques allow the patient to experience the quality-of-life improvements associated with a functioning INV but they also allow patients to preemptively experience the expectations from a proper surgical intervention prior to the actual surgery.[31,32]

16.6 Invasive Techniques: Suspension Sutures

The first group of invasive modalities includes suturing techniques used to lateralize and/or strengthen the lateral component of the nasal valve region.[6,7,8,9,10,11] In most techniques, the suture is placed at the site of maximum dysfunction through the upper or lower lateral cartilage and fixed to a rigid anchor point located lateral to the nasal valve. The surgical approach and the site of incision are different in every technique. When placing suspension sutures, care should be taken to avoid alar rim lifting.[7] Additionally, suspension sutures should not be used to restore the nasal contour if such is needed.[6] Bone anchoring systems[33,34] are not discussed in this chapter given the need for specialized equipment that is not readily available to all reconstructive surgeons.

16.6.1 Nasal Valve Suspension toward the Orbital Rim

Originally, Paniello[8] described a technique in which a 3–0 polypropylene suture was introduced endonasally at the site of maximum dysfunction and in the direction of a transconjunctival incision via a Keith needle (▶ Fig. 16.3). Once the needle appeared through the conjunctival incision, the suture was affixed to the infraorbital periosteum with a French eye needle.[8] Unfortunately, this technique was noted to have a few drawbacks with a reported complication rate of approximately 25%, including pain, inflammation, suborbital swelling, loss of suspension and nasal facial fullness, and facial scarring.[14,35,36,37,38] Lee and Glasgold[9] modified this technique by using a 4–0 polypropylene suture and an infraorbital incision through the skin to expose the infraorbital periosteum. Both of these techniques are corrective methods that can be used if postoperative INV dysfunction occurs.[8,9]

16.6.2 Nasal Valve Suspension toward the Lateral Side of the Nasal Bone

In 2003, Rizvi and Gauthier[11] described a technique in which a 3–0 polypropylene suture is passed medially and laterally to the ULC with a Keith needle and is firmly secured to the periosteum superficial musculoaponeurotic system over the lateral nasal bone (▶ Fig. 16.4). This method simultaneously addresses both the medial displacement of the caudal border of the ULC and weakness of the lateral nasal wall.[11] It is also claimed to be technically easier than the Paniello[8] technique and is reported

to have an approximately 90% improvement rate of nasal airway breathing over a 10-year follow-up period.[39] Like the Paniello[8] and Lee and Glasgold[9] techniques, this technique is a corrective method for postoperative INV dysfunction.[11]

16.6.3 Nasal Valve Suspension toward Local Tissue

Although some surgeons use the Paniello[8] technique to avoid major skin incisions, in the setting of MMS, where deeper tissues are already exposed, many reconstructive surgeons suggest securing the nasal valve laterally to adjacent local tissue preventively. This modified suspension suture pulls the nasal side wall tissue anteriorly and superolaterally.[6,7,10] It can be performed with a single suture or two sutures for greater security and further widening of the INV.[10] In contrast to traditional nasal valve suspension, the modified suspension stitch does not pass through the nasal mucosa and is anchored to adjacent local tissue, often maxillary periosteum, instead of the distant orbital rim (▶ Fig. 16.5).[6,7,10] Additionally, this modified nasal suspension suture uses standard surgical instruments and does not require a Keith needle.[6,7,10] Wang et al[10] have used this technique on hundreds of patients and have found it to be useful in combination with flaps, grafts, and linear closures.

Another similar technique involving local tissue is the buried 3-point stitch that can be placed during repair of the nasal sidewall or dorsum, extending to the alar groove or coming 1 mm from it (▶ Fig. 16.6).[6] The first point of the stitch includes the soft tissue of the alar groove overlying the nasal valve, and the second and third points are the medial and lateral edges of the overlying dermis, respectively.[6] Special attention is given to

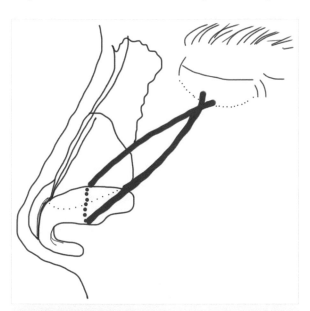

Fig. 16.3 Lateral suspension suture toward orbital rim. (Image courtesy of Dr. Parth Patel.)

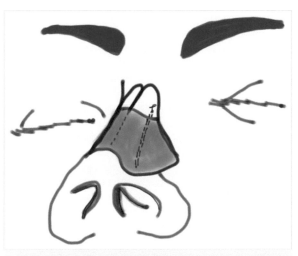

Fig. 16.4 Suspension toward the lateral side of the nasal bone. (Image courtesy of Dr. Parth Patel.)

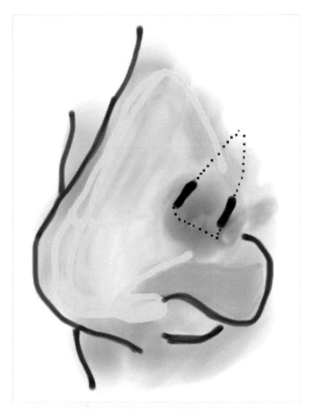

Fig. 16.5 Lateral suspension suture toward local tissue. (Image courtesy of Dr. Parth Patel.)

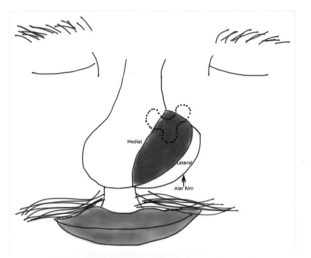

Fig. 16.6 Three-point stitch. (Image courtesy of Dr. Parth Patel.)

avoid pulling on the free margin of the alar rim and to ensure symmetry.[6]

16.7 Invasive Techniques: Cartilage Grafts

The second group of invasive treatment modalities includes the placement of autologous cartilage grafts in nonanatomical locations.[1] In most reconstructions in the area of the INV, batten grafts are utilized to add structural rigidity and resist dysfunction.[12,13,14] Batten grafts involve a strip of cartilage that typically spans the area between the pyriform aperture and lateral crura, and is placed at the point of maximal lateral nasal wall dysfunction, which can vary slightly per defect (▶ Fig. 16.7).[12,13,14] Autologous cartilage grafts are often taken from an auricular source, such as the conchal bowl or antihelix due to the inherent curvature of the cartilage, but can less preferably be taken from a septal or costal source.[40] Regardless of the cartilage source, all can be successfully combined with primary closures, flaps, and full-thickness grafts.[40] As a side note, in contrast to typical surgery in otolaryngology and plastic surgery, the use

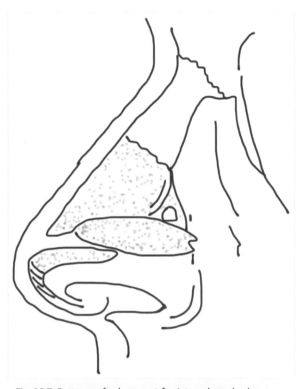

Fig. 16.7 Batten graft placement for internal nasal valve dysfunction. (Image courtesy of Dr. Parth Patel.)

of alloplastic implants for INV dysfunction in MMS is limited, and the long-term safety and success of alloplastic materials in this setting is not known.

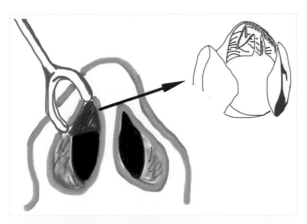

Fig. 16.8 Z-plasty for stenotic tissue. (Image courtesy of Dr. Parth Patel.)

16.8 Invasive Techniques: Repositioning and Reallocation of Scar Tissue

The last group of invasive techniques primarily involves the Z-plasty technique, which is utilized when there is significant stenotic scarring/webbing from secondary mucosal healing after a prior procedure, trauma, or inflammation (▶ Fig. 16.8).[3] The Z-plasty technique can be performed via the endonasal approach to reorient scarred stenotic tissue and widen the INV aperture.[15,16] Mucosal scarring can be prevented by repairing mucosal defects preferentially via a primary repair or internal nasal mucosal flap, or in certain cases split-thickness grafts or hinge flaps.[3]

16.9 Postoperative Instructions

Instructions for postoperative care for the invasive techniques include general wound care, preventing nasal trauma, and limiting nasal strain/high intranasal pressures. Notably, patients should avoid rubbing, wiping or blowing their nose, and if patients have to sneeze, it is recommended to do so with the mouth open.

16.10 Potential Complications and their Management

Complications of techniques used to prevent or repair INV dysfunction are specific to the technique utilized. Whereas treatments using external nasal dilators and nasal clips are low-risk options, filler injections into the nose with hyaluronic acid, and to a greater extent calcium hydroxylapatite, are risky treatment options due to the possibility of vascular occlusion, most worrisome of which is retinal or ophthalmic artery occlusion leading to visual impairment.[41] The primary treatment for filler occlusion is the same regardless of location, but in the case of ophthalmic involvement, emergency ophthalmology consultation is also warranted. When using suspension sutures, complications include slipped or broken sutures and neuralgia due to nerve impingement by suture material. Treatment options for the former include re-suturing or attempting an alternative technique, while for the latter, an attempt can be made for pain control with neuromodulatory medications (e.g., gabapentin, amitriptyline, etc.), or the suture can be removed or replaced. When using cartilage grafts, complications to consider include graft migration, and recipient or donor chondritis/infection. Treatment options for graft migration include removal or repositioning, and those for chondritis include nonsteroidal anti-inflammatory diseases, and antibiotics with possible debridement if also infected. Finally, complications of scar revision with the Z-plasty technique include flap necrosis, flap infection, recurrent stenotic scarring/webbing, as well as additional scar formation. Treatment for flap necrosis is continued wound care. Treatment for flap infection is antibiotics with possible debridement, and treatment for persistent or additional scarring is further scar revision and/or intralesional steroids.

16.11 Pearls/Pitfalls

Reconstructive surgeons would do well to realize that repairs of defects in the INV area have not only aesthetic but also functional consequences. In certain situations, it may be prudent to refer patients to those more experienced in rhinology. This includes patients with preexisting nasal obstruction that worsened after MMS or patients who may benefit from a rhinoplasty,[42] septoplasty,[43] turbinoplasty/turbinectomy,[43] spreader graft/flap,[21,44] butterfly graft,[45] splay graft,[46] flaring suture,[47] bone anchored system,[33,34] endoscopic/fibroscopic evaluation,[21] radiofrequency ablation,[48,49,50,51] or novel lateral implant (Latera, Spirox Inc., Redwood City, California, United States).[52]

As with many surgical issues, it is easier to prevent INV dysfunction rather than treat the ensuing complication. Unfortunately, there are no well-randomized trials to compare the outcomes of different techniques used to prevent and treat INV dysfunction. Most studies are based on heterogeneous groups of patients with a mixture of pathologies. In this respect, there is not a single surgical solution to all cases of potential INV dysfunction, and each case must be considered uniquely.

Risk factors for INV dysfunction include bulky flaps; large defects of the nasal ala, alar crease, and/or lateral sidewall; inadequate structural support; and inappropriate use of secondary healing for cutaneous and/or mucosal defects.[2,3] Armed with an understanding of the nasal valve, recent refinements in surgical techniques, and an accompanying thorough preoperative and postoperative evaluation, findings of INV dysfunction may be identified, prevented, and treated for improved outcomes and patient satisfaction.

References

[1] Samra S, Steitz JT, Hajnas N, Toriumi DM. Surgical management of nasal valve collapse. Otolaryngol Clin North Am. 2018; 51(5):929–944

[2] Robinson JK, Burget GC. Nasal valve malfunction resulting from resection of cancer. Arch Otolaryngol Head Neck Surg. 1990; 116(12):1419–1424

[3] Reynolds MB, Gourdin FW. Nasal valve dysfunction after Mohs surgery for skin cancer of the nose. Dermatol Surg. 1998; 24(9):1011–1017

[4] Schlosser RJ, Park SS. Surgery for the dysfunctional nasal valve. Cadaveric analysis and clinical outcomes. Arch Facial Plast Surg. 1999; 1(2):105–110

[5] Timmer FC, Roth JA, Börjesson PK, Lohuis PJ. The lateral crural underlay spring graft. Facial Plast Surg. 2013; 29(2):140–145

[6] Miladi A, McGowan JW, IV, Donnelly HB. Two suturing techniques for the prevention and treatment of nasal valve collapse after Mohs micrographic surgery. Dermatol Surg. 2017; 43(3):407–414

[7] Orseth ML, Nijhawan RI. Managing nasal valve compromise with suspension sutures. Dermatol Surg. 2018; 44(6):878–881

[8] Paniello RC. Nasal valve suspension. An effective treatment for nasal valve collapse. Arch Otolaryngol Head Neck Surg. 1996; 122(12):1342–1346

[9] Lee DS, Glasgold AI. Correction of nasal valve stenosis with lateral suture suspension. Arch Facial Plast Surg. 2001; 3(4):237–240

[10] Wang JH, Finn D, Cummins DL. Suspension suture technique to prevent nasal valve collapse after Mohs micrographic surgery. Dermatol Surg. 2014; 40(3):345–347

[11] Rizvi SS, Gauthier MG. Lateralizing the collapsed nasal valve. Laryngoscope. 2003; 113(11):2052–2054

[12] Toriumi DM, Josen J, Weinberger M, Tardy ME, Jr. Use of alar batten grafts for correction of nasal valve collapse. Arch Otolaryngol Head Neck Surg. 1997; 123(8):802–808

[13] Cervelli V, Spallone D, Bottini JD, et al. Alar batten cartilage graft: treatment of internal and external nasal valve collapse. Aesthetic Plast Surg. 2009; 33(4):625–634

[14] Mendelsohn MS, Golchin K. Alar expansion and reinforcement: a new technique to manage nasal valve collapse. Arch Facial Plast Surg. 2006; 8(5):293–299

[15] Varadharajan K, Choudhury N, Saleh HA. Modified Z-plasty of the internal nasal valve-to treat mechanical nasal obstruction: how we do it. Clin Otolaryngol. 2019; 44(6):1203–1204

[16] Dutton JM, Neidich MJ. Intranasal Z-plasty for internal nasal valve collapse. Arch Facial Plast Surg. 2008; 10(3):164–168

[17] Kiyohara N, Badger C, Tjoa T, Wong B. A comparison of over-the-counter mechanical nasal dilators: a systematic review. JAMA Facial Plast Surg. 2016; 18(5):385–389

[18] Nyte CP. Spreader graft injection with calcium hydroxylapatite: a nonsurgical technique for internal nasal valve collapse. Laryngoscope. 2006; 116(7):1291–1292

[19] Nyte CP. Hyaluronic acid spreader-graft injection for internal nasal valve collapse. Ear Nose Throat J. 2007; 86(5):272–273

[20] Rhee JS, Weaver EM, Park SS, et al. Clinical consensus statement: diagnosis and management of nasal valve compromise. Otolaryngol Head Neck Surg. 2010; 143(1):48–59

[21] Goudakos JK, Fishman JM, Patel K. A systematic review of the surgical techniques for the treatment of internal nasal valve collapse: where do we stand? Clin Otolaryngol. 2017; 42(1):60–70

[22] Murrell GL. Components of the nasal examination. Aesthet Surg J. 2013; 33(1):38–42

[23] Villwock JA, Kuppersmith RB. Diagnostic algorithm for evaluating nasal airway obstruction. Otolaryngol Clin North Am. 2018; 51(5):867–872

[24] Fung E, Hong P, Moore C, Taylor SM. The effectiveness of modified cottle maneuver in predicting outcomes in functional rhinoplasty. Plast Surg Int. 2014; 2014:618313

[25] Bloching MB. Disorders of the nasal valve area. GMS Curr Top Otorhinolaryngol Head Neck Surg. 2007; 6:Doc07

[26] Patel B, Virk JS, Randhawa PS, Andrews PJ. The internal nasal valve: a validated grading system and operative guide. Eur Arch Otorhinolaryngol. 2018; 275(11):2739–2744

[27] Woodard CR, Park SS. Reconstruction of nasal defects 1.5 cm or smaller. Arch Facial Plast Surg. 2011; 13(2):97–102

[28] Yong JS, Christophel JJ, Park SS. Repair of intermediate-size nasal defects: a working algorithm. JAMA Otolaryngol Head Neck Surg. 2014; 140(11):1027–1033

[29] Park SS. Reconstruction of nasal defects larger than 1.5 centimeters in diameter. Laryngoscope. 2000; 110(8):1241–1250

[30] Ezzat WH, Liu SW. Comparative study of functional nasal reconstruction using structural reinforcement. JAMA Facial Plast Surg. 2017; 19(4):318–322

[31] Gruber RP, Lin AY, Richards T. Nasal strips for evaluating and classifying valvular nasal obstruction. Aesthetic Plast Surg. 2011; 35(2):211–215

[32] Gelardi M, Porro G, Accettura D, Quaranta VN, Quaranta N, Ciprandi G. The role of an internal nasal dilator in athletes. Acta Biomed. 2019; 90 2-S:28–30

[33] Friedman M, Ibrahim H, Syed Z. Nasal valve suspension: an improved, simplified technique for nasal valve collapse. Laryngoscope. 2003; 113(2):381–385

[34] Friedman M, Ibrahim H, Lee G, Joseph NJ. A simplified technique for airway correction at the nasal valve area. Otolaryngol Head Neck Surg. 2004; 131(4):519–524

[35] André RF, Vuyk HD. Nasal valve surgery; our experience with the valve suspension technique. Rhinology. 2008; 46(1):66–69

[36] Wittkopf M, Wittkopf J, Ries WR. The diagnosis and treatment of nasal valve collapse. Curr Opin Otolaryngol Head Neck Surg. 2008; 16(1):10–13

[37] Apaydin F. Nasal valve surgery. Facial Plast Surg. 2011; 27(2):179–191

[38] Bae JH, Most SP. Cadaveric analysis of nasal valve suspension. Allergy Rhinol (Providence). 2012; 3(2):e91–e93

[39] Rizvi SS, Gauthier MG. Lateralizing the collapsed nasal valves simplified: 10-year survey of a simple concealed suture technique. Laryngoscope. 2011; 121(3):558–561

[40] Adams DC, Ramsey ML. Grafts in dermatologic surgery: review and update on full- and split-thickness skin grafts, free cartilage grafts, and composite grafts. Dermatol Surg. 2005; 31(8, Pt 2):1055–1067

[41] Beleznay K, Carruthers JDA, Humphrey S, Carruthers A, Jones D. Update on avoiding and treating blindness from fillers: a recent review of the world literature. Aesthet Surg J. 2019; 39(6):662–674

[42] Ballert JA, Park SS. Functional rhinoplasty: treatment of the dysfunctional nasal sidewall. Facial Plast Surg. 2006; 22(1):49–54

[43] Clark DW, Del Signore AG, Raithatha R, Senior BA. Nasal airway obstruction: prevalence and anatomic contributors. Ear Nose Throat J. 2018; 97(6):173–176

[44] Teymoortash A, Fasunla JA, Sazgar AA. The value of spreader grafts in rhinoplasty: a critical review. Eur Arch Otorhinolaryngol. 2012; 269(5):1411–1416

[45] André RF, Vuyk HD. The "butterfly graft" as a treatment for internal nasal valve incompetence. Plast Reconstr Surg. 2008; 122(2):73e–74e

[46] Guyuron B, Michelow BJ, Englebardt C. Upper lateral splay graft. Plast Reconstr Surg. 1998; 102(6):2169–2177

[47] Rasic I, Pegan A, Kosec A, Ivkic B, Bedekovic V. Use of intranasal flaring suture for dysfunctional nasal valve repair. JAMA Facial Plast Surg. 2015; 17(6):462–463

[48] Brehmer D, Bodlaj R, Gerhards F. A prospective, non-randomized evaluation of a novel low energy radiofrequency treatment for nasal

obstruction and snoring. Eur Arch Otorhinolaryngol. 2019; 276(4): 1039–1047

[49] Jacobowitz O, Driver M, Ephrat M. In-office treatment of nasal valve obstruction using a novel, bipolar radiofrequency device. Laryngoscope Investig Otolaryngol. 2019; 4(2):211–217

[50] Seren E. A new surgical method of dynamic nasal valve collapse. Arch Otolaryngol Head Neck Surg. 2009; 135(10):1010–1014

[51] Weissman JD, Most SP. Radiofrequency thermotherapy vs bone-anchored suspension for treatment of lateral nasal wall insufficiency: a randomized clinical trial. JAMA Facial Plast Surg. 2015; 17(2):84–89

[52] Sanan A, Most SP. A bioabsorbable lateral nasal wall stent for dynamic nasal valve collapse: a review. Facial Plast Surg Clin North Am. 2019; 27(3):367–371

Index

Note: Page numbers set **bold** or *italic* indicate headings or figures, respectively.